Lewis's Child and Adolescent Psychiatry Review

1,400 QUESTIONS TO HELP YOU PASS THE BOARDS

Lewis's Child and Adolescent Psychiatry Review

1,400 QUESTIONS TO HELP YOU PASS THE BOARDS

A Board Review
and
Companion Guide

Yann B. Poncin, MD and
Prakash K. Thomas, MD

Child Study Center
Yale University School of Medicine
New Haven, Connecticut

Wolters Kluwer | Lippincott Williams & Wilkins
Health

Philadelphia · Baltimore · New York · London
Buenos Aires · Hong Kong · Sydney · Tokyo

Acquisitions Editor: Lisa McAllister
Product Manager: Tom Gibbons
Vendor Manager: Alicia Jackson
Senior Manufacturing Manager: Benjamin Rivera

Marketing Manager: Brian Freiland
Design Coordinator: Steve Druding
Production Service: Thomson Digital

530 Walnut Street
Philadelphia, PA 19106 USA
LWW.com

Printer: Strategic Content Imaging

978-0-7817-9507-4

0-7817-9507-9

Library of Congress Cataloging-in-Publication Data

Poncin, Yann B.
  Lewis's child and adolescent psychiatry review book: a board review and companion guide/Yann B. Poncin and Prakash K. Thomas.
      p. ; cm.
  Companion guide to: Lewis's child and adolescent psychiatry: a comprehensive textbook/editors, Andres Martin, Fred R. Volkmar. 4th ed. c2007.
  Includes bibliographical references and index.
  ISBN-13: 978-0-7817-9507-4 (pbk. : alk. paper)
  ISBN-10: 0-7817-9507-9 (pbk. : alk. paper)
  1. Child psychiatry—Examinations, questions, etc. 2. Adolescent psychiatry—Examinations, questions, etc. I. Thomas, Prakash K. II. Lewis, Melvin, 1926–2007. III. Lewis's child and adolescent psychiatry. IV. Title. V. Title: Child and adolescent psychiatry review book.
  [DNLM: 1. Mental Disorders—Examination Questions. 2. Adolescent. 3. Child. 4. Infant. WM 18.2 P795L 2010]
  RJ499.32.P66 2010
  618.92'890076—dc22   2009028698

10 9 8 7 6 5

We would like to thank the editors of Lewis's Textbook, fourth edition: Andrés Martin, MD, MPH and Fred R. Volkmar, MD whose support and mentorship made this book possible.

Yann's dedication—
To Shem, Jana and Forrest.

Prakash's dedication—
To Alice.

Foreword

New Developments

In keeping with the tradition of a parent textbook that has spanned four editions over two decades, this new addition to the *Lewis* series is all about development. These complementary books mark more than the simple progression from an encyclopedic source to its manageable distillation: taken together, they embody development quite concretely.

For starters, there is the development of the science of human development itself. In a relatively short period, our understanding of development has grown rapidly, moving from an almost entirely observational discipline to one firmly grounded in the neurosciences. Genetic underpinnings have been described for a range of illnesses; genes are increasingly understood through their interplay with ever-present external influences; temperamental traits are being related to specific pathways in brain circuitry; and developmental milestones traced to the orderly maturation of brain cortex, which, in turn, has been pegged to molecular signals. As our understanding of the remarkable underpinnings of developmental psychopathology has unfolded, the observational earlier stage of the discipline has not been supplanted but rather deepened. Along the best lines of developmental maturation, earlier stages—of the science as much as of the *Textbook*—have not been discarded, but served as a foundation to build upon.

Quite apart from the many advances visible in its content, the format of the *Textbook* has likewise progressed. This transition was most readily apparent with the Fourth Edition—the first to come accompanied by a fully searchable, web-based clone. And with this new Review and Companion Guide, the *Lewis* "brand" breaks new ground by providing an interactive approach to the original source. Although the print-to-electronic transition reflects broader trends in academic publishing, this companion book underscores the importance of the actively engaged reader it is intended to reach.

The title of this new volume suggests that it is actually two books rolled into one. Taking this implicit suggestion one step further, I would propose that the two parts of the title provide distinct ways to elicit the "actively engaged" potential of its audience. By taking the Companion Guide approach, the interested reader can take the book one chapter at a time, a piecemeal strategy well-suited to the trainee encountering the material for the first time or to the instructor looking for objective and measurable learning targets. For those readers at the later developmental stage of wanting to review it all in one fell swoop—typically in preparation for certification or recertification examinations—the *Review* option may be the more relevant one to pursue. Both strategies have the common goals of making an otherwise imposing tome more approachable and of bringing down the barriers that so often relegate large textbooks to a classic yet premature entombment.

A final developmental domain worth noting concerns the editors of this book. In compiling and organizing *Lewis's Child and Adolescent Psychiatry Review*, Yann Poncin and Prakash Thomas have moved their teachers' work forward—just as Fred Volkmar and I had had the earlier privilege of advancing our own teacher's work by editing the Fourth Edition. But the word "teacher," with whatever hierarchical implications it carries, does not quite do justice to what these collaborations have entailed. A better approximation would be *From Generation to Generation*, the words inscribed at the entrance of the Yale Child Study Center, the institution that has housed and nurtured each one of us over so many years. It thus seems fitting to end where it all started, with the late Melvin Lewis we each knew, respected and came to emulate. This newest addition to his legacy speaks to the enduring example of scholarship he left us with. Yann and Prakash—and the colleagues they lassoed into this truly collective effort—are the next generation of Yale Child Study Center faculty and friends carrying on with the life's work of our elder. Mel would have been delighted to see these new developments.

Andrés Martin
Yale Child Study Center
New Haven, Connecticut

Preface

What is this book? First and foremost, we consider it a companion guide to *Lewis's Child and Adolescent Psychiatry: A Comprehensive Textbook, Fourth Edition*. The 1400 questions summarize the material covered in the textbook. Where we encountered key points representative of a chapter, we formed questions from them, and avoided the temptation to stray into esoteric information. As only brief explanations, if any, are provided in the answer section, and as the included page references are intended to spur further reading, this book is best used while having *Lewis's Textbook* an arm's length away for easy perusal. Although it can be used alone, the true value of the questions derives from the consideration of *why* your answer was right or wrong upon reading the textbook.

Secondly, this Review aids in preparation for the child and adolescent specialty boards, recertification, and the Child Psychiatry Resident-In-Training Examination (CHILD PRITE®). We did not specifically write questions to reflect the content and emphasis of the boards; however, the comprehensive scope of the 1400 questions addresses many, if not all, of the subject areas tested. To correspond to the written boards examination, the book is divided into seven tests, composed of 200 questions each, and followed by the respective answer section. Considering how these questions cover the great range of topics in child and adolescent psychiatry, you should be able to gauge your areas of strength and expertise as well as areas requiring further study.

A few caveats will preempt assumptions that these questions have a direct similarity to those encountered in the boards. For example, a number of questions concern the history of child and adolescent psychiatry, a topic not tested in the written examination. Regardless, we felt that practitioners in the discipline should be aware of the historical influences that continue to shape our present-day practice. In addition, the true/false and matching terms questions are not found on the boards, but these formats allow access to topics that were not easily covered by the standard multiple-choice template. Finally, in our estimation, the difficulty of these questions is greater than what you will encounter on the boards, but we hope this challenge will encourage further reading and solid preparation.

For each of the seven tests, we designed a random distribution of questions covering nearly all of the chapters in *Lewis's Textbook*. However, some readers may want to focus on a particular topic in their studies, such as clinical pharmacology, in which case they can refer to the Appendix to locate all questions pertaining to the subject. This section may also help identify topics that require further study after the completion of a test and the consideration of which questions were incorrect. Finally, true to its nature as a companion guide, the Appendix can also facilitate a quick review after reading a chapter in *Lewis's Textbook*.

We would like to acknowledge those who helped make this book possible. We thank Andrés Martin for his gracious introduction of the book in the foreword, as well as for his inspiration and guidance in this project. We are grateful for the work of the additional contributors in composing questions. We thank the team from Lippincott Williams and Wilkins, especially Lisa McAllister, Tom Gibbons, Charley Mitchell, Sirkka Howes, and Jennifer LaGreca, for their coordination of this enterprise. We found great pleasure in the opportunity to work with *Lewis's Textbook* and rediscover the impressive breadth of its introduction to child and adolescent psychiatry, made possible by a multitude of authors. We hope you make use of these questions and discover the same.

Prakash K. Thomas
Yann B. Poncin
Yale Child Study Center
New Haven, Connecticut

List of Additional Contributors

Heather Goff, MD (Chapters 3.1.2, 3.1.3, 3.1.4)
Assistant Professor
Department of Psychiatry
Yale University School of Medicine
New Haven, Connecticut

Kamilah Jackson, MD (Chapters 2.3.1, 2.3.2, 2.3.3)
Child & Adolescent Psychiatry Fellow
Child Study Center
Yale University School of Medicine
New Haven, Connecticut

Dana Kober, MD (Chapters 5.1.1, 5.6, 6.3.1)
Assistant Professor
Texas Children's Hospital
Houston, Texas

Christina Lee, MD (Chapters 5.1.2, 5.1.3, 5.1.4)
Child & Adolescent Psychiatry Fellow
Child Study Center
Yale University School of Medicine
New Haven, Connecticut

Marian Moca, MD (Chapters 5.15.1, 5.15.3, 5.15.4, 5.15.5)
Child & Adolescent Psychiatry Fellow
Child Study Center
Yale University School of Medicine
New Haven, Connecticut

Sunanda Muralee, MD (Chapters 1.7.1, 1.7.2, 1.7.3, 5.3)
Child & Adolescent Psychiatry Fellow
Child Study Center
Yale University School of Medicine
New Haven, Connecticut

Christopher Raczynski, MD (Chapters 6.2.2, 6.2.5, 6.2.6)
Child & Adolescent Psychiatry Fellow
Child Study Center
Yale University School of Medicine
New Haven, Connecticut

Edwin Williamson, MD (Chapters 5.7.1, 5.7.2, 5.7.3)
Child & Adolescent Psychiatry Fellow
Child Study Center
Yale University School of Medicine
New Haven, Connecticut

Contents

All page references in the Answer sections correspond to *Lewis's Child And Adolescent Psychiatry: A Comprehensive Textbook, fourth edition.*

Questions

1. Glutamatergic neurons and *N*-methyl-D-aspartate receptors in the hippocampus are important in the creation of long-term potentiation, which is integral to which of the following?
   A. Fight or flight response
   B. Memory
   C. Hunger and satiety
   D. Homeostatic equilibrium
   E. Body temperature control

2. The National Youth Risk Behavior Surveillance System of 2007 found that in the past 12 months prior to the survey the percentage of high school students who "seriously considered attempting suicide" was:
   A. 3%
   B. 6%
   C. 10%
   D. 15%
   E. 20%

3. What are the most common causes of psychogenic nonepileptic seizures in children, listed in order of descending frequency?
   A. Sexual abuse, family discord, separation anxiety with school refusal
   B. Separation anxiety with school refusal, sexual abuse, family discord
   C. Family discord, sexual abuse, separation anxiety with school refusal
   D. Family discord, separation anxiety with school refusal, sexual abuse
   E. Sexual abuse, separation anxiety with school refusal, family discord

4. The odds ratio in a case–control study is expressed as odds ratio = 2.2 (95% confidence interval: 1.5–3.4). Here the null hypothesis is:
   A. Rejected
   B. Not rejected
   C. 1.5
   D. 3.4
   E. 2.2

5. ALL of the following are interventional strategies for children and adolescents with conduct problems and oppositional behaviors, including aggression EXCEPT:
   A. Parent management training (PMT)
   B. Parent–child interaction training
   C. School and community-based programs
   D. Dialectical-behavior therapy
   E. Individual cognitive-behavioral treatments

6. True or False: When compared to children returned to their families of origin or to children raised in long-term foster care, adoption is clearly beneficial.
   A. True
   B. False

7. Research indicates strong links between early loss, trauma, and disturbance in the family with which of the following?
   A. Alcoholism
   B. Firesetting
   C. Interpersonal dysfunction
   D. Intrapsychic conflict

8. In studies of adults what percentage of those diagnosed with substance abuse go on to develop substance dependence?
   A. 10%
   B. 20%
   C. 30%
   D. 50%
   E. 75%

9. True or False: Projective techniques are one method of accessing the "inner life" of the child or adolescent.
   A. True
   B. False

10. True or False: Child psychiatry residency programs do not provide trainees with significant instruction in disaster intervention.
    A. True
    B. False

11. Who originally described a patient group as having "early infantile autism"?
    A. Kraepelin
    B. Freud
    C. Kernberg
    D. Chess
    E. Kanner

12. True or False: In psychiatric formulation, there are two distinct goals: that of understanding the patient and that of explaining the patient's symptoms, conditions, and concerns.
    A. True
    B. False

13. Which of the following captures the neuroendocrine response of those individuals who are resilient in the face of adversity?
    A. Excessive activation of the hypothalamic-pituitary-adrenal axis
    B. Chronic levels of cortisol
    C. Relatively quick return to baseline levels of cortisol
    D. Sensitive startle reflex

14. True or False: According to the 1998 Current Population Survey, children under 6 years of age living with a single mother were twice as likely to be poor than those living with both parents.
    A. True
    B. False

15. Which protein is affected in Fragile X?
    A. Methyl CpG binding protein 2 (MECP2)
    B. Signaling Nested Reservation Protocol
    C. Hypoxanthine–guanine phosphoribosyltransferase
    D. Fragile X mental retardation-1
    E. Cyclic AMP response element binding

16. Which of the following represents a key strategy or technique of Structural Family Therapy?
    A. Creation of a holding environment
    B. Strengthening of parental hierarchy
    C. Use of a genogram
    D. Use of "miracle" questions
    E. None of the above

17. Human leukocyte antigen (HLA) testing in patients with narcolepsy often reveals positivity for what alleles?
    A. HLA-A
    B. HLA-DP
    C. HLA-DQ
    D. HLA-B
    E. HLA-C

18. True or False: Federal regulations state that the assent of children is a necessary condition in the case of therapeutic interventions or procedures.
    A. True
    B. False

19. What is the recommended maximum dose of clonidine (in mg) in prepubertal children for the treatment of psychiatric disturbances?
    A. 0.1
    B. 0.2
    C. 0.3
    D. 0.4
    E. None of the above

20. Which edition of the International Classification of Diseases (ICD) first separated research diagnostic criteria from clinical descriptions?
    A. ICD-3
    B. ICD-5
    C. ICD-6
    D. ICD-8
    E. ICD-10

21. ALL of the following are true of early neural development EXCEPT:
    A. Environmental factors can influence brain development
    B. Instructions contained in the genetic code drives development
    C. Neuronal connections are strengthened through pruning of synaptic connections
    D. Neuronal activity may be required for proliferation and refinement of connections
    E. Neuronal connections can be made throughout life

22. What is criterion-related validity?
    A. The extent to which an instrument is representative of the universe of empirical indicators that are related to the concept measured
    B. The most empirical form of validity; it allows an index to be compared to an independent external criterion thought to assess the same concept
    C. The extent to which individual items or measures intercorrelate or group together to produce derived higher order constructs
    D. None of the above

23. In a study, what type of variable represents the predictors, antecedents, presumed causes, or influences under investigation?
    A. Active independent variable
    B. Independent variable
    C. Dependent variable
    D. Attribute independent variable
    E. Extraneous variable

24. Which infant assessment tool, appropriate for children from birth to 36 months, is useful in providing schemata for organizing information from caregiver interviews, medical and developmental records, and behavioral observations?
    A. Gesell Development Schedules
    B. Vineland Adaptive Behavior Scales
    C. Brazelton Neonatal Behavioral Assessment Scale
    D. Infant–Toddler Developmental Assessment
    E. Battelle Developmental Inventory

25. The majority of students with learning disabilities are identified in:
    A. Preschool
    B. Kindergarten to third grade
    C. Fourth or fifth grade
    D. Middle school or high school
    E. College

26. Seminal research by Sir Michael Rutter has revealed that when discrete risk factors faced by children (e.g., community violence, poverty, parent mental illness) coexist with other risks, as they often do in the real world, the effects on children tend to be:
    A. Additive
    B. Synergistic
    C. Compounded
    D. Minimized
    E. Resilient

27. Clinicians are susceptible to a number of collection biases in the process of interviewing and diagnosing a patient. Which of the following biases is the definition of a confirmatory bias?
    A. Arriving at a diagnostic determination before collecting all the relevant information
    B. Focusing on collecting information to confirm a diagnosis
    C. Making judgments based on the most readily available cognitive patterns
    D. Seeing correlations where none exist
    E. Ignoring disconfirming information

28. The monozygotic concordance rate for schizophrenia is approximately:
    A. 10%
    B. 25%
    C. 50%
    D. 75%
    E. 90%

29. True or False: Carbamazepine can induce its own metabolism.
    A. True
    B. False

30. The school consultation model, which includes problem identification, problem analysis, plan implementation, and problem evaluation, is best characterized by which consultation model?
    A. Mental Health Consultation
    B. Organizational Consultation
    C. Behavioral Consultation
    D. System Consultation
    E. Administrative Consultation

31. A neuropsychological battery can assess ALL of the following functional domains of the brain EXCEPT:
    A. Alertness/arousal
    B. Sensory perception
    C. Latent dynamic content
    D. Attention
    E. Information processing

32. Who was the author of the first text on child psychiatry in the United States?
    A. Arnold Gesell
    B. Benjamin Spock
    C. Leo Kanner
    D. Sigmund Freud

33. Which group prescribes the majority of psychoactive substances to children and adolescents?
    A. Child and adolescent psychiatrists
    B. General psychiatrists
    C. Primary care physicians
    D. Nurse practitioners
    E. Physician assistants

34. Which of the following interventions in the context of reactive attachment disorder is MOST LIKELY associated with injuries:
    A. Infant–parent psychotherapy
    B. Rebirthing
    C. Foster care placement
    D. Speech and occupational therapy
    E. The "strange situation" procedure

35. Animal and human studies provide indisputable evidence that this part of the brain plays an important role in fear conditioning:
    A. Caudate
    B. Striatum
    C. Amygdala
    D. Mesocortex
    E. All of the above

36. Prevalence in epidemiology is calculated as:
    A. Number of new onsets of disease divided by the population or sample size
    B. Number of subjects with the disease divided by the population or sample size
    C. Number of subjects with the disease divided by the disease-free population
    D. Number of subjects with the disease divided by the incidence rate

37. What is the minimum duration requirement for symptoms to be present to diagnose posttraumatic stress disorder?
    A. 1 day
    B. 5 days
    C. 30 days
    D. 60 days
    E. 90 days

38. True or False: Marriages of parents of children with cancer remain surprisingly stress free.
    A. True
    B. False

39. Which of the following assessment team structures is a team made up of professionals from different disciplines with formal communication channels and services coordinated by a case manager among the disciplines?
    A. Multidisciplinary
    B. Interdisciplinary
    C. Transdisciplinary
    D. Subdisciplinary
    E. Postdisciplinary

40. The two most important conditions for a group therapy setting are privacy for the duration of each meeting and:
    A. Developmentally appropriate furnishings and equipment
    B. Seating of members and coleaders at a circular or square table
    C. Coleaders seated in positions where they can easily make eye contact
    D. Coleaders seated in positions that do not block the door
    E. Positioning of a clock in view of all members

41. True or False: If a man is involved in the physical care of his child prior to age 3, there is a decreased probability that he will be involved with sexual abuse of his own or other children.
    A. True
    B. False

42. Troiden examined the typical development of sexual minorities. Which of the following is true of Troiden's model of homosexuality?
    A. It was based on prospective data
    B. It was based on openly identified gay men
    C. It begins with a stage of identification
    D. It correlates more strongly for women than men
    E. All of the above

43. Which of the following databases is operated by the American Psychological Association (APA)?
    A. Cochrane Library
    B. PubMed
    C. Journal of the American Academy of Child & Adolescent Psychiatry
    D. PsycINFO
    E. None of the above

44. What is the current view on selective serotonin reuptake inhibitors and suicidal thinking and behaviors when compared to placebo?
    A. Their effect is equal to placebo
    B. They decrease suicidal thinking compared to placebo
    C. They increase suicidal thinking compared to placebo
    D. They should not be used in children with suicidal thoughts

45. Which part of the serotonergic neuron is the primary target site for atypical neuroleptics such as risperidone, ziprasidone, and olanzapine?
    A. $5\text{-}HT_2$ receptor
    B. $5\text{-}HT_1$ receptor
    C. Serotonin transporter
    D. $5\text{-}HT_3$ receptor
    E. None of the above

46. When medications are used for the treatment of drug naive patients with obsessive–compulsive disorder (OCD), which is the most accurate statement?
    A. Up to 50% of patients experience a 25% to 45% reduction in severity in symptoms
    B. Up to 90% of patients experience at least a 25% reduction in severity of symptoms
    C. Up to 50% of patients experience a remission and an additional 50% experience a reduction of 25% to 45% severity in symptoms
    D. Up to 90% of patients experience at least a 50% reduction in symptoms

47. Synaptic pruning:
    A. Terminates around the age of 7
    B. Continues through adolescence
    C. Represents another form of myelinization
    D. Ends by the time of birth
    E. Occurs only in the basal ganglia

48. ALL of the following have been described as a category of encopresis EXCEPT:
    A. Children who have adequate bowel control and volitionally deposit feces in inappropriate places
    B. Children who are either unaware that they are soiling or are aware but unable to control the process
    C. Situations where the soiling is due to excessive fluid, which may be caused by diarrhea, anxiety, or retentive overflow
    D. Children who have short bowel syndrome

49. True or False: A recent multisite study found that children with pervasive developmental disorders appeared to be at higher risk for adverse events when prescribed stimulant medications compared to typically developing children with attention deficit hyperactivity disorder (ADHD).
    A. True
    B. False

50. Child care provider depression has been associated with ALL of the following EXCEPT:
    A. Less sensitive child care
    B. More intrusive or negative child care
    C. Low levels of job turnover
    D. Higher rates of expulsion of preschoolers

51. True or False: Rates of schizophrenia or psychosis in persons with an intellectual disability are higher than the rates of schizophrenia in the general population.
    A. True
    B. False

52. Functional dysphagia is defined as:
    A. A burning sensation in the epigastric area
    B. An inability to chew
    C. A subjective feeling of difficulty with speaking
    D. Weight loss due to a mental disorder
    E. A subjective experience of difficulty or discomfort associated with the act of swallowing

53. Current recommendations for lithium management include repeat laboratory testing at which time-interval after obtaining baseline or initial levels?
    A. 12 months
    B. 8 months
    C. 6 months
    D. 3 months
    E. 2 months

54. True or False: The same susceptibility genes of the associated clinical disorder influence endophenotypes.
    A. True
    B. False

55. ALL of the following conditions are more frequently found in persons with Tourette's syndrome compared to the general population EXCEPT:
    A. ADHD
    B. Disinhibited behavior
    C. Schizophrenia
    D. OCD
    E. Disinhibited speech

56. Which technique of operant conditioning reinforces approximations of a behavior?
    A. Token economy
    B. Differential reinforcement of other behavior
    C. Shaping
    D. Time out
    E. None of the above

57. The use of play in a therapeutic environment is:
    A. Most effective when the therapist simply joins the child's play
    B. A straightforward, accurate account of a child's past experiences
    C. A means of expression of a child's anxieties or worries
    D. A child's conscious use of characters and themes to reflect his experience
    E. A marker for delayed cognitive development

58. Imaging studies in OCD tend to indicate increased activity in the:
    A. Amygdala
    B. Hippocampus
    C. Medulla
    D. Caudate nucleus

59. For bipolar disorder in children, clear consensus does not exist for any of the following EXCEPT:
    A. The existence of bipolar disorder in children
    B. The necessity of cardinal symptoms (e.g., elated mood and/or grandiosity)
    C. The role of irritable mood
    D. The requirement of clearly demarcated mood episodes
    E. The best way to attribute potential symptoms of mania that also commonly present in other disorders

60. True or False: In 1997, the U.S. Congress enacted the State Children's Health Insurance Program (SCHIP) to expand health insurance coverage for children. This program provided states with federal matching funds to insure low-income children in addition to their Medicaid coverage.
    A. True
    B. False

61. Interpersonal psychotherapy for depressed adolescents has three primary components of treatment that are evident in the three phases of treatment: initial, middle, and termination. Which of the following is NOT one of the three primary components?
    A. Perspective-taking
    B. Education
    C. Affect identification
    D. Interpersonal skills building

62. Each of these refers to a sexual minority group, EXCEPT:
    A. Gay-Straight Alliance (GSA)
    B. Feminist Research Group (FRG)
    C. Gay, Lesbian Straight Education Network
    D. Gay Lesbian Bisexual Transgender/Transsexual (GLBT)
    E. Parents, Friends and Families of Lesbians and Gays

63. True or False: Defense is a term describing ego efforts to protect against external dangers.
    A. True
    B. False

64. Children with enuresis and behavioral problems usually have which of the following?
    A. Higher bladder capacity and developmental delays
    B. Marked structural anomalies
    C. Lower functional bladder volumes and developmental delays
    D. Parents who use a punishment-based approach
    E. None of the above

65. What is the leading cause of death from disease for children ages 1 to 14 years?
    A. Cancer
    B. Suicide
    C. Homicide
    D. Premature birth
    E. Neglect

66. Which of the following mechanisms describes lithium's main effect on the brain?
    A. Postsynaptic antagonism
    B. Intracellular signaling
    C. Presynaptic antagonism
    D. Reuptake inhibition
    E. Selective agonism

67. In response to critiques of poor internal validity attributed to early efficacy studies of child and adolescent therapies, the design of these studies evolved into the experimental clinical trial, which is characterized by ALL of the following EXCEPT:
    A. Explicit inclusion and exclusion criteria
    B. Random assignment
    C. Blinded and standardized diagnostic assessment
    D. Heterogeneous samples undergoing intervention
    E. Manual-based treatments

68. True or False: Research in resilience shows that positive adaptation in the early years is the determining factor for success in the later stages of life.
    A. True
    B. False

69. How do research assessments measure resilience?
   A. Cohen's *d*
   B. Kappa statistic
   C. Correlation, *r*
   D. Resilience is only a clinical assessment
   E. Resilience cannot be measured

70. What is the strongest risk factor for youth suicide?
   A. Major depression
   B. Bipolar disorder
   C. Substance use disorder
   D. Prior history of a suicide attempt
   E. Borderline personality disorder

71. Which term denotes the paradigm used in functional magnetic resonance imaging studies, which uses a series of single trials at a relatively slow rate of stimulus presentation to reduce the overlap of the hemodynamic responses evoked by consecutive individual trials?
   A. Event-related design
   B. Blocked design
   C. Region of interest
   D. Parcellation
   E. Subtraction paradigm

72. Which of the following statements is true?
   A. There is an equal sex distribution of OCD
   B. Males appear to have an earlier onset of OCD
   C. More females than males have OCD
   D. A and B
   E. B and C

73. True or False: Males and females have equal rates of night terrors.
   A. True
   B. False

74. Which of the following terms describes the number of patients that must be treated with an intervention to prevent one additional bad outcome?
   A. Absolute risk reduction
   B. Number needed to treat
   C. Correlation, *r*
   D. Cohen's *d*
   E. Number needed to harm

75. All of the following seem to contribute to the risk of developing borderline personality disorder in children and adults. Which experience is more discriminatory for borderline personality disorder compared to other personality disorders?
   A. Trauma
   B. Neglect
   C. Maltreatment
   D. Sexual abuse
   E. Physical abuse

76. In the treatment of autism, which type of applied behavior analysis model is structured and requires the child to work one-on-one with a therapist?
   A. Discrete trial training
   B. Pivotal response training
   C. Incidental teaching
   D. All of the above
   E. None of the above

77. True or False: Most children who develop posttraumatic stress disorder meet criteria for acute stress disorder within the first month after the traumatic event.
   A. True
   B. False

78. What is the primary underlying assumption of interpersonal psychotherapy?
    A. The quality of one's intrapsychic life can cause, maintain, or buffer against depression
    B. The quality of interpersonal relationships can cause, maintain, or buffer against depression
    C. The interpersonal relationship between therapist and patient can cause, maintain, or buffer against depression
    D. The transference relationship between patient and therapist can cause, maintain, or buffer against depression

79. In the Four Ps model of psychiatric formulation, which domain of factors is concerned with the features that make the presenting condition endure, such as the severity of the condition and compliance issues?
    A. Predisposing
    B. Precipitating
    C. Perpetuating
    D. Protective

80. True or False: It is always most effective to phrase verbal limits in positive terms.
    A. True
    B. False

81. True or False: Children with oppositional defiant disorder (ODD) alone compared to children with ODD and ADHD together, are equally likely to develop conduct disorder.
    A. True
    B. False

82. Codeine or morphine can be detected in the urine for how long?
    A. Less than 24 hours
    B. 24 to 72 hours
    C. 3 to 5 days
    D. 1 week
    E. More than 10 days

83. In general, what is the treatment for manic and mixed episodes in youth?
    A. Lithium monotherapy
    B. Valproate monotherapy
    C. Atypical antipsychotic monotherapy
    D. None of the above
    E. All of the above

84. The strongest risk factor of childhood and adolescent obesity is:
    A. Maternal smoking
    B. Fast food intake
    C. Parental neglect
    D. Parental obesity
    E. Time spent watching TV

85. Among normal metabolizers, the blood levels of nortriptyline are close in absolute value to which of the following?
    A. Half the daily oral dosage
    B. Three-quarters of the daily oral dosage
    C. Twice the daily oral dosage
    D. Daily oral dosage
    E. Weekly oral dosage

86. Premature terminations occur when there is a decision to end the therapy before the treatment goals have been accomplished. Child psychodynamic psychotherapy describes two types of premature terminations. Which TWO terms describe these types?
    A. Suspension
    B. Disruption
    C. Absconding
    D. Interruption
    E. Pause

87. In which year did Congress pass The Mental Health Act that provided funds for the training of child psychiatrists?
    A. 1898
    B. 1914
    C. 1946
    D. 1968
    E. 1984

88. When an adolescent expresses intent to harm seriously another person at school, what should you do?
    A. First and foremost, maintain the adolescent's confidentiality or he may not disclose information in the future
    B. Tell the adolescent's parents
    C. Protect the potential victim
    D. Call your malpractice insurer
    E. Discuss the matter with school personnel

89. Red and blue leading to purple is an example of which of the following?
    A. Associativity
    B. Composition
    C. Decentration
    D. Reversibility
    E. Seriation

90. According to the U.S. Office of Education, the term "specific learning disability" includes children who have learning problems from the result of which of the following conditions?
    A. Brain injury
    B. Emotional disturbance
    C. Hearing handicap
    D. Mental retardation
    E. Visual handicap

91. What is the goal of null hypothesis significance testing?
    A. To make inferences from the sample of subjects to the target population
    B. To reject the null hypothesis in favor of an alternative hypothesis
    C. To prove the statistical significance of the null hypothesis
    D. To ensure the randomization of subjects into control and experimental groups
    E. None of the above

92. Neuroendocrine side effects of anorexia nervosa include ALL of the following EXCEPT:
    A. Increased corticotropin-releasing hormone
    B. Hyposecretion of gonadotropin-releasing hormone
    C. Amenorrhea
    D. Increased luteinizing hormone by overstimulation of pituitary cells
    E. Low levels of leptin

93. Clinicians who express concern about the diagnostic category of somatoform disorders have argued ALL of the following EXCEPT:
    A. The category is inherently dualistic (physical vs. mental) and culturally limited
    B. The diagnoses are unreliable because of poorly defined symptom thresholds
    C. The diagnoses are unreliable because of ambiguities in the symptom criteria
    D. The included subgroupings are not coherent
    E. The diagnoses are too readily accepted by patients and adopted by colleagues in general medicine

94. True or False: Persons with autism tend to focus on mouths rather than eyes when they observe social interaction.
    A. True
    B. False

95. True or False: The use of child care by parents may interfere with the mother–child attachment bond.
    A. True
    B. False

96. Which of the following appears to predict the onset of functional somatic symptoms and somatoform disorders in children and adolescents?
    A. Borderline intellectual functioning
    B. Sexual maltreatment
    C. A specific learning disorder
    D. Obesity

97. ALL of the following descriptors are associated with systems of care EXCEPT:
    A. Deficit model
    B. Culturally competent
    C. Strength-based
    D. Child and family empowered
    E. Community-based

98. Which of these does NOT belong to the microsystem in Kazak's social–ecological model of children with pediatric illness?
    A. Ill child
    B. Disease
    C. Parents
    D. Extended family
    E. Social class
    F. Siblings

99. What is a simple alternative to the bell and pad method for the treatment of enuresis?
    A. Waking up the child using a bullhorn
    B. Setting an alarm clock after 2 to 3 hours of sleep, when the bladder may be reaching maximal capacity
    C. Keeping the lights on at night to aid arousal when the bladder signals full capacity
    D. Restricting fluids after 4 PM
    E. None of the above

100. The psychiatric problems that most commonly co-occur with language disorders include ALL of the following EXCEPT:
    A. ADHD
    B. Conduct disorder
    C. ODD
    D. Psychosis
    E. Selective mutism

101. ALL of the following are examples of concrete operational thinking EXCEPT:
    A. Ordering and rituals
    B. A child's coin collection
    C. Favorite or lucky numbers
    D. Obeying the golden rule
    E. Strictly following the rules in a game

102. ALL of the following psychosocial interventions have good empirical support EXCEPT:
    A. Clown-based therapy
    B. Interpersonal therapy
    C. Parent management training
    D. Parent-child interaction therapy
    E. Cognitive-behavioral family interventions

103. There is evidence for the success of prevention strategies for the initial onset of each of the following EXCEPT:
    A. Somatization
    B. Depression
    C. Anxiety
    D. Psychosis

104. True or False: The psychoanalytic concept of the superego constitutes a set of standards epitomizing the individual's belief of what is right, good, or desirable.
    A. True
    B. False

105. In addition to clinical and family history, a near confirmatory diagnostic test for tic disorders is:
    A. Magnetic resonance imaging
    B. Single photon emission computed tomography
    C. Electroencephalogram
    D. Blood dopamine level
    E. None

106. True or False: As most cognitive and intelligence tests yield a single intelligence quotient (IQ) score, this suggests that intelligence is a unitary construct.
    A. True
    B. False

107. True or False: The presence of children in a marriage is a deterrent for divorce.
    A. True
    B. False

108. ALL of the following are true about Rett's disorder EXCEPT:
    A. Head circumference is normal at birth
    B. Early development is typical
    C. Hand movements develop that resemble hand washing
    D. Language skills deteriorate
    E. Mental retardation develops

109. In psychoanalytic thought which of the following terms refer to all the factors that keep a patient in treatment and enable the patient to remain in treatment despite phases of resistance and hostile transference?
    A. Transference
    B. Countertransference
    C. Working alliance
    D. Observing ego
    E. Projection

110. True or False: On average, women have larger brains than men do.
    A. True
    B. False

111. Activities to develop resilience (empowerment) in communities affected by disasters include ALL of the following EXCEPT:
    A. Volunteer services
    B. Job fairs
    C. Arts and sports
    D. Free medical services
    E. Educational programs

112. Which of the following is the normal milestone for speech development regarding a child's ability to speak in two-word combinations and follow simple directions?
    A. 9 months
    B. 12 months
    C. 18 months
    D. 24 months
    E. 26 months

113. When a parent who has physical custody decides to move away, the noncustodial parent:
    A. Can stop the move by request in writing
    B. Can be granted immediate custody
    C. Is entitled to a full evidentiary hearing
    D. Must make a showing of detriment to the child
    E. Must accede to the move

114. Which of the following is the best approach in assessing youth who use illicit substances?
    A. Rogerian client-centered
    B. Cognitive-behavioral
    C. Psychodynamic
    D. Motivational interviewing
    E. Interpersonal therapy

115. True or False: Complaints by patients or their parents to state licensing boards and professional ethics committees for clinical care or for the Health Insurance Portability and Accountability Act violations require that harm to the patient be demonstrated for the complaint to be found justified.
    A. True
    B. False

116. True or False: Tic disorders were first identified in the late 19th century.
    A. True
    B. False

117. True or False: Both the Diagnostic and Statistical Manual of Mental Disorders-Fourth Edition-Text Revision (DSM-IV-TR) and ICD-10 require the absence of conduct disorder to allow a diagnosis of ODD.
    A. True
    B. False

118. The first psychiatric inpatient units dedicated to children and adolescents served:
    A. A custodial role for children with postencephalitic brain disorders
    B. As housing for the vast numbers of orphaned children due to the 1918 influenza pandemic
    C. As treatment centers for primarily well-off families that sent their "unruly teenagers"
    D. As housing for children removed from families by protective services due to abuse or neglect
    E. As learning centers for children with savant skills

119. Behavioral inhibition to the unfamiliar, a temperamental characteristic seen in infants as young as 21 months, has been associated with which of the following?
    A. OCD
    B. Panic disorder
    C. Major depressive disorder
    D. Specific phobia
    E. Social anxiety disorder

120. Which of the following is the correct characterization of children's ability to describe pain?
    A. Children can identify the presence and location of pain by age 2, pain intensity by age 4, can participate in formal pain ratings by age 5, and describe the quality of the pain experience by age 8
    B. Children can identify the presence and location of pain by age 4, pain intensity by age 4, participate in formal pain ratings by age 7, and describe the quality of the pain experience by age 9
    C. Children can identify the presence and location of pain by age 1, pain intensity by age 3, can participate in formal pain ratings by age 4, and describe the quality of the pain experience by age 8
    D. Children can identify the presence and location of pain by age 3, pain intensity by age 5, can participate in formal pain ratings by age 7, and describe the quality of the pain experience by age 9

121. Although most psychotropic medications reach steady-state concentration, the psychostimulants do not. Which TWO of the following statements state the reason why?
    A. They induce their own metabolism
    B. They have a very short half-life
    C. They have negligible blood serum levels
    D. They have therapeutic effectiveness at low concentrations
    E. They inhibit their own metabolism

122. Which of the following is NOT an element proposed by Himelstein and others as essential to pediatric palliative care?
    A. Physical concerns
    B. Psychosocial concerns
    C. Spiritual concerns
    D. Advance care planning
    E. Athleticism
    F. Practical concerns

123. Which one of the following was the most enduring of Freud's metapsychological frameworks, which divides mental functions into id, ego, and superego?
    A. The topographical model
    B. The tripartite model
    C. Object constancy
    D. Psychic determinism
    E. Internalization

124. True or False: Child abuse or neglect account for most cases of failure to thrive.
    A. True
    B. False

125. You are seeing a 9-year-old boy with ADHD and decide that stimulant medications are indicated to address his symptoms. In a shared custody arrangement, which option for obtaining parental consent for medications is the BEST?
    A. Attempt to contact both parents regarding the treatment decision
    B. Obtain consent from the primary parent (usually the mother)
    C. Attempt to contact the guardian ad litem regarding the treatment decision
    D. Obtain consent from the parent who has physical custody of the child

126. Which of the following statistical approaches to the classification of psychiatric disorders can be used to establish which symptoms and symptom combinations are more strongly related to a particular diagnosis?
    A. Cluster analysis
    B. Factor analysis
    C. Latent class analysis
    D. Latent trait analysis
    E. Signal detection analysis

127. What is the typical starting dose of sertraline for children?
    A. 12.5 to 25 mg
    B. 25 to 50 mg
    C. 50 to 62.5 mg
    D. 50 to 75 mg
    E. 75 to 100 mg

128. ALL of these are potentially useful agents to treat an acutely agitated patient in the emergency room EXCEPT:
    A. Lorazepam
    B. Chlorpromazine
    C. Diphenhydramine
    D. Benztropine
    E. Haloperidol decanoate

129. ALL of the following statements describe 20th-century dynamic psychiatry EXCEPT:
    A. Emphasis on the patient's subjective experience
    B. Emphasis on the workings of the unconscious psychological processes
    C. Emphasis on the patient's unique inner life
    D. Emphasis on categorizing patients according to observable behavior

130. For complex child psychiatric disorders it is assumed that rare, gross chromosomal anomalies are unlikely to account for the risk in most of the affected population. Given this assumption, what would be the potential advantage in looking for such anomalies?
    A. Genetic mutations are difficult to discern indicating the need for replication
    B. Rare chromosomal abnormalities as one pathway to a disease can provide clues to disease mechanisms and novel therapeutic insights
    C. Child psychiatric disorders occur within a developmental context and gene activation may occur at different stages of development
    D. Child psychiatric disorders may have common final pathways emanating from divergent genetic influences

131. True or False: One is required to disclose one's HIV-positive status to a sexual partner.
    A. True
    B. False

132. True or False: Juveniles who commit arson tend to have heightened suicidal thinking and an increased risk of suicide attempts.
    A. True
    B. False

133. The psychiatric assessment of the child commonly differs from the assessment of adults in ALL of the following ways EXCEPT:
    A. The child and clinician are at different developmental levels, such that they may have difficulties in communication
    B. The clinician need only focus on the assessment and treatment of the child
    C. The child may function differently in different settings
    D. The child's presenting problems must be examined in a developmental context
    E. There are developmental differences in the presentation of mental illness as categorized in the DSM-IV-TR

134. ALL of the following tasks are characteristic of preschool aged children EXCEPT:
    A. Parallel play
    B. Indiscriminately positive self-image
    C. Temper tantrums
    D. Object constancy
    E. Chumship

135. Executive function is a term generally used to encompass several higher order cognitive functions and is composed of a set of abilities including ALL of the following EXCEPT:
    A. Inhibition
    B. Set shifting
    C. Planning
    D. Sensory perception
    E. Working memory

136. ALL of following symptoms of ADHD are more likely to persist into adulthood EXCEPT:
    A. Inattention
    B. Distractibility
    C. Disorganization
    D. Hyperactivity
    E. Failure to finish things

137. Of the following treatments utilized in inpatient treatment settings, which is limited by the need for multidisciplinary staff training?
   A. Behavioral treatment through "token economies"
   B. PMT
   C. Cognitive-behavioral therapy
   D. Psychopharmacology
   E. Dialectical-behavior therapy

138. Which TWO of the four functionally distinct pharmacokinetic phases are primarily responsible for determining the speed of onset of drug effect?
   A. Absorption
   B. Metabolism
   C. Distribution
   D. Excretion

139. The conditions in which catatonia is expressed include ALL of the following EXCEPT:
   A. Mood disorders
   B. Psychotic disorders
   C. Medical disorders
   D. Somatization disorders

140. Which of the following medical conditions is associated with regression?
   A. Central nervous system infection
   B. Phenylketonuria
   C. Hypothyroidism
   D. Seizure disorder
   E. All of the above

141. True or False: Parents of boys with gender identity disorder have the prenatal desire for a girl.
   A. True
   B. False

142. Children with autism have increased rates of epilepsy. Its onset has a bimodal distribution best characterized by:
   A. First peak before age 5 years and the other after age 10 years
   B. First peak before age 10 years and the other after age 20 years
   C. First peak before age 15 years and the other after age 20 years
   D. First peak before age 20 years and the other after age 25 years

143. Which of the following is the BEST description of transference?
   A. The ability to take account of one's own and others' mental states in understanding why people behave in specific ways
   B. The unconscious displacement onto the therapist of patterns of feelings, thoughts, and behavior originally experienced in relation to significant figures during childhood
   C. The internalization of a positive representation of the parent by the child
   D. The attribution of internal conflicts to the external environment and a search for external solutions

144. Home and community-based interventions for youths served by the mental health sector have their origins in:
   A. The systems of care movement
   B. Wraparound services
   C. Women and children experiencing the loss of husbands and fathers in the Vietnam War
   D. The number of "baby boomer" births
   E. The emergence of eastern religious thought and its emphasis on interdependence

145. True or False: Treatment for ODD and conduct disorder is more likely to be effective when administered early in the course of the disorder.
    A. True
    B. False

146. How many standard deviations below the mean qualify for interventional services when assessing infant performance on developmental testing?
    A. One standard deviation
    B. Two standard deviations
    C. Three standard deviations
    D. Four standard deviations

147. Critics of the gender identity diagnosis generally believe what about children who demonstrate a preference for being the opposite sex of their birth?
    A. The child was "born this way"
    B. There is too much coddling of children
    C. Parents should be more traditional in their roles
    D. Children will be confused as long as their parents are confused
    E. None of the above

148. True or False: All selective serotonin reuptake inhibitors have relatively long half-lives, permitting single daily dosing.
    A. True
    B. False

149. What may be the responsible factor for a child who has a dystonic reaction, such as oculogyric crisis, while receiving a combination of paroxetine and risperidone?
    A. Risperidone's inhibition of paroxetine metabolism
    B. Paroxetine's inhibition of risperidone metabolism
    C. Risperidone's induction of paroxetine metabolism
    D. Paroxetine's induction of risperidone's metabolism
    E. Paroxetine and risperidone's dual inhibition of the other's metabolism

150. In the disclosure of cancer to a child patient, what does the International Society of Pediatric Oncologists recommend?
    A. Limit the information revealed to the child about his or her condition
    B. Share information if and when the child asks for information
    C. Tell the child without the parents present so that the parents' distress does not overwhelm the child
    D. Full disclosure to the child after or during a conference with the parents
    E. Have the parents tell the child

151. The elderly are thought to be more vulnerable to delirium because of diminished cholinergic reserve. Children are thought to be more vulnerable because of which of the following?
    A. Greater brain-to-body ratio
    B. Imagination and its role in development
    C. Media exposure, which involves fantasy-based themes
    D. Immature and evolving structural and biochemical brain development
    E. All of the above

152. Autism has been associated with ALL of the following medical conditions EXCEPT:
    A. Seizures
    B. Tuberous sclerosis
    C. Spina bifida
    D. Fragile X syndrome
    E. Maternally inherited deletions

153. True or False: Parents and caretakers are notoriously poor at identifying internalizing symptoms in children under their care.
    A. True
    B. False

154. ALL of the following organizations allow you to file an ethical complaint against a colleague who is engaging in questionable activities with a patient EXCEPT:
    A. The district branch of the APA
    B. The local medical society
    C. The Assembly of the APA
    D. The state licensing board

155. Which of the following statements about maturation in boys is most accurate based on research findings?
    A. Early maturation leads to an increased vulnerability to depression and anxiety
    B. Early maturation is advantageous in terms of popularity and self-esteem
    C. Late maturation is related to increased risk for delinquency or problem behaviors
    D. None of the above

156. The "Early Intervention Foster Care Program" includes ALL of the following EXCEPT:
    A. 24/7 emergency availability of staff
    B. Daily telephone contact with the foster parents
    C. Weekly visits to the foster home
    D. Weekly school visits
    E. Weekly group sessions with other foster care providers

157. True or False: Graft versus host disease is a common occurrence in transplant medicine.
    A. True
    B. False

158. True or False: Among children between the ages of 3 to 12, girls are referred clinically more often than boys for concerns regarding their gender identity.
    A. True
    B. False

159. For a child with severe expressive language delay or dysfunction, or absence of language, ALL of the following augmentative communication modalities may be taught to the child as an alternative or complement to vocal communication EXCEPT:
    A. Occupational therapy
    B. Sign language
    C. Picture board
    D. Electronic speech aid

160. True or False: In adolescent mothers of low socioeconomic status, the Brazelton Neonatal Behavioral Assessment Scale, second edition (NBAS-2), serves as an effective intervention tool for increasing maternal involvement and responsiveness.
    A. True
    B. False

161. Following the development of the IQ test, two basic approaches were used in exploring the intellectual development of infants. Which TWO choices describe these approaches?
    A. Anna Freud's concept of developmental lines
    B. Infant IQ
    C. Gesell model of development schedules
    D. Engels' biopsychosocial model
    E. Margaret Mahler's theories including separation-individuation

162. Which of the following is TRUE of the precocity of babies?
    A. The precocity of babies is described in industrialized societies
    B. Precocity has been linked with reports of precocity in parents
    C. Precocity has been linked with reports of precocity in older siblings
    D. Precocity is largely correlated with environmental factors
    E. None of the above

163. In every infant assessment one must especially consider:
    A. Whether the infant is breast-fed or bottle-fed
    B. The other individuals involved in the infant's life
    C. The details of the mother's period of pregnancy, labor, and delivery
    D. The family history of the maternal and paternal lineage of the infant

164. Which edition of the DSM recognized ADHD for the first time as an official diagnosis, but called it "hyperkinetic reaction" based on the prevailing psychodynamic philosophy that mental disorders are reactions to a stressor?
    A. DSM-I
    B. DSM-II
    C. DSM-III
    D. DSM-III-R
    E. DSM-IV

165. Which of the following is among the most common projective techniques used in a child psychiatric interview in order for the child to express concerns indirectly?
    A. Asking questions about specific symptoms
    B. Drawing
    C. Having the child climb stairs to assess gross motor development
    D. Asking the child how he feels
    E. Assessing fund of knowledge

166. Complications of binging and purging behavior include ALL of the following EXCEPT:
    A. Dental enamel erosion and caries
    B. Subconjunctival hemorrhaging
    C. Esophageal or gastric rupture
    D. Renal failure
    E. Hyperchloremic acidosis

167. True or False: A follow-up study of child care in four states confirmed that children who are in poor quality care experience developmental problems that persist when the children are of school age.
    A. True
    B. False

168. What case established due process for juveniles and the standards for transfer of juveniles to adult criminal court?
    A. *Jones v. United States*
    B. *Sboket v. United States*
    C. *Kent v. United States*
    D. *Seohs v. United States*
    E. Juveniles do not have due process rights

169. True or False: Use of disulfiram (Antabuse) in the treatment of alcohol dependence is based on the principles of operant conditioning.
    A. True
    B. False

170. True or False: An Institutional Review Board allows for the determination of the specific information that must be divulged to prospective subjects when conducting research on human subjects.
    A. True
    B. False

171. True or False: The Early Periodic Screening Detection and Treatment mandate for Medicaid mandates periodic health and mental health screening for covered children as well as medical necessity authorization for treatment and services to address abnormal findings.
    A. True
    B. False

172. Developmental factors that may contribute to an increased risk of depression after puberty include ALL of the following EXCEPT:
    A. Early-onset puberty in girls
    B. Experimentation with tobacco, drugs, and alcohol
    C. Decreased adult supervision and contact
    D. Greater physiological need for sleep
    E. Poor academic success

173. Malpractice litigation is one way of holding physicians to appropriate standards and compensating patients who have been negligently harmed. The use of litigation to achieve these particular goals can be a problem for ALL of the following reasons EXCEPT:
    A. Many patients who have been harmed do not sue
    B. Many patients who have suffered damage were not harmed by negligence
    C. The practice of defensive medicine becomes more likely
    D. Psychiatrists may avoid taking on more complicated patients
    E. Child psychiatry is a high-risk specialty and fear of litigation exacerbates the shortage of child psychiatrists

174. ALL of these factors differentiate pediatric medical services and pediatric psychology or psychiatry services EXCEPT:
    A. Biomedical versus biopsychosocial model
    B. Pace of work
    C. Privacy
    D. Empathy

175. Since 1989 what is the country of origin of the largest group of international adoptees?
    A. China
    B. Guatemala
    C. Sweden
    D. Russia
    E. Korea

176. A measurement is considered reliable when the correlation coefficient, r, ranges from +0.7 to +1.0. However, what minimal value of reliability is usually required for measures that are used to make clinical decisions on patients?
    A. +0.6
    B. +0.7
    C. +0.8
    D. +0.9
    E. +1.0

In the following questions, match the MEDIAN age during which the following oppositional defiant and conduct symptoms occur in children.

177. Stubbornness

178. Defiance and temper tantrums

179. Argumentativeness

180. Lying

181. Bullying

182. Stealing
    A. 9 years
    B. 5 years
    C. 8 years
    D. 6 years
    E. 12 years
    F. 3 years

183. Which one of the following cytochrome P450 (CYP) families is MOST involved in hepatic drug metabolism, responsible for metabolizing half of the psychotropic drugs?
    A. CYP 1A
    B. CYP 2B
    C. CYP 2C
    D. CYP 2E
    E. CYP 3A

184. True or False: Patients with trichotillomania often have a family history of OCD.
    A. True
    B. False

185. Which of the following statements about stuttering is FALSE?
    A. Girls are more likely than boys to experience unassisted recovery from stuttering
    B. The prevalence of stuttering is about one in 30 children, but this number drops to one in 100 adolescents
    C. Psychotherapy alone has been shown to be an effective treatment for stuttering
    D. The ratio of boys to girls who begin to stutter between the ages of 2 and 4 is approximately equal
    E. The ratio of boys to girls who persist in stuttering increases to approximately three to one in adolescence

186. Two important factors affecting the distribution of drugs in the body change substantially during child and adolescent development in comparison with adults. Which TWO of the following comprise these factors?
    A. Fat stores
    B. The ratio of total body water to extracellular water
    C. Serum albumin levels
    D. Alpha-1-acid glycoprotein levels
    E. Platelet count

187. What would be an appropriate initial approach to the education of a child who has cancer and is returning to school?
    A. Reintegrate normally without specific planning for reentry to normalize the experience
    B. Develop a 504 plan
    C. Establish special education programming
    D. Communicate with the school
    E. Establish homebound schooling

188. ALL of the following were found in the studies by Asarnow and colleagues for children with childhood onset schizophrenia EXCEPT:
    A. Children performed normally on simple perceptual processing skills
    B. Children performed poorly on rote language skills
    C. Children performed poorly on tasks involving fine motor coordination
    D. Children performed poorly on tasks involving short-term memory
    E. Children performed poorly on tasks involving working memory

189. Which of the following is a respondent-based interview that covers a wide range of childhood and adolescent disorders, and is suitable for use with 9- to 18-year-olds?
    A. Anxiety Disorders Interview Schedule
    B. Diagnostic Interview Schedule for Children
    C. Interview Schedule for Children and Adolescents
    D. Kiddie-Schedule for Affective Disorders and Schizophrenia
    E. Child and Adolescent Psychiatric Assessment

190. Which of the following is accurate?
    A. Growth factor receptors lie in the cell nucleus
    B. Hormone receptors lie in the cell nucleus
    C. Growth factor receptors lie on the cell membrane
    D. A and B
    E. B and C

191. In the United States, which of the following groups of children have the highest rate of reactive attachment disorder?
    A. Children who are homeless
    B. Children in foster care
    C. Children in Head Start
    D. Children who live in residential treatment centers
    E. Children in state custody

192. Neuroleptic malignant syndrome is characterized by ALL of the following signs and symptoms EXCEPT:
    A. High fever
    B. Nausea and vomiting
    C. Autonomic instability
    D. Muscle breakdown
    E. Elevated creatine phosphokinase titers

193. Which of the following primary preventions have been demonstrated to be most effective for preventing suicide?
    A. Physician education in the recognition of depression and its treatment
    B. Restricting lethal methods of suicide
    C. No primary preventions are effective
    D. A and B

194. In a female with borderline personality disorder who has a history of being sexually abused, what role may promiscuity play?
    A. It affords the opportunity to turn around and gain control of the helplessness associated with being abused
    B. Sublimation
    C. Altruism
    D. Idealization
    E. It affords the opportunity to punish the self, which affirms and reenforces the feelings of worthlessness that are present

195. Atomoxetine has which mechanism of action?
    A. Selective norepinephrine reuptake inhibition
    B. Selective serotonin reuptake inhibition
    C. Selective dopamine reuptake inhibition
    D. Serotonin postsynaptic antagonism
    E. Norepinephrine postsynaptic antagonism

196. In the development of the brain, neurogenesis of the cerebral cortex occurs by neurons migrating past earlier born cells to reach their final destination. Disruption of the normal migration of cells causes several disorders. The most common of these, which lack the normal pattern of gyri and sulci, are called:
    A. The lissencephalies
    B. The cortical degeneration diseases
    C. The spongiform encephalopathies
    D. The central nervous system matrix diseases
    E. The Wile E. Coyote brain

197. Which of the following agents may be used in the treatment of opiate dependence?
    A. Buprenorphine
    B. Bupropion
    C. Naltrexone
    D. A and C
    E. B and C

198. ALL of the following have been found in children with profound visual impairment EXCEPT:
    A. Increased rates of autism or autism-like behaviors
    B. Increased rates of psychiatric disorders
    C. Increased rates of schizophrenia
    D. Increased rates of intellectual disabilities
    E. Increased rates of loneliness

199. Intensive home-based services have ALL of the following common elements
     EXCEPT:
     A. Services are provided in the home and community with appointment times con-
        venient to the family
     B. Treatment is time limited, of 1 to 5 months' duration
     C. Therapists have caseloads of 2 to 6 families
     D. Team members are available around the clock to travel to the home to respond
        to crises
     E. Therapists make multiple weekly visits

200. Piaget's stage of formal operations includes ALL of the following EXCEPT:
     A. The ability to construct "contrary to fact" propositions
     B. The growth in hypothetico-deductive problem solving ability
     C. Increased understanding of propositional logic and probability
     D. Improvement in mathematics test scores
     E. Greater capacity for abstraction

1. **Answer: B.** Page 243.

2. **Answer: D.** This answer reflects 2007 Youth Risk Behavior Surveillance System (YRBSS) data and not the YRBSS data in the Lewis textbook, which dates from 2005. 7% of high school students reported having attempted suicide in the last 12 months and 2% reported needing attention by a nurse or physician as a result. The YRBSS includes a national school-based survey conducted by the Centers for Disease Control and Prevention and local surveys conducted by state, territorial, community education and health agencies, and tribal governments. Page 900.

3. **Answer: C.** The point of this question is to highlight the key triggers for nonepileptic seizure disorder (NESD) in children. NESD is the preferred term for pseudoseizures. Environmental stress is the number one cause of NESD, which includes sexual abuse and family discord (such as parental conflict or divorce or death in the family). A family history of epilepsy is also found commonly. Page 963.

4. **Answer: A.** In the question, the null hypothesis is rejected at the 0.05 significance level. To explain the converse: A value of 1.0 indicates no association between an exposure and disease, and represents the expected value of the null hypothesis. If the confidence interval around a point estimate includes 1.0 the null hypothesis is not rejected. Page 154.

5. **Answer: D.** Page 478.

6. **Answer: A.** Adoption itself poses low absolute risks for emotional and behavioral problems. The relative risk is increased compared to controls, but is decreased compared to children living in long-term foster care or children returned to their families of origin. Page 1015.

7. **Answer: C.** Attachment studies have indicated how malign early life influences can contribute to persisting (and perpetuating) interpersonal dysfunction. Page 3.

8. **Answer: A.** The question is unanswered for adolescents. Page 616.

9. **Answer: A.** These assessment techniques, such as drawing, completing sentences, and providing narratives to pictures, may be more engaging and less confrontational than direct questioning, especially for children and adolescents. Page 365.

10. **Answer: A.** Most teaching programs are not committed to disaster intervention training. Page 728.

11. **Answer: E.** Leo Kanner first described a group of 11 children as having similar characteristics he termed "early infantile autism" in 1943. Hans Asperger described a similar group as having "autistic psychopathy" in 1944. Page 384.

12. **Answer: A.** The psychiatric formulation organizes the clinician's interactions with patients into a concise form that makes an argument for further investigation and intervention. Page 377.

13. **Answer: C.** Chronic exposure to stressful experiences tends to lead to hypercorticolism due to excessive activation of the hypothalamic-pituitary-adrenal axis that can have damaging effects on neural functioning; however, resilient individuals may avoid the damage conferred by hypercorticolism by their quick return to baseline levels of cortisol. Page 296.

14. **Answer: B.** Children under 6 years of age living with a single mother were FIVE times more likely to be poor than those living with both parents. Other contributing factors include cuts in public assistance and the decline in the real value of family income. Page 37.

15. **Answer: D.** Page 201.

16. **Answer: B.** Page 856.

17. **Answer: C.** HLA-DQB1*0602 and HLA-DR2 alleles are found in 85% of patients with narcolepsy compared to 12% to 38% in the general population. Page 630.

18. **Answer: B.** The assent of children is not a necessary condition for a therapeutic intervention as per federal regulations. Page 145.

19. **Answer: B.** Generally, for psychiatric treatment, doses higher than 0.2 mg in prepubertal children and 0.3 mg in older children are considered 'maximum' doses; however, much higher doses are used to treat hypertension. Page 781.

20. **Answer: E.** Page 305.

21. **Answer: C.** The proper neuronal connections are strengthened throughout early infancy by the expansion of functioning synaptic contacts. Genetic as well as environmental factors (drugs, alcohol, altered nutrition, etc.) and infectious illness all affect brain development. Neuronal connections can be made throughout life, although the greatest amount of change occurs during the early childhood years and again during puberty. Page 186.

22. **Answer: B.** This can be either concurrent (high stress predicts cortisol levels) or predictive (intelligence quotient [IQ] predicts later academic achievement). Page 160.

23. **Answer: B.** Page 105.

24. **Answer: D.** Page 312.

25. **Answer: D.** The majority of students with learning disabilities are identified in middle school and high school; the early years of schooling might be insufficient for exposing and making evident a deficit in a particular academic domain. Page 415.

26. **Answer: B.** This cumulative risk approach shows the effect of synergy, as the effect of multiple risks on children produces outcomes far poorer than when any one of these risks exists in isolation. Page 292.

27. **Answer: B.** Page 345.

28. **Answer: C.** Given that monozygotic twins share all their genetic material but only 50% are concordant for schizophrenia, suggests that influences apart from the DNA sequence contribute to the disease. These influences may be environmental or involve inheritable genetic mechanisms not coded for in the DNA (i.e., epigenetic factors). Page 190.

29. **Answer: A.** This can result in decreased efficacy of the medication. Page 772.

30. **Answer: C.** Behavioral Consultations explore problematic behaviors exhibited by students or staff. Elements include direct observation in the classroom and counting frequency and duration of behavior. The consultant provides recommendations to alter and shape student responses that lead to the problem behavior. Table 7.2.2 in Lewis describes the other school models, Mental Health Consultation and Organizational Consultation. Page 981.

31. **Answer: C.** Other domains include memory, motor activity, and intentional or goal-directed activity. Page 359.

32. **Answer: C.** Kanner was not only the first author on child psychiatry with a textbook published in 1935 (which indicates the relative youth of this discipline), but is also credited for the first recognition and description of autism in children. Page 15.

33. **Answer: C.** Primary care physicians. Page 923.

34. **Answer: B.** Holding therapy and other alternative approaches, including rebirthing are associated with high risk and death. Page 717.

35. **Answer: C.** The amygdala is part of the limbic system. For example, children and adults with anxiety disorders show greater amygdala activity in response to face stimuli. The orbital frontal cortex and anterior cingulate cortex are also thought to be involved in the neural circuitry of anxiety. Page 543.

36. **Answer: B.** In psychiatry, prevalence rates often refer to specific time periods. The most commonly used prevalence rates are 3-, 6-, and 12-month periods. Page 151.

37. **Answer: C.** In acute stress disorder (ASD), posttraumatic symptoms are present between 2 and 30 days after the traumatic event. Page 701.

38. **Answer: B.** Studies have shown conflicting results; some show profound changes and marital discord, whereas others show that marital relationships remain stable or improve over the course of the child's cancer. However, they are seldom stress free. Page 701.

39. **Answer: B.** Page 372.

40. **Answer: A.** Some wear and tear in the environment must be a realistic expectation in working with children and adolescents. It would be too difficult to carry out the work of the group if leaders were faced with constant worry about protecting a more adult-oriented room that contained objects or interior decorations of great value. Page 845.

41. **Answer: A.** This is one of the more notable findings in father–infant care research, as a father's physical involvement in their child's life during infancy and toddlerhood is correlated with a dramatic decreased probability of subsequent perpetration of child sexual abuse. Page 7.

42. **Answer: B.** In Troiden's model, development begins with a stage of sensitization. Sensitization is described in the literature as a sense of being different from peers. This sense of being different often stems from nonconforming gender roles and correlates with later same-sex orientation more strongly for men than for women. Identity confusion and identity assumption are subsequent stages in Troiden's model. Page 81.

43. **Answer: D.** Page 132.

44. **Answer: C.** By about two-fold, from approximately two out of 100 for placebo to four out of 100 for selective serotonin reuptake inhibitors. Page 535.

45. **Answer: A.** In addition to their blocking properties at dopamine receptors, these atypical antipsychotics target serotonergic receptors; and it appears that their effects at cortical 5-HT$_{2a}$ receptors help mediate the antipsychotic effects. Page 239.

46. **Answer: A.** This statistic would be beneficial to communicate for informed consent and to help patients understand that they may continue to experience symptoms after treatment. Page 558.

47. **Answer: B.** Synaptic pruning in the prefrontal cortex continues as an ongoing process through adolescence. Page 268.

48. **Answer: D.** Page 663.

49. **Answer: A.** Page 755.

50. **Answer: C.** Page 266.

51. **Answer: A.** Rates of schizophrenia or psychosis in persons with an intellectual disability range from 1% to 9% among nonreferred samples and 2.8% to 24% in referred samples. Although variable, these rates are much higher than the 0.5% to 1% seen in the general population with schizophrenia. Page 404.

52. **Answer: E.** Functional dysphagia is an eating disorder characterized by a subjective experience of difficulty or discomfort associated with the act of swallowing that is not primarily due to an organic medical condition. Page 589.

53. **Answer: C.** These laboratories include complete blood cell count, electrolytes, blood urea nitrogen, creatinine, and thyroid indices; lithium levels can be obtained routinely at 3 to 6 month intervals. Page 769.

54. **Answer: A.** Endotypes are phenotypes that are assumed to be less complex in presentation and etiology than signs and symptoms of the associated clinical disorder. Page 433.

55. **Answer: C.** Page 571.

56. **Answer: C.** Page 798.

57. **Answer: C.** Child psychiatrists need to learn how to use play therapeutically to communicate with young children and is different from simply joining in with the play. Child psychiatrists may be more effective by staying "within the play" and working within the child's story to help him expand his expression of feelings and beliefs in a way that helps the therapist to better understand him. Page 263.

58. **Answer: D.** Neuroimaging studies indicate increased activity in the head of the caudate nucleus. Increased activity in the orbital frontal cortex is also found. Page 553.

59. **Answer: A.** That the diagnosis exists is not a controversy. Page 513.

60. **Answer: B.** The programs were designed for children of low-income families who were NOT eligible for Medicaid. Page 52.

61. **Answer: A.** Perspective-taking is one of the skills that adolescent patients learn in the primary component of interpersonal skills building. Page 821.

62. **Answer: B.** GSA (Gay-Straight Alliance) exists in over 2,000 schools across the United States. PFLAG (Parents, Friends and Families of Lesbians and Gays) has chapters and support groups in all 50 states. GLSEN stands for Gay, Lesbian and Straight Education Network. GLBT (or LGBT) refers to gay lesbian bisexual and transgender/transsexual people. Page 85.

63. **Answer: B.** The ego functions to restrain prohibited expressions of inner urges and likewise promote approved expressions—the ego protects against internal dangers. Page 829.

64. **Answer: C.** Page 656.

65. **Answer: A.** Page 928.

66. **Answer: B.** Lithium has specific effects on the phosphatidylinositol and protein kinase C pathways of intracellular signaling. Page 769.

67. **Answer: D.** One of the critiques of early efficacy studies was how their samples of children were too heterogeneous in terms of diagnoses and developmental levels, making interpretation of any results problematic. Page 790.

68. **Answer: B.** Although early relationships are extremely important in influencing how people view subsequent interactions, a "faulty lens" can be corrected to some degree; that is, early life experiences and adaptation are a probabilistic rather than deterministic indicator of success at later stages. Page 294.

69. **Answer: E.** Resilience cannot be directly measured. It is inferred by the presence of two fundamental conditions: the existence of significant risk or adversity and positive adaptation. Page 293.

70. **Answer: D.** Prior suicide attempts increase the risk by 50- to 90-fold. Substance use is more common in young victims than adults. Page 531.

71. **Answer: A.** Event-related designs isolate individual trials, which provide clearer images of transient neuronal changes from cognitive and sensory processes. Page 222.

72. **Answer: D.** Thirty five percent of males have their onset between 5 and 15, compared to 20% of females. Page 550.

73. **Answer: B.** There is a predominance of males to females and a strong positive family history. Page 628.

74. **Answer: B.** The number needed to treat (NNT) is calculated as:

    NNT = 1/ARR (absolute risk reduction). Page 127.

75. **Answer: D.** Page 683.

76. **Answer: A.** Page 811.

77. **Answer: B.** Most do not meet ASD criteria; however, the presence of ASD is a potent predictor of later posttraumatic stress disorder. Page 706.

78. **Answer: B.** Interpersonal psychotherapy assumes that if one improves the relationships in the patient's life, one can change the course of the depressive episode. Page 819.

79. **Answer: C.** Page 379.

80. **Answer: A.** Page 848.

81. **Answer: A.** However, children with these comorbidities display a progression to conduct disorder much earlier, and this predicts worse outcomes. Page 471.

82. **Answer: B.** Page 619.

83. **Answer: E.** If a youth does not respond to one agent, trying another not previously tried is recommended. For those with severe agitation or partial response, two agents are indicated. If psychosis is present, an atypical antipsychotic, singly or in combination, can be tried. Page 521.

84. **Answer: D.** There is a general consensus that parental obesity is by far the strongest risk factor for childhood and adolescent obesity. The risk is influenced by the degree of parental obesity. Pages 606–607.

85. **Answer: D.** This means that 75 mg of nortriptyline a day is expected to yield a steady-state trough level of about 75 ng/mL in a normal metabolizer. When a major discrepancy from this correspondence occurs, the clinician can consider noncompliance or ultrafast or slow metabolism of the medication. Page 764.

86. **Answer: B and D.** Disruption refers to the decision to end treatment due to external factors affecting the parents, child, or therapist. Interruption refers to a unilateral decision by one of the parties to end the treatment primarily attributed to intrapsychic factors or conflicts. Page 836.

87. **Answer: C.** In 1946, World War II was over and there was political momentum to provide for the children of the new baby boom. Page 23.

88. **Answer: C.** The most well-known consideration of this issue is the Tarasoff decision in California. Jurisdictions vary and you should know your state's requirements. However, generally, when an identifiable victim is named, you have a duty to protect, which may take the form of warning the potential victim, informing the police, hospitalizing the patient (if psychiatric treatment is indicated), or a combination of these. Clinically it is often best to let the adolescent know what your obligations are and even enlist them in the process of addressing Tarasoff concerns. Page 906.

89. **Answer: B.** Composition is combining elements to lead to another class. It is one of Piaget's concrete logical operations. Page 270.

90. **Answer: A.** According to this definition, specific learning disability includes such conditions as perceptual handicaps, brain injury, minimal brain dysfunction, dyslexia, and developmental aphasia. The term does not include children who have learning problems which are primarily the result of visual, hearing, or motor handicaps, of intellectual disability, or emotional disturbance, or of environmental, cultural, or economic disadvantage. Page 411.

91. **Answer: B.** Page 115.

92. **Answer: D.** It is well established that pituitary cells producing luteinizing hormone are understimulated in patients with anorexia nervosa because of hyposecretion of gonadotropin-releasing hormone by the hypothalamus. Page 597.

93. **Answer: E.** The diagnoses are not well accepted by patients and not well adopted by general medicine. Page 634.

94. **Answer: A.** Individuals with autism have difficulty processing facial information. It has been demonstrated that people with autism have decreased levels of responsiveness to the human face in the fusiform face area of the temporal lobe. Pages 387–388.

95. **Answer: B.** Although an earlier study suggested the statement is true, later research did not find this association with childcare use independently but only in conjunction with low maternal sensitivity and responsiveness when this interacted with poor quality childcare, multiple childcare arrangements, and larger quantities of childcare. Page 255.

96. **Answer: B.** Page 638.

97. **Answer: A.** The deficit model, which focuses on uncovering problems and prescribing solutions—the traditional approach to mental health delivery—is not part of a system of care (SOC), which approaches issues via a strength-based model. Page 891.

98. **Answer: E.** Kazak's model has a microsystem, mesosystem, exosystem, and macrosystem to help organize thinking which examines multiple layers of influence and bidirectionality of influence. The Disability-Stress-Coping Model of adjustment is another model. Page 914.

99. **Answer: B.** Success rates of 61.8% (2–3 hours sleep method) and 77.1% (maximal capacity method) have been found, with 6-month relapse rates of 14.7% and 24.1%, respectively. Page 660.

100. **Answer: D.** The psychiatric problems that most commonly co-occur with language disorders include attention deficit hyperactivity disorder, conduct, oppositional, and anxiety disorders. Page 421.

101. **Answer: D.** The Golden Rule (do unto others as you would have them do unto you) is an example of Kohlberg's theory of conventional morality (not concrete operational thinking), the first part of which is interpersonal concordance—the idea that a child measures behavior and bases it on whether it pleases those he looks up to. This stage of morality is followed by orientation toward authority, in which the greater social system or society, rather than the proximal family or school standards, sets the child's moral compass. Page 271.

102. **Answer: A.** Page 894.

103. **Answer: A.** Page 172.

104. **Answer: B.** The concept of the ego ideal constitutes this function; the superego can be effective in controlling behavior in conformance with this ideal, depending on the developmental status of the ego. Page 830.

105. **Answer: E.** There are no confirmatory tests for tic disorders. Diagnosis is made by obtaining a history, observation, neurological examination, and by ruling out other disorders. Page 576.

106. **Answer: B.** Instead, the IQ or ability score is typically composed of a variety of subtests measuring a range of functions. Moreover, tests are based on different theories of intelligence and may differ markedly in terms of content and emphasis. Page 363.

107. **Answer: B.** Roughly 60% of all current divorces involve children. Page 39.

108. **Answer: B.** ALL are true except that early development is unremarkable. Head growth, though initially normal, begins to decelerate sometime between 5 and 48 months of age. Page 393.

109. **Answer: C.** Treatment alliance is another term referring to this descriptor. Page 831.

110. **Answer: B.** The difference in brain size is primarily attributable to larger body size. This question is intended to obliquely refer to the difficulty of statistically analyzing anatomical magnetic resonance imaging data given individual and group differences in brain morphology. Page 230.

111. **Answer: D.** Programs to enhance resilience may include the arts, sports, gardening, decorating, continuing-education, job clubs, and volunteer recruitment and training in a number of areas. Page 735.

112. **Answer: D.** Page 371.

113. **Answer: D.** This is an area of evolving case law. In the state of California, which has a number of landmark cases, a noncustodial parent must show that there is detriment to the child after which the parent can receive a full evidentiary hearing. Page 1010.

114. **Answer: D.** Resources are available at www.motivationalinterview.org. Page 618.

115. **Answer: B.** Neither a doctor–patient relationship nor harm is required for complaints to go forward. For example, any parent in a custody evaluation may launch a complaint. Many insurers cover attorney costs in licensing board investigations. Page 1029.

116. **Answer: B.** References to tics in the literature have been noted as far back as 1482. Page 569.

117. **Answer: A.** This criterion implies a hierarchical relationship. Page 455.

118. **Answer: A.** The first child and adolescent inpatient psychiatric units were created in the 1920s and 1930s. During the mid-1980s the private sector grew and advertised to families worried about their teens. Page 866.

119. **Answer: E.** Page 540.

120. **Answer: A.** Page 974.

121. **Answer: B and D.** Page 743.

122. **Answer: E.** Palliative care is not just about death. The American Academy of Pediatrics states in its guidelines: "the components of palliative care are offered at diagnosis, and continued throughout the course of illness, whether the outcome ends in cure or death." Page 973.

123. **Answer: B.** Page 828.

124. **Answer: B.** Failure to thrive was previously believed to be the result of abuse or neglect. The best available evidence now suggests that child abuse and neglect are implicated in failure to thrive in less than 10% of all cases. Child abuse and neglect should be ruled out, but not assumed to be of etiological significance. Page 692.

125. **Answer: A.** In arrangements of shared custody, joint decision-making is usually part of the agreement, so both parents should be contacted for consent of treatment. However, when there is disagreement between the guardians, some states allow for the parent with physical custody to make the decision. Page 18.

126. **Answer: E.** Note that all of the choices are different statistical approaches to the classification of disorders. Page 305.

127. **Answer: A.** The usual dosage range is 50 to 150 mg daily. Page 763.

128. **Answer: E.** This is the long-acting depot formulation of haloperidol and would not be suited to treat an acutely agitated patient. Page 905.

129. **Answer: D.** Descriptive psychiatry, not dynamic psychiatry, strives to categorize patients according to observable behaviors. Page 826.

130. **Answer: B.** The other options may be true, but do not answer the question. Page 196.

131. **Answer: A or B.** It depends on the state. Currently about half the states have established criminal penalties for knowingly exposing or transmitting HIV to someone else. Some states do not require disclosure if protection is used. What are the laws in your state?

132. **Answer: A.** Page 486.

133. **Answer: B.** In fact, the clinician needs to form alliances with multiple parties, including but not limited to the parents and the school, to best assess and treat the child. Pages 323–324.

134. **Answer: E.** "Chumship," or an intimate friendship with a peer of the same sex, is typical of school-aged children. Object constancy, as it pertains to people, begins in preschool. Pages 263–265.

135. **Answer: D.** Self-monitoring is also an executive function ability. However, most cognitive or intelligence tests do not comprehensively assess executive function. Page 368.

136. **Answer: D.** Page 441.

137. **Answer: E.** Dialectical-behavior therapy requires a large commitment from staff. The other treatments listed are generally directed by single disciplines within the milieu staff. Page 867.

138. **Answer: A and C.** Page 743.

139. **Answer: D.** Page 651.

140. **Answer: E.** All of the listed medical conditions are associated with regression, highlighting the importance of an appropriate medical workup in the assessment of children with possible pervasive developmental disorders. Page 397.

141. **Answer: B.** Page 675.

142. **Answer: A.** The incidence of epilepsy in autism ranges from 5% to 30%. Rett's disorder and childhood disintegrative disorder carry the highest rates at 90% and 70%, respectively. Any seizure type can be associated with autism and there is no gender difference. Page 966.

143. **Answer: B.** Choice D is a description of externalization, a defense commonly exhibited by children in psychodynamic psychotherapy. Pages 827 and 829.

144. **Answer: A.** The beginnings of the SOC movement are attributed in part to the seminal publication of *Unclaimed Children* in 1982, which uncovered the inadequacies of the mental health care system in addressing the problems of seriously emotionally disturbed children and their families. The SOC approach emphasizes a full spectrum of care and family involvement, hence the emergence of home-based treatment as one element of SOC. Page 883.

145. **Answer: A.** When maladaptive behaviors are continually reinforced over time, negative perceptions, emotions, and patterns of relating become more entrenched and resistant to intervention. Page 461.

146. **Answer: B.** Page 315.

147. **Answer: A.** Critics of the gender identity diagnosis, who may use the term gender-variant, can be viewed as displaying "essentialism" by those who support the diagnosis: the child is "born this way" and there are no psychosocial, psychodynamic, or other factors that may be involved in either a causal or perpetuating manner. Treatment will often follow one's conceptual framework, with the essentialist group generally supporting and encouraging transition to a cross-gender identity and role at an earlier age. Page 678.

148. **Answer: A.** Page 763.

149. **Answer: B.** Paroxetine inhibits the CYP2D6 pathway, a major pathway for the metabolism of risperidone. This can be a problem with fluoxetine as well. Page 764.

150. **Answer: D.** Page 934.

151. **Answer: D.** Page 648.

152. **Answer: C.** Autism has been associated with a number of medical conditions, but not spina bifida. Other associated conditions are phenylketonuria and duplications of chromosome 15q11-q13. Approximately 20% of children with autism develop seizures, with the onset occurring either in early childhood or adolescence. Page 390.

153. **Answer: A.** Children are usually the better informants for symptoms of anxiety and depression. Page 705.

154. **Answer: C.** The Assembly is a national component of the American Psychiatric Association and is not appropriate for filing a local ethics complaint. Page 21.

155. **Answer: C.** Page 281.

156. **Answer: D.** The Early Intervention Foster Care Program is a comprehensive program aimed at promoting permanency for children who have been maltreated. Page 698.

157. **Answer: B.** This is rare in modern transplant medicine but still a possibility, especially with bone marrow transplantation. It can be associated with significant delirium and encephalopathy. Page 945.

158. **Answer: B.** Boys are referred more frequently; however, the ratio of boys to girls who are referred narrows with adolescence. Studies have demonstrated that there is a higher threshold for cross-gender behavior in girls. Page 671.

159. **Answer: A.** The intent of this question is to promote an awareness of the types of alternative and augmentative communication modalities. Page 373.

160. **Answer: A.** Page 316.

161. **Answer: B and C.** The infant cognition model sought to extend IQ testing to children younger than school age, whereas the Gesell model examined child development from infancy onward. Page 310.

162. **Answer: D.** Precocity to a large degree is correlated with environmental factors. Page 59.

163. **Answer: B.** All of the options are worthy of being addressed; however, as the dyadic relationship between primary caregiver and infant is crucial in a child's development, this consideration cannot be missed in the psychiatric assessment of an infant. Page 253.

164. **Answer: B.** Page 432.

165. **Answer: B.** Commonly, the child is asked to draw a picture of himself or herself or the family doing something. Page 338.

166. **Answer: E.** Hypochloremic *alkalosis* is a possible side effect of binging and purging behavior and not hyperchloremic acidosis. Page 594.

167. **Answer: A.** Page 41.

168. **Answer: C.** *Kent v. United States* was an opinion rendered in 1966. The other options are made up. Page 1005.

169. **Answer: B.** The ill effect of drinking while on Antabuse is an example of aversive counterconditioning, which is based on principles of classical conditioning. Page 805.

170. **Answer: A.** Page 141.

171. **Answer: A.** Page 889.

172. **Answer: E.** There has been no correlation of increased risk of depression and poor grades thus far. Page 504.

173. **Answer: E.** Child psychiatry is considered a low-risk specialty, and when sued most child psychiatrists prevail. Some insurers give discounted premiums to child psychiatrists. Page 1018.

174. **Answer: D.** Page 912.

175. **Answer: A.** The purpose of this question is to highlight the key countries involved in international adoption. Romania, India, and Colombia are others. Page 1014.

176. **Answer: D.** Page 107.

177–182. **Answers:** 177-F; 178-B; 179-D; 180-C; 181-A; 182-E. Page 457.

183. **Answer: E.** CYP 3A constitutes 30% of total CYP hepatic content and 70% of intestinal CYP content. Page 747.

184. **Answer: A.** Page 567.

185. **Answer: C.** Psychotherapy alone has not been shown to be an effective treatment for stuttering, but counseling is often helpful for overcoming the secondary effects of stuttering on self-concept, thoughts, and feelings. All of the other statements are true. Page 424.

186. **Answer: A and B.** Although albumin and alpha-1-acid glycoproteins are reduced in the neonate and infant, this does not appear to be an important developmental factor in older children and adolescents. Page 746.

187. **Answer: D.** The parents (or clinical team) communicating with the school about a child's needs is a reasonable first step. A child whose medical problems adversely affect their educational performance may require a 504 plan to accommodate their disability; or if academic deficits or learning problems are present, they may qualify for special education services under the rubric of "other health impaired." Children may need homebound services, especially if infection is a concern; however, homebound is remembered by treatment survivors as an isolating and academically inadequate experience. Page 933.

188. **Answer: B.** The studies by Asarnow and colleagues demonstrated that rote language skills and simple perceptual processing are not impaired in children with childhood onset schizophrenia, but such children perform poorly on tasks involving fine motor coordination, attention, short-term memory, and working memory. Page 496.

189. **Answer: B.** Although each of the choices represents a clinical interview, the DISC (The Diagnostic Interview Schedule for Children) best fits the question. Page 349.

190. **Answer: E.** Hormone receptors lie in an inactive state. When a hormone binds, a series of events happen and the transcription of genes required by the cell at that moment occurs. Page 182.

191. **Answer: B.** In the United States, rates of reactive attachment disorder (RAD) parallel the environmental or family risk of adverse caregiving. Children in foster care had the highest rate of RAD, followed by homeless children and then children in Head Start. In addition, being exposed to maltreatment and institutionalization does not necessarily create sufficient conditions for the development of RAD. Up to 70% of children postinstitutionalization may show no attachment disorder behaviors. Page 714.

192. **Answer: B.** The elevated creatine phosphokinase titers are due to the muscle breakdown. Page 778.

193. **Answer: D.** Page 175.

194. **Answer: A.** Page 686.

195. **Answer: A.** Unlike desipramine, which has a similar mechanism of action, atomoxetine does not appear to prolong cardiac conduction times. Page 766.

196. **Answer: A.** Although the cortex normally has six layers, cortices of affected individuals have only four. Page 210.

197. **Answer: D.** Page 623.

198. **Answer: C.** Some children with profound visual impairment may have autism by virtue of brain damage (e.g., caused by rubella or cytomegalovirus). There may also be an overlap of children with congenital visual impairment and autism by virtue of the deprivation of social–emotional experiences. Pages 74–75.

199. **Answer: D.** Although team members or their proxies are available 24/7 to respond to crises and treatment needs, travel to the home 24/7 is not a common element. Page 879.

200. **Answer: D.** There is general consensus that adolescents' cognitive abilities are characterized by growing complexity, the ability to think about possibilities, and increased speed and efficiency of information processing. Page 282.

Test Two

Questions

1. True or False: Duplications and deletions in the human genome are quite frequent in normal individuals, except for regions known to contain genes with important biological functions.
   A. True
   B. False

2. When is the anticipated publication date of the fifth edition of the Diagnostic and Statistical Manual of Mental Disorders (DSM-V)?
   A. 2001
   B. 2012
   C. 2010
   D. 2016
   E. 2014

3. True or False: Despite popular perception, exceedingly few school districts actively avoid the mandates of federal laws such as the Individual with Disabilities Education Act.
   A. True
   B. False

4. In psychoanalytic thought, which of the following terms refers to the psychological mechanisms that cling to the intrapsychic status quo and seek to prevent change?
   A. Transference
   B. Countertransference
   C. Observing ego
   D. Resistance
   E. Working alliance

5. Which of the following is least likely to be seen on imaging studies in childhood onset schizophrenia?
   A. Increased lateral ventricular volume
   B. Decreased gray matter volume
   C. Decreased volume of the cerebellum
   D. Reduced volumes of temporal lobe structures
   E. Increased basal ganglia volume

6. How many genes are on the 46 chromosomes typically found in humans?
   A. 100
   B. 500
   C. 15,000
   D. 35,000
   E. 100,000

7. Review of studies of delirium in adults suggests EACH of the following is a core symptom of delirium EXCEPT:
   A. Perceptual disturbances
   B. Attentional deficits
   C. Memory deficits
   D. Thought process abnormalities
   E. Sleep–wake cycle disturbances

8. True or False: The Brazelton Neonatal Behavioral Assessment Scale, second edition (NBAS-2), has been shown to predict infant–parent attachment and subsequent infant development within the first year.
   A. True
   B. False

9. Which of the following is a primary parameter in assessing rapid eye movement or nonrapid eye movement sleep?
   A. Cardiac
   B. Respiratory
   C. Episodic limb movement
   D. Muscle tone

10. Neuroleptic malignant syndrome has a mortality rate of up to 9% in children and adolescents. Which step is necessary when the syndrome is identified?
    A. Administration of dantrolene
    B. Starting intravenous fluids, specifically normal saline
    C. Application of cooling blankets
    D. Discontinuation of the antipsychotic medication
    E. Administration of an antipyretic

11. In the Four Ps model of psychiatric formulation, which domain of factors is concerned with the features that describe a patient's strengths, resilience, and supports?
    A. Predisposing
    B. Precipitating
    C. Perpetuating
    D. Protective

12. ALL of the following have been implicated in obsessive–compulsive disorder (OCD), EXCEPT:
    A. Serotonin
    B. Dopamine
    C. Glutamate
    D. Choline

13. Chronic medical illnesses associated with weight loss include ALL of the following EXCEPT:
    A. Crohn's disease
    B. Hyperthyroidism
    C. Prader-Willi syndrome
    D. Diabetes mellitus
    E. Addison's disease

14. Family systems theorists have sometimes viewed pediatric somatoform disorders as:
    A. Disrupting the parental hierarchy
    B. Oppositional defiance
    C. A conflict between the superego and the id
    D. A way to avoid conflict

15. How is narcolepsy diagnosed definitively?
    A. A good history
    B. Observation in the home, with recording by parents, if possible
    C. Treatment response to stimulants
    D. Multiple Sleep Latency Test

16. Having a child wash their soiled clothing after a toileting accident is an example of:
    A. Overcorrection
    B. Response cost
    C. Negative reinforcement
    D. Extinction
    E. Classical conditioning

17. Smyke and Zeanah developed which of the following approaches in assessing attachment disorders?
    A. Disturbances of Attachment Interview
    B. Preschool Assessment of Attachment
    C. Attachment Q-Set
    D. Child Attachment Interview
    E. Narrative Story Stem Techniques

18. What is the genetic mutation in Fragile X?
    A. Point mutation
    B. Small deletion
    C. Large deletion
    D. Gene duplication
    E. Triplet repeat

19. Amphetamine use can be detected in the urine for how long?
    A. Less than 24 hours
    B. 24 to 72 hours
    C. 3 to 5 days
    D. 1 week

20. Research reveals how teachers rate boys and girls from families with an absent father as more _____ compared with children from intact mother–father families.
    A. shy
    B. depressed
    C. aggressive
    D. inattentive

21. What is a well recognized problem of retrospective case–control studies?
    A. Selection bias
    B. Recall bias
    C. Missing data
    D. Sampling errors
    E. Sampling size

22. Borderline personality disorder is often comorbid with ALL of the following EXCEPT:
    A. Major depression
    B. Schizotypal personality disorder
    C. Posttraumatic stress disorder (PTSD)
    D. Eating disorders
    E. Substance use

23. True or False: Resilience is evident when an individual achieves success in a single domain despite the presence of significant risk or adversity.
    A. True
    B. False

24. Which part of the neuron is responsible for synthesizing nearly all cell-specific proteins, including transporters, receptors, and the enzymes needed for neurotransmitter production?
    A. Axon
    B. Dendrites
    C. Cell body
    D. Nerve terminal
    E. Synapse

25. What is the overlap of epileptiform and nonepileptiform seizure disorders?
    A. Up to 20% of children with intractable epilepsy also have nonepileptic seizures
    B. Up to 15% of children on a pediatric epilepsy unit will have nonepileptic seizures
    C. Up to 50% of children on a pediatric epilepsy unit who have nonepileptic seizures will also have epileptic seizures
    D. Nonepileptic seizures in children can be difficult to delineate from true epilepsy
    E. All of the above

26. In which year did the American Board of Psychiatry and Neurology recognize child psychiatry as a subspecialty and establish standards for its training?
    A. 1876
    B. 1911
    C. 1945
    D. 1957
    E. 1982

27. The term "learning disabled" refers to children who have ALL of the following disorders in development EXCEPT:
    A. Attention
    B. Communication skills
    C. Language
    D. Reading
    E. Speech

28. What is the treatment of encopresis?
    A. Psychoeducation and bowel catharsis
    B. Psychoeducation, bowel catharsis, daily dose of laxatives or mineral oil, and parent management training
    C. Psychoeducation, bowel catharsis, daily dose of laxatives or mineral oil, and daily timed intervals on the toilet with rewards for success
    D. Psychoeducation, bowel catharsis, and morning timed intervals on the toilet with rewards for success

29. Which one of the following is true of PTSD in children according to Sack et al.?
    A. Diagnostic status does not relate to functional status
    B. Children with PTSD never show a delayed onset of symptoms
    C. In most children with PTSD, symptoms dissipate within 1 year
    D. In children with PTSD, symptoms of depression worsen over time
    E. All of the above

30. The most common formulation used in psychiatry is the biopsychosocial model developed by whom?
    A. Meyer
    B. Engel
    C. Kraepelin
    D. Freud
    E. Jaspers

31. Often, the major source of mental health referrals to the emergency department is:
    A. Parents
    B. Child protective services
    C. Schools
    D. Outpatient psychiatrists
    E. Community agencies

32. Which of the following is the normal milestone for speech development regarding a child's ability to speak in sentences?
    A. 5 years
    B. 4 years
    C. 3 years
    D. 2 years
    E. 1 year

33. True or False: A diagnosis of acute stress disorder within the first month is necessary for the diagnosis of PTSD.
    A. True
    B. False

34. True or False: In several studies, researchers have concluded that there is a powerful, though indirect, link between poverty and mental health disorders in children.
    A. True
    B. False

35. True or False: A psychoanalytic finding indicates that the harshness and rigidity of a person's superego is directly proportional to the parental severity during childhood.
    A. True
    B. False

36. True or False: The mother and father's attitudes and behaviors toward their child is the key element that fosters the development of gender identity disorder (GID).
    A. True
    B. False

37. For patients with GID seen for the first time in adolescence, there are two subgroups. Select answer D or E.
    A. Male and female youth who have very clear childhood onset of GID, which has persisted into adolescence. Almost all the youth in this group have a homosexual orientation (sexually attracted to members of their own birth sex)
    B. Male and female youth who have very clear childhood onset of GID, which has persisted into adolescence. Almost all the youth in this group have a heterosexual orientation (sexually attracted to members of the opposite birth sex)
    C. Male youth without cross-gender history in childhood who express the desire to be the opposite sex, voiced only during the beginning of adolescence or later. These youth often have a heterosexual, bisexual, or asexual orientation
    D. A and B
    E. A and C

38. True or False: The response rates of selective serotonin reuptake inhibitors (SSRIs) in OCD are comparable, and clomipramine is superior by a significant margin.
    A. True
    B. False

39. True or False: Placement in a long-term residential facility serves as one way to achieve permanency in children who were removed from their homes.
    A. True
    B. False

40. True or False: Trichotillomania is more common in females.
    A. True
    B. False

41. The pruning of cortical synapses that occurs in adolescence:
    A. Can lead to the loss of up to 30,000 synapses per second
    B. Results in the loss of 95% of the cortical synaptic connections present before puberty
    C. Affects inhibitory synapses preferentially
    D. Is accompanied by increases in brain glucose metabolism, oxygen utilization, and blood flow

42. Which of the following models of classification focuses on the total context of the individual person?
    A. Dimensional
    B. Categorical
    C. Ideographic
    D. Archetypal

43. Regarding Tourette's syndrome (TS) and comorbid conditions, which of the following is TRUE?
    A. Children with combined TS and attention deficit hyperactivity disorder (ADHD) have less psychiatric morbidity than those with ADHD alone
    B. Children with combined TS and ADHD are at greater risk for disruptive behaviors and impairments than those with TS alone
    C. There is no qualitative difference between TS comorbid with OCD and OCD without TS
    D. Tic-related OCD tends to have a later age of onset compared with nontic-related OCD
    E. Tic-related OCD tends to be less responsive to antipsychotics and more responsive to serotonin reuptake inhibitors

44. True or False: Females with ADHD have a higher rate of unwed pregnancy than those who do not.
    A. True
    B. False

45. Multiple lines of evidence support the role of which neurotransmitter in the etiology of ADHD and in the response to treatment?
    A. Serotonin
    B. Substance P
    C. Dopamine
    D. Norepinephrine
    E. Glutamate

46. Which of the following is an example of policy?
    A. Federal or state legislation
    B. Position statements from American Academy of Child & Adolescent Psychiatry
    C. Governmental procedures developed to guide provision of services
    D. Governing rules of the American Psychiatric Association (APA)
    E. All of the above

47. If the APA confirms an ethical violation by a psychiatrist, there are four possible sanctions that the APA can issue, including ALL of the following EXCEPT:
    A. Admonishment
    B. Reprimand
    C. Suspension
    D. Expulsion
    E. Appeal

48. Which of the following *best* describes child psychiatric emergencies?
    A. Emergencies can be characterized as a mismatch between needs and resources
    B. Emergencies represent a parent's inability to provide adequate support
    C. Emergencies usually have an element of school dysfunction as a contributing factor
    D. Emergencies represent the lack of outpatient resources
    E. None of the above

49. True or False: In psychoanalytic thought, drive is a term that encompasses the mental representations of the instinctual forces.
    A. True
    B. False

50. Logical operations are a crucial developmental stage because
    A. They are necessary for conducting social interactions
    B. They are necessary to mastering basic reading skills
    C. They are necessary to mastering basic mathematics skills
    D. A and C only
    E. A, B, and C

51. Which of the following statements about stuttering is false?
    A. Most cases of stuttering are due to learned behavior rather than due to a biological component
    B. Most children recover within the first 1 to 2 years after their stuttering was first noted
    C. People who stutter have been found to show laryngeal behavior different from that in normal speakers
    D. The risk of stuttering among first-degree relatives is more than three times the population risk
    E. Treatments for stuttering, like anti-anxiety medications, have not been found to be effective

52. The periods of infancy and toddlerhood are defined as the first 3 years of postpartum life. Infancy refers to specifically what period in a child's life?
    A. The period up to 6 months before object permanency begins
    B. The period up to 18 months before expressive verbal communication begins
    C. The period up to 12 months before independent walking begins
    D. The period up to 24 months before toilet training begins

53. What was a conclusion of the Fort Bragg study, a large, randomized trial of a system-of-care approach?
    A. Children who received intensive, coordinated services fared no better than children who received traditional services
    B. Children who received intensive, coordinated services fared better than children who received traditional services
    C. Children who received intensive, coordinated services displayed more acting-out behaviors than those who received traditional services
    D. Children who received intensive, coordinated services displayed fewer acting-out behaviors than those who received traditional services

54. The blockade of which part of the dopaminergic neuron is the major mechanism of action of most antipsychotic medications?
    A. D1 receptor
    B. D2 receptor
    C. Dopamine transporter
    D. Monoamine oxidase
    E. D3 receptor

55. A patient has experienced a major depressive episode during the past 12 months but has now remitted. The patient will:
    A. Be best characterized as partially remitted, given duration of time criteria
    B. Contribute to the numerator in an incidence study
    C. Contribute to the numerator in a 12-month prevalence study
    D. Is likely to experience another depressive episode
    E. All of the above

56. Which of the following enzymes are involved in Phase II metabolic reactions?
    A. CYP 1A
    B. UGT 1
    C. CYP 2C
    D. CYP 2E
    E. CYP 3A

57. Which TWO of the four functionally distinct pharmacokinetic phases are primarily responsible for terminating the action of the pharmacological agent?
    A. Absorption
    B. Metabolism
    C. Distribution
    D. Excretion

58. A child psychiatrist reports suspected abuse by a father and tells the mother she should withhold visitations from the father. The father could sue the clinician:
    A. True
    B. False

59. What are common potential errors in documentation from a liability perspective?
    A. Raising a diagnostic question and not following through or not following up on the results
    B. Overlooking discrepancies among professionals in the progress notes; for example, a nurse's suicide assessment that differs from the child psychiatrist's
    C. Signing off on a trainee's note by declaring "agree with the above"
    D. Recording psychodynamic considerations in the progress notes
    E. All of the above

60. Which TWO of the following side effects are relatively common with lithium treatment?
   A. Glomerular damage
   B. Polyuria
   C. Hypothyroidism
   D. Polydipsia
   E. Seizures

61. True or False: There is only one standardized measure that specifically assesses for symptoms of acute stress disorder in children.
   A. True
   B. False

62. Which of the following is true of suicides in sexual minority youth in the United States?
   A. Suicide is the third leading cause of death among sexual minority youth
   B. About 10% of sexual minority youth commit suicide annually
   C. Gay minority youth are two to three times more likely to commit suicide than other youth
   D. Sexual orientation has an independent association with suicide attempts for female minority youth
   E. All of the above

63. If a child is deaf and her family chooses to proceed with cochlear implants, when is the best age to undergo the procedure?
   A. Under 2 years
   B. Under 3 years
   C. Under 4 years
   D. Under 5 years
   E. Under 6 years

64. According to Thabet and Vostanis, which one of the following is the most important predictor of general mental health problems in children exposed to conflict in the Gaza strip?
   A. Parental alcohol consumption
   B. Low socioeconomic status
   C. Parental mental illness
   D. Living in the inner city
   E. Single parent family

65. True or False: Academically, children with nonverbal learning disability (NLD or NVLD) show better arithmetic skills relative to reading and spelling skills.
   A. True
   B. False

66. The half-life of lithium in adults is approximately 24 hours, but in children what is the approximate half-life?
   A. 36 hours
   B. 32 hours
   C. 28 hours
   D. 26 hours
   E. 18 hours

67. True or False: Brains of toddlers with autism have been observed to be smaller in size than toddlers without autism.
   A. True
   B. False

68. True or False: Issues of confidentiality between children and parents should not be emphasized in child psychiatric treatment.
   A. True
   B. False

69. What percentage of children diagnosed with cancer in the United States are expected to survive their disease and treatment?
    A. 15%
    B. 30%
    C. 45%
    D. 60%
    E. 75%

70. Which of the following represent(s) goal(s) of Bowen family systems?
    A. Increased differentiation
    B. Detriangulation
    C. Improved ability to manage anxiety
    D. Resolution of cutoff
    E. All of the above

71. Which of the following is true of aggressive behavior in preschool children?
    A. Verbal aggression increases as children gain more language skills
    B. Aggression is typically focused on social situations
    C. Physically aggressive behavior usually subsides by age 3 or 4
    D. A and C
    E. None of the above

72. Which of the following statements describes the minimal effective concentration of a drug?
    A. The blood plasma concentration likely to produce a toxic effect
    B. The blood plasma concentration needed to achieve steady-state levels
    C. The blood plasma concentration likely to produce a clinical effect
    D. The blood plasma concentration found with minimal dosing

73. Between 1965 and 1998, the father's share of child care in the home has:
    A. Doubled
    B. Halved
    C. Remained the same
    D. Tripled

74. ALL of the following statements are true EXCEPT:
    A. Pornographic photography of children is generally considered a form of sexual abuse
    B. About one-third of child maltreatment reports are substantiated
    C. "False memories" during the interview of an abused child can be minimized by using open-ended questions
    D. Screening for abuse/neglect is not a necessary part of all mental health evaluations
    E. It is a good practice to notify the guardian about the clinician's decision to report suspected maltreatment

75. ALL of the following are obsessions typically found in adolescents EXCEPT:
    A. Dirt and germs
    B. Fear of an ill fate befalling loved ones
    C. Exactness or symmetry
    D. Religious scrupulosity
    E. Sexual preoccupations

76. Which publication of Sigmund Freud is considered the beginning of the discipline of psychodynamic psychotherapy for children?
    A. Totem and Taboo
    B. Little Hans
    C. The Rat Man
    D. The Interpretation of Dreams
    E. Civilization and Its Discontents

77. True or False: Every human being is capable of self-determination.
    A. True
    B. False

78. True or False: In psychoanalytic thought, the psychological maneuver by which the ego accomplishes inhibition against an internal danger is termed repression.
    A. True
    B. False

79. The *crisis intervention model*, exemplified by the Home-builders approach emphasizes among other elements:
    A. Concrete services, such as food and clothing
    B. Aversive conditioning
    C. Negative reinforcement
    D. Punishment
    E. Shaping

80. Which of the following statements is FALSE regarding the cultural formulation in the DSM-IV?
    A. It is a key component of the biopsychosocial assessment and diagnosis of mental disorders
    B. It has five main themes
    C. It serves as a sensitive instrument for culturally diverse and multicultural groups
    D. It includes the cultural identity of the patient
    E. It includes the cultural explanations of the patient's illness

81. True or False: Oxcarbazepine like carbamazepine can induce its own metabolism.
    A. True
    B. False

82. In which year did the American Academy of Child Psychiatrists expand to include the treatment of adolescents in its scope and influence, hence becoming the American Academy of Child & Adolescent Psychiatry, as it is known today?
    A. 1942
    B. 1959
    C. 1963
    D. 1974
    E. 1989

83. What provides for most of the biosynthetic capacity in the early human embryo?
    A. mRNA synthesized by the mother
    B. mRNA synthesized by the father
    C. Maternal DNA
    D. Paternal DNA
    E. mRNA synthesized by the mother and father

84. In 1925, Arnold Gesell published the Gesell Development Schedules to assess normal maturational development systematically in infants and toddlers. This groundbreaking research was different from prior efforts in ALL of the following ways EXCEPT:
    A. Infant cognition tests sought to identify deviance, whereas Gesell's work sought to document normal development
    B. Gesell's model conceptualized development as occurring simultaneously in multiple domains as opposed to a singular test for intelligence quotient (IQ)
    C. Gesell's model took into account environmental influences upon the developmental trajectory as opposed to viewing IQ as a static and stable trait
    D. Gesell Development Schedules were able to predict infant IQ at later stages in development

85. In a study of child care centers in four states, one major finding was that most centers are mediocre in quality and "sufficiently poor to interfere with children's emotional and intellectual development." Moreover, what percentage of infants and toddlers in center-based care were found to be at risk because of poor health and safety standards?
    A. 40%
    B. 30%
    C. 20%
    D. 10%
    E. 5%

86. Which of the following definitions best describes the statistic of absolute risk reduction?
    A. The number of patients that needs to be treated with an intervention to prevent one additional bad outcome
    B. Proportion of patients with an undesired consequence in the intervention group compared with the control group
    C. Proportion of patients in the control group with bad outcome compared to patients in the intervention group with bad outcome
    D. None of the above

87. True or False: The DSM-IV diagnosis of pyromania represents a category of firesetting that is somewhat common in children.
    A. True
    B. False

88. True or False: Projective techniques in psychological testing are based on the premise that responses to and interpretations of ambiguous stimuli provide insight into the examinee's unconscious mental processes, such as needs, motives, and conflicts.
    A. True
    B. False

89. What is construct validity?
    A. The extent to which an instrument is representative of the universe of empirical indicators that are related to the concept measured
    B. The most empirical form of validity, which allows an index to be compared with an independent external criterion thought to assess the same concept
    C. The extent to which individual items or measures intercorrelate or group together to produce derived higher order constructs
    D. None of the above

90. What is one of the primary sources of psychological pain for children with cancer?
    A. Their siblings
    B. Their pets
    C. Their grandparents
    D. Their parents
    E. School reentry

91. Which of the following is the only Food and Drug Administration approved, non-stimulant medication for the treatment of ADHD?
    A. Desipramine
    B. Guanfacine
    C. Clonidine
    D. Atomoxetine
    E. Bupropion

92. True or False: The relative volume of extracellular water is higher in children and tends to decrease with development.
    A. True
    B. False

93. ALL of the following brain areas have been implicated in the symptomatology of autism EXCEPT:
    A. Frontal lobe
    B. Temporal lobe
    C. Amygdala
    D. Limbic system
    E. Occipital lobe

94. In which part of the night are night terrors most likely to occur?
    A. First third
    B. Second third
    C. Last third
    D. At any time of night
    E. Just before waking after a night's sleep

95. On average, what percentage of students ages 14 and older diagnosed with learning disabilities graduate with a regular high school diploma?
    A. 40%
    B. 50%
    C. 60%
    D. 70%
    E. 80%

96. Which answer captures the DSM-IV-TR diagnostic criteria for somatization disorder?
    A. Pain in at least four body sites, at least two gastrointestinal symptoms, one sexual or reproductive symptom, and one pseudoneurological symptom
    B. Pain in at least four body sites, at least two gastrointestinal symptoms, two sexual or reproductive symptoms, and one pseudoneurological symptom
    C. Pain in at least four body sites, at least one gastrointestinal symptom, one sexual or reproductive symptom, and one pseudoneurological symptom
    D. Pain in at least four body sites, at least two gastrointestinal symptoms, and one sexual or reproductive symptom
    E. None of the above

97. What is the typical starting dose of fluvoxamine for children?
    A. 5 to 10 mg
    B. 25 to 50 mg
    C. 12.5 to 25 mg
    D. 10 to 20 mg
    E. 75 to 100 mg

98. Which of the following statements BEST describes the goal of the discipline of neuropsychoanalysis?
    A. Trace the psychodynamic roots of many neurological disorders such as pseudo-seizures
    B. Improve understanding of the brain substrates of psychoanalytic constructs
    C. Provide commentary on the psychoanalytic aspects of neurological disorders
    D. The transformation of psychoanalysis into a more scientific, neurologically based discipline

99. Environmental factors that have been associated with childhood and adolescent obesity include ALL of the following EXCEPT:
    A. Maternal smoking during pregnancy
    B. Breastfeeding
    C. Increased TV viewing
    D. Shorter duration of sleep

100. What percentage of children before the age of 15 years will lose a parent to death?
    A. 1%
    B. 2%
    C. 3%
    D. 4%
    E. 5%

101. Clinicians are susceptible to a number of collection biases in the process of interviewing and diagnosing a patient. Which of the following biases is the definition of the availability heuristic?
    A. Arriving at a diagnostic determination before collecting all the relevant information
    B. Focusing on collecting information to confirm a diagnosis
    C. Making judgments based on the most readily available cognitive patterns
    D. Seeing correlations where none exist
    E. Ignoring disconfirming information

102. True or False: IQ scores are generally stable in children 5 years of age and older.
    A. True
    B. False

103. Which of the following agents has over 40 double-blind studies showing its efficacy for the treatment of enuresis?
    A. Imipramine
    B. Desipramine
    C. Desmopressin
    D. Amitriptyline
    E. Synthroid

104. International Classification of Diseases (ICD)-10 describes three subtypes of conduct disorder, which include ALL of the following EXCEPT:
    A. Confined to the family context
    B. Confined to the legal context
    C. Unsocialized
    D. Socialized

105. Teachers' reports indicate that most oppositional symptoms such as arguing, screaming, disobedience, and defiance peak between what ages?
    A. 14 and 18
    B. 12 and 14
    C. 14 and 16
    D. 20 and 24
    E. 8 and 11

106. Which of the following is a strong predictor of patient traumatic reaction in pediatric transplant surgery?
    A. Parental substance use
    B. Parental divorce
    C. Parental trauma
    D. Peer rejection
    E. Schizophrenia

107. The National Comorbidity Survey has found that approximately what percentage of all mental health disorders have their onset at or before age 14?
    A. 10%
    B. 20%
    C. 30%
    D. 50%
    E. 75%

108. Of individuals arrested for arson in the mid-1990s, approximately what fraction were under 18 years of age?
    A. Two-thirds
    B. Half
    C. One-quarter
    D. One-third
    E. Three-quarters

109. Among child and adolescent psychiatric outpatients with a diagnosis of major depressive disorder, what percentage report suicidal ideation or attempts?
    A. 20%
    B. 40%
    C. 70%
    D. 95%

110. In one test of anxiety disorders, subjects are required to name the color of potentially threatening words such as "snake." This type of test or task is known as:
    A. Tower of London test
    B. Wisconsin card sorting task
    C. Continuous performance task
    D. Stroop task
    E. Controlled work oral association test

111. Twelve million cases of sexually transmitted diseases occur each year in the United States. Teenagers account for what percentage of these sexually transmitted diseases?
    A. 10%
    B. 20%
    C. 25%
    D. 33%
    E. 66%

112. Once a child has been diagnosed with communication deficits, a speech–language pathologist begins a detailed assessment of the child's functioning using THREE main goals as a guide. Which of the following is NOT one of those goals?
    A. Establish baseline function
    B. Establish a psychiatric diagnosis
    C. Identify goals for intervention
    D. Monitor progress in the therapy

113. Which of the following tests should be obtained prior to starting any of the tricyclic antidepressants?
    A. Electrocardiogram
    B. Blood pressure
    C. Heart rate
    D. A and B
    E. All of the above

114. Which of the following statements is true:
    A. Girls' brains are about 10% larger than boys' brains
    B. Boys show a greater growth in the hippocampus than girls
    C. As frontal lobes develop, children become increasingly less able to inhibit cognitively
    D. The speed of information processing increases significantly between ages 6 and 12
    E. At birth, the brain is estimated to be about 90% of adult volume

115. Which of the following atypical antipsychotics is the one best studied in pediatric populations?
    A. Aripiprazole
    B. Quetiapine
    C. Clozapine
    D. Risperidone
    E. Olanzapine

116. True or False: The analgesic ladder of the World Health Organization, which steps pain management from the initial use of acetaminophen and nonsteroidal anti-inflammatory drugs to a mild opioid (codeine ± adjuvant) and then to a strong opioid (morphine, fentanyl ± adjuvant) is not appropriate for children.
    A. True
    B. False

117. Approximately how many children are infected with HIV worldwide?
    A. 500,000
    B. 2 million
    C. 5 million
    D. 10 million
    E. 20 million

118. What is the problem with the assertion by some authors that adoption is in itself always a loss or an injury to a child's self-esteem?
    A. It encourages rescue fantasies
    B. It reenforces negative attributions
    C. It neglects the impact of intrapsychic processes
    D. We do not have evidence that this is indeed so

119. Psychosocial dwarfism is characterized by ALL of the following EXCEPT:
    A. Deceleration of linear growth
    B. Frontal bossing
    C. Sleep disorder
    D. Reversible by a change in the psychosocial environment
    E. Absence of weight gain deceleration
    F. Bizarre eating habits

120. Which of the following is/are true regarding use of a physical limit?
    A. When inappropriate behavior persists despite all efforts, a physical limit is mandatory to guarantee the group's safety
    B. Permanent group removal should be imposed only if the danger to the group is pronounced and no alternative is available
    C. There is always irreparable damage to the group when a member is removed, regardless of the justifications for the removal
    D. All of the above
    E. None of the above

121. What is the DSM-IV-TR definition of personality disorder?
    A. An enduring pattern of behaviors, cognitions, and thoughts that deviates from the culture, is stable, and manifests itself across psychosocial contexts
    B. An enduring pattern of disturbed temperament, manifesting itself over time, and stabilizing in adolescence
    C. An enduring pattern of inner experiences and behavior that deviates markedly from the expectations of the individual's culture
    D. An enduring pattern of behavior and thoughts that is perceived as atypical by members of the same culture

122. True or False: Depression in children can be decreased with interventions that include them in the treatment of their depressed parent.
    A. True
    B. False

123. Which of the following theories of group therapy was developed by Wilfred Bion to assist the British military during World War II?
    A. Cognitive behavioral
    B. Psychodynamic
    C. Gestalt
    D. Group-as-a-whole
    E. None of the above

124. Which of the following statements describe what the null hypothesis primarily states?
    A. The mean of the population of those who receive the intervention is greater than the mean of the population of those who do not
    B. The mean of the population of those who receive the intervention is less than the mean of the population of those who do not
    C. The mean of the population of those who receive the intervention is equal to the mean of the population of those who do not
    D. The median of the population of those who receive the intervention is equal to the median of the population of those who do not
    E. The median of the population of those who receive the intervention is less than the median of the population of those who do not

125. Attainment of formal operational thinking in adolescence results in the following:
    A. A decline in childhood egocentrism
    B. More simplistic moral reasoning
    C. A decrease in interpersonal skills
    D. Consistent decision-making regardless of affect, stress, or peer influence
    E. None of the above

126. When was fluoxetine, the first SSRI antidepressant, introduced?
    A. The late 1960s
    B. The late 1970s
    C. The late 1980s
    D. The late 1990s
    E. 2001

127. True or False: Evidence for the effectiveness of wilderness programs and boot camps for oppositional defiant disorder and conduct disorder is strong.
    A. True
    B. False

128. In the United States when were the first consultation–liaison/psychosomatic medicine units formally founded?
    A. 1900
    B. 1930
    C. 1950
    D. 1970
    E. 2000

129. Epilepsy is best defined as:
    A. Two or more seizures in the absence of provoking stimuli
    B. A seizure in the absence of provoking stimuli
    C. Recurrent seizures that have a known underlying pathology, such as infection or fever
    D. Video electroencephalogram captured seizure activity

130. Which of the following structured interviews do researchers typically use to assess diagnosis in children?
    A. Kiddie-Schedule for Affective Disorders and Schizophrenia
    B. Child Behavior Checklist
    C. Diagnostic Interview Schedule for Children—IV
    D. Behavior Assessment System for Children
    E. A and C

131. You are a child psychiatrist consulting with a school and are asked to interview a student who has trouble functioning in class. The parents do not give you permission to interview the child. Which of the following is most appropriate?
    A. You interview the student based on the student's assent to the interview
    B. Send a letter by mail explaining the objectives of the interview
    C. Observe the student unobtrusively and consult to staff on their questions about how to work with the student
    D. Inform the school that you are unable to consult because the parents have not given you permission to speak to their child
    E. None of the above

132. If after an initial evaluation for catatonia there is no clear etiology, it is diagnostically helpful to administer which of the following agents?
    A. Lorazepam
    B. Haloperidol
    C. Hydroxyzine
    D. Perphenazine
    E. None of the above

133. The statistic usually used to interpret test–retest reliability for categorical data such as diagnoses is called what?
    A. Cronbach's α
    B. Intraclass correlation coefficient
    C. Cohen's κ
    D. Correlation, r

134. Which of the following is true about aggression in children?
    A. Physically aggressive behavior generally begins to subside by age 3
    B. Verbal aggression increases between the ages of 2 and 4
    C. Both physical and verbal aggression diminish by age 5 or 6
    D. Older children tend to focus aggression on social situations and needs
    E. All of the above

135. There is little evidence comparing the effectiveness of inpatient hospitalization versus intensive in-home services for children with serious clinical problems. To address this issue, the National Institute of Mental Health funded a randomized trial of 156 families to examine multisystemic therapy (MST) as a feasible alternate strategy to emergency psychiatric hospitalization. What were the main findings regarding overall outcome?
    A. In the short term, there was little difference between the two treatments
    B. In the long term, there was little difference between the two treatments
    C. No child in the MST arm, over the course of treatment, required inpatient hospitalization
    D. In the long term, the children treated with inpatient hospitalization had better functional outcomes
    E. The MST population had higher rates of suicide attempts

136. Which of the following is the most well validated and widely disseminated treatment for childhood PTSD?
    A. Dialectical-behavior therapy
    B. Mentalization-based treatment
    C. Parent–child therapy
    D. Trauma-focused cognitive-behavioral therapy
    E. Habit reversal training

Questions 137–139. Match the type of prevention with its proper description:

137. Primary prevention

138. Secondary prevention

139. Tertiary prevention
    A. An intervention designed to decrease the amount of disability associated with existing illness
    B. An intervention designed to lower the rate of established cases of a disorder or illness
    C. An intervention designed to decrease the number of new cases of a disorder or illness

140. What type of variable is not of interest in a particular study but could influence the dependent variable and needs to be controlled?
    A. Active independent variable
    B. Independent variable
    C. Extraneous variable
    D. Attribute independent variable
    E. None of the above

141. In infant assessments using standardized testing, the normative data based on populations of children should be no more than how many years old to keep pace with intergenerational escalation in test performance?
    A. 2 years
    B. 5 years
    C. 10 years
    D. 15 years
    E. 20 years

142. The DSM-IV-TR criteria for mental retardation include ALL of the following essential features EXCEPT:
    A. Subnormal intellectual functioning
    B. Commensurate deficits in adaptive functioning
    C. Onset before 18 years of age
    D. IQ less than 75

143. How are the fears of a school-aged child different from the fears of a preschool child?
   A. School-aged children are less likely to witness catastrophic events
   B. School-aged children develop an understanding of the irreversibility of death
   C. Preschool children's dreams often reflect efforts to master their fears by setting themselves up as heroes who save whole families or communities
   D. Preschool children are more likely than school-aged children to feel inferior after evaluating themselves and measuring themselves against others
   E. School-aged children do not have any significant fears

144. True or False: Psychopharmacological agents are the optimal initial treatment of tics.
   A. True
   B. False

145. True or False: A high school girl with end-stage cystic fibrosis is assessed as part of a pretransplant evaluation. She has declined recommendations to have a G-tube placed because she says she could not tolerate it, and she has not worn a nasal cannula for oxygen because she is embarrassed to wear one in public. Based on the information presented, it is reasonable to deny her candidacy for a transplant.
   A. True
   B. False

146. Barbiturates can be detected in the urine for how long?
   A. Less than 24 hours
   B. 24 to 48 hours
   C. 3 to 5 days
   D. 1 week
   E. More than 10 days

147. At what age does the infant begin to develop object permanence, the understanding that people and objects continue to exist even when not seen or heard?
   A. $3\frac{1}{2}$ to 6 months
   B. $9\frac{1}{2}$ to 11 months
   C. $4\frac{1}{2}$ to 7 months
   D. $7\frac{1}{2}$ to 8 months

148. A measurement is considered reliable when the correlation coefficient, r, ranges from +0.7 to +1.0. However, what minimal value of reliability is usually acceptable for research purposes?
   A. +0.6
   B. +0.7
   C. +0.8
   D. +0.9
   E. +1.0

149. True or False: Longitudinal studies indicate that the occurrence of early oppositional defiant disorder in a child's life confers heightened risk for an adolescent mood disorder.
   A. True
   B. False

150. True or False: Epidemiological studies have found a correlation between psychological disturbance and enuresis.
   A. True
   B. False

151. True or False: Children with a microdeletion on chromosome 7 typically exhibit indiscriminate behavior.
   A. True
   B. False

152. True or False: It appears that generalized anxiety disorder in adolescence tends to precede later depression.
   A. True
   B. False

153. True or False: Autism is a homogeneous disorder.
   A. True
   B. False

154. Empirical studies of youths who attempt suicide and are seen in the emergency department and referred for outpatient therapy have found what proportion makes it to at least one outpatient appointment?
   A. One-fifth
   B. One-fourth
   C. One-third
   D. One-half
   E. Two-thirds

155. True or False: The effect of shared environment is at least as potent as heritable factors in influencing the outcome of a depressive disorder.
   A. True
   B. False

156. Regardless of diagnosis, the daily dose of bupropion should not exceed which of the following amounts in children?
   A. 50 mg
   B. 100 mg
   C. 150 mg
   D. 300 mg
   E. 450 mg

157. Which of the following statements about selective mutism is FALSE:
   A. It is most often seen in school settings
   B. It only affects children who have cultural and linguistic differences from others in the classroom
   C. Children who are selectively mute have the ability to comprehend and use spoken language
   D. Seventy five percent of children who are selectively mute have been found to have articulation disorders and expressive language problems
   E. There is a higher prevalence in girls than boys

158. Group therapy for mothers who are exposed to disasters might be an indirect tool in also helping:
   A. Infants
   B. Preschool children
   C. School age children
   D. Adolescents
   E. Young adults

159. A 9-year-old boy has been under your care for the treatment of anxiety. A major source of anxiety appears to be the father's verbally and emotionally abusive actions toward his wife, the boy's mother. You have met the father and you suspect he has antisocial personality traits. Several months into treatment the mother announces that she and her husband are divorcing. She asks that you write a letter of support for full custody. You think that indeed, she may be the better parent. Your best approach is to:
   A. Inform her that you are not comfortable with the request and explain that it would be unethical for you to write such a letter
   B. Inform her that you will write a letter of support
   C. Inform her that you will be glad to testify in court during a custody determination
   D. Inform her that joint custody would be best
   E. Inform that you will write a letter of support, but that this is not billable to the insurance company

160. ALL of the following are true about tics EXCEPT:
    A. Tics tend to occur in clusters and wax and wane in frequency and severity
    B. Tics are involuntary, sudden movements or vocal utterances that usually resemble normal behavior
    C. Tics are motor movements or noises that are unconsciously made to manipulate the environment
    D. Solitary tics can occur
    E. Multiple tics may occur simultaneously

161. True or False: Regardless of the ages of group members, it is always better to have more rather than fewer materials available in a group therapy setting.
    A. True
    B. False

162. The ability to engage in pretend play requires which of the following:
    A. Play materials
    B. Object permanence
    C. The ability to symbolize
    D. Peer acceptance
    E. Extremely rigid thinking

163. True or False: The potential for suicidal behavior has been documented to occur within 2 weeks after media presentations of actual or fictional suicide.
    A. True
    B. False

164. Comorbidities of bulimia include ALL of the following EXCEPT:
    A. Weight below 15th percentile
    B. Substance abuse
    C. Depression
    D. Problems with interpersonal relationships
    E. High levels of anxiety and compulsivity

165. Placebo-controlled studies have shown the efficacy of which tricyclic antidepressant in children with ADHD?
    A. Desipramine
    B. Clomipramine
    C. Imipramine
    D. Amitriptyline
    E. Nortriptyline

166. True or False: Height and intelligence follow a mendelian pattern of inheritance.
    A. True
    B. False

167. In a review of the research, Emery found four salient points regarding the impact of divorce and remarriage on children. Which one of the following is FALSE?
    A. Divorce is a source of great stress for children
    B. Divorce can lead to the emotional isolation from one parent
    C. Divorce makes psychological problems as much as twice as likely for children
    D. Despite the risks, most children from divorced families function as well as those from married families
    E. Children experience difficult feelings despite coping well

168. What is the ICD-10 equivalent of the DSM-IV diagnosis of ADHD?
    A. Hyperkinetic disorder
    B. ADHD
    C. Hyperactive disorder
    D. Hyperkinetic conduct disorder

169. Which symptoms of mania, from a meta-analysis of pediatric bipolar studies, are displayed in the correct descending order of frequency with the most common symptom first?
    A. Hypersexuality, flight of ideas, poor judgment, euphoria/elation, decreased need for sleep
    B. Increased energy, distractibility, pressured speech, irritability, grandiosity, racing thoughts
    C. Racing thoughts, decreased need for sleep, euphoria/elation, poor judgment, flight of ideas
    D. Pressured speech, irritability, grandiosity, racing thoughts, decreased need for sleep

170. Which TWO hypotheses drive the general approaches to investigating the genetic contributions to complex neuropsychiatric disorders?
    A. The common disease–common variant hypothesis, which holds that most of the risk for complex disorders will be accounted for by variations, or alleles, that are common in the population
    B. The rare genetic variant hypothesis, which holds that there are rare mutations within one or a small number of genes or rare mutations in any of a larger number of genes, resulting in a similar or overlapping phenotype
    C. The common disease–common variant hypothesis, which holds that most of the risk for complex disorders will be accounted for by variations, or alleles, under the influence of environmental factors
    D. A and B
    E. B and C

171. In disaster management, evacuation of the population is an event that occurs in what stage of a disaster:
    A. Predisaster
    B. First
    C. Second
    D. Third
    E. Fourth

172. Which of the following statements best describes diffusion tensors as used in the relatively new modality of diffusion tensor imaging?
    A. The degree of directional dependence of water diffusion in the brain
    B. Ellipsoid geometrical representations of the diffusional properties of water at a given voxel in the brain
    C. The orientation of an ellipsoid's longest axis representing the local orientation of brain fibers
    D. The connectivity of white matter in the brain by reconstructing the pathways of nerve fiber bundles based on the principal direction of water diffusion
    E. None of the above

173. Which of the following SSRIs has the shortest half-life?
    A. Sertraline
    B. Fluvoxamine
    C. Fluoxetine
    D. Citalopram
    E. Paroxetine

174. When a research study uses a more conservative p value in testing the null hypothesis such as 0.01 instead of 0.05, the probability of making what kind of error decreases?
    A. Selection bias
    B. Sampling error
    C. Type I
    D. Type II

175. Psychomotor development encompasses ALL of the following milestones EXCEPT:
   A. Standing
   B. Verbal skills
   C. Walking
   D. Jumping
   E. Skipping

176. Theorists have claimed that parents of future individuals with borderline personality disorder reward each of the following EXCEPT:
   A. Passivity and dependence
   B. Helplessness
   C. Dependence
   D. Striving for mastery

177. Cognitive behavioral interventions in the treatment of ADHD have demonstrated efficacy in which of the following?
   A. Increased learning
   B. Improved academic performance
   C. Reduced impulsivity
   D. Improved attention and concentration
   E. All of the above

178. True or False: In neuropsychological testing, qualitative observations must be integrated with test scores to provide a more complete understanding of the results and the conditions under which they were obtained.
   A. True
   B. False

179. True or False: Relative to the general population, people with mental retardation are more likely to show autism, behavior disorders, substance abuse, and affective disorders.
   A. True
   B. False

180. Each of these medications or class of medications is considered a first-line treatment for bipolar depression EXCEPT:
   A. Lithium
   B. Lamotrigine
   C. Valproate
   D. Bupropion
   E. Atypical antipsychotic

181. What is custody of care?
   A. When middle class families that do not qualify for Medicaid transfer custody of their children to child welfare or other government services to obtain mental health care
   B. When parents undergoing a contentious divorce transfer court custody of the child to the guardian ad litem
   C. When the state's child and family services suspend parental rights of a child during an investigation of abuse or neglect
   D. When one of the parents undergoing a contentious divorce is ultimately deemed the "psychological parent" and given physical custody of a child

182. Secure attachment behaviors include ALL of the following EXCEPT:
   A. Using the parent as a secure base from which to explore
   B. Evidence of trust and delight in the parent
   C. Eager seeking of contact after separation or when frightened
   D. Prolonged crying after a brief separation

183. True or False: In persons who were adopted and who have a high genetic risk for schizophrenia, disordered adoptive rearing can predict schizophrenia-spectrum disorders.
   A. True
   B. False

184. In custody evaluations, ALL of the following are generally indicated EXCEPT:
  A. Interview of each parent alone
  B. Interview of the child alone
  C. Interview of the child with each parent
  D. Psychological testing of each parent
  E. Referral from attorneys of each parent and the judge

185. In child and adolescent psychiatry, what is the primary role of classification systems of psychiatric disorders?
  A. To provide an explanation for a child's symptoms
  B. To facilitate communication for both clinical and research purposes
  C. To provide a prognosis
  D. To provide a current procedural terminology code for billing purposes

186. Which of the following statements regarding Rett's disorder is TRUE?
  A. It occurs more often in males
  B. It is lethal *in utero* to females
  C. It is the result of high peripheral ammonia levels
  D. It is associated with a genetic defect
  E. There are no associated medical conditions

187. True or False: Confidentiality refers to how private information is managed.
  A. True
  B. False

188. Which of the following assessment team structures is a team made up of members who are encouraged to share information and skills across disciplines, where assessment is collaborative in that one individual may do all or most of the interaction with the child patient, whereas others observe or make suggestions for the professional to use during the assessment process, and where team members train and receive training from each other in reciprocal interactions?
  A. Multidisciplinary
  B. Interdisciplinary
  C. Transdisciplinary
  D. Subdisciplinary
  E. Postdisciplinary

189. The International Algorithm Project put forth a simple method for ranking available treatments according to their level of empirical support. Medications with fair empirical support showing positive, but inconsistent, results in randomized control trials, or positive results from small sample trials would receive what classification?
  A. Class A
  B. Class B
  C. Class C
  D. None of the above

190. The prevalence of lifetime marijuana use by 12th grade is:
  A. 20%
  B. 30%
  C. 45%
  D. 60%
  E. 75%

191. What is the typical starting dose of guanfacine in children?
  A. 0.25 mg
  B. 0.5 mg
  C. 1 mg
  D. 2 mg
  E. None of the above

192. What is the most common metric used in meta-analytic studies to assess efficacy of psychotherapy interventions?
    A. Cohen's d
    B. Multiple regression analysis
    C. Analysis of variance
    D. PATH analysis
    E. Correlation, r

193. Habit reversal in the treatment of trichotillomania involves ALL of the following stages EXCEPT:
    A. Awareness training
    B. Training in an incompatible competing response
    C. Aversive counterconditioning
    D. Social support

194. Which TWO of the following constructs are considered integral to "good parenting"?
    A. Warmth
    B. Attachment
    C. Appropriate control
    D. Communication
    E. Sharing

195. The parents of a 13-year-old adolescent who are in the midst of a conflicted divorce seek your services because they would like you "to teach her some manners" as she is verbally abusive to both parents and staying out late at night. Moreover, they would like you "to stop her whining" as she is having frequent tearful episodes. Which ethical term best fits your pursuit of the parents' agenda without regard to the child's best interests?
    A. Breach of confidentiality
    B. Conflict of interest
    C. Role confusion
    D. Double agentry
    E. Fiduciary relationship

196. How many total students will the average middle school teacher have?
    A. 25
    B. 50
    C. 75
    D. 100
    E. 150

197. To establish malpractice, the plaintiff must demonstrate at least which of the following?
    A. The clinician had duty of reasonable care to the patient
    B. There was a dereliction of duty
    C. The patient sustained damage
    D. The damage was a direct result of the clinician's failure to exercise a reasonable standard of care
    E. All of the above

198. Interpersonal psychotherapy can trace its emphasis on the connection between relationships and mental health to which THREE of the following psychological theorists?
    A. Harry Stack Sullivan
    B. Anna Freud
    C. Adolf Meyer
    D. John Bowlby
    E. Eric Erikson

199. In the initial phase of interpersonal psychotherapy for depressed adolescents (IPT-A), the therapist conducts the Interpersonal Inventory, which is a detailed review of the adolescent's significant relationships. This inventory facilitates the understanding of the interpersonal context of the depressive symptoms. Which of the following tasks is helpful in conducting an Interpersonal Inventory?
   A. Self-soothing skills
   B. Habit-reversal training
   C. Exposure-response prevention
   D. Closeness circle
   E. Core belief identification

200. In infant and toddler assessments, observations of play can be important in obtaining additional information about the child including ALL of the following EXCEPT:
   A. Intellectual development
   B. Cognitive development
   C. Symbolic/linguistic development
   D. Social development
   E. Motor development

Test Two

1. **Answer: B.** Duplications and deletions are common even in regions known to contain genes with important biological functions. Page 197.

2. **Answer: B.** Page 305.

3. **Answer: B.** This is false. Many school districts, for a number of reasons—budgetary, resource—do find themselves temporizing services and underidentifying children with disabilities. Page 890.

4. **Answer: D.** Page 831.

5. **Answer: C.** Decreased cerebellar volume is not seen on imaging studies of patients with childhood onset schizophrenia. Page 497.

6. **Answer: D.** Ten thousand of these are thought to be expressed within the central nervous system. Page 177.

7. **Answer: A.** Associated, or noncore, symptoms include illusions, hallucinations, delusions, and affective changes. This idea of core versus noncore symptoms might be "splitting hairs" clinically; often, a patient with delirium comes to attention because of perceptual disturbances. Page 648.

8. **Answer: A.** However, studies have not shown that the Brazelton Neonatal Behavioral Assessment Scale, second edition, can accurately predict infant development beyond the first year of life. Page 316.

9. **Answer: D.** The key parameters are peripheral muscle tone, assessed by submental muscle EMG (electromylogram), EOG (electrooculogram), from electrodes placed periorbitally, and EEG (electroencephalogram), which help to diagnose specific sleep disorders. Page 625.

10. **Answer: D.** Discontinuation of the medication may be all that is required to halt the progression of neuroleptic malignant syndrome, which highlights the importance of early identification of the condition. Page 778.

11. **Answer: D.** Page 379.

12. **Answer: D.** Page 555.

13. **Answer: C.** Prader-Willi syndrome is associated with overeating and weight gain. The other choices are frequently associated with weight loss. Page 598.

14. **Answer: D.** Especially marital conflict, thus preserving family homeostasis. Other ideas are that somatic symptoms serve as a communicative function in the family on the order of body language, or are a plea for help. Page 637.

15. **Answer: D.** This test is used for a definitive diagnosis of narcolepsy. Page 630.

16. **Answer: A.** Page 798.

17. **Answer: A.** The use of a semistructured interview such as the Disturbances of Attachment Interview may be helpful to assess attachment disorder behaviors in a systematic manner. Page 715.

18. **Answer: E.** Typical individuals have 6 to 50 cytosine–guanine–guanine (CGG) repeats in their FMR-1 gene. Affected individuals have 200 to 1,000 CGG repeats. Carriers have 50 to 200 CGG repeats. FMR protein is thought to be necessary for synaptic plasticity and its absence affects spine morphology (spines in neurons not the spinal cord). Page 203.

19. **Answer: B.** Page 619.

20. **Answer: C.** This question emphasizes the psychological impact of a father's presence in the home, although this protective factor was not as apparent in low-income families. Page 8.

21. **Answer: B.** Recall bias is also known as differential misclassification. One well-known example: In a case–control study of severe birth abnormality of unknown origin, mothers of cases reported significantly more psychosocial stressors during pregnancy. Later, it turned out that the abnormality was Down syndrome; the chromosomal abnormality was discovered only in the months that followed the study. The only explanation for the spurious association lies in the differential reporting of mothers. Page 154.

22. **Answer: B.** Page 687.

23. **Answer: B.** Doing well in one domain cannot be considered resilience as this limited or narrowed success may convey a false picture of the whole. For example, adolescents with a history of significant adversity may be socially successful with their peers but at the same time perform poorly academically or even demonstrate conduct disorder traits. Page 293.

24. **Answer: C.** Page 235.

25. **Answer: E.** Nonepileptic seizure disorder, the preferred term for pseudoseizures, can overlap true epilepsy. An event that lasts longer than 10 minutes, has no postictal state, and is neuroanatomically incongruent with a seizure is likely to be nonepileptic. Disorders to be considered when nonepileptic seizure disorder is present are conversion disorder, factitious disorder, or malingering. Page 963.

26. **Answer: D.** Child psychiatry is a young subspecialty with much progress in the discipline occurring in the course of the last century. Page 15.

27. **Answer: A.** The term learning disabled refers to children who have disorders in development of language, speech, reading, and associated communication skills. In common practice, a learning disorder as established in DSM-IV is equivalent to a "specific learning disability." Page 411.

28. **Answer: C.** Regarding diagnosis, a plain abdominal x-ray reveals evidence of retention. Generally, a positive rectal examination is sufficient to determine retention but a negative examination does not rule it out. Page 664.

29. **Answer: A.** According to Sack et al., diagnostic status does not relate to functional status. Children not only show persistence of posttraumatic stress disorder (PTSD) symptoms but also demonstrate, at times, a delayed onset of symptoms. Even in those demonstrating delayed symptoms of PTSD, symptoms of depression diminish over time. Page 93.

30. **Answer: B.** The biopsychosocial approach is attributed to Engel, but Meyer should also be given credit for developing the psychobiological approach. Engel advocated for the approach to formulation as a "way of thinking that enables the physician to act rationally in areas now excluded from a rational approach." Page 378.

31. **Answer: C.** Families are second to schools as the source of referrals to emergency departments. Page 870.

32. **Answer: C.** Page 371.

33. **Answer: B.** The diagnosis of acute stress disorder is not necessary for the subsequent diagnosis of PTSD. Page 702.

34. **Answer: A.** The researchers have concluded that poverty is one of the major risk factors in mental health disorders in children. Page 37.

35. **Answer: B.** The severity of a child's superego, instead of being related to parental severity or the child's experiences with the parents, is rather related to the intensity of the aggressive wishes in face of the relative weakness and immaturity of the individual's ego and defenses. Page 830.

36. **Answer: B.** A number of theories have been advanced regarding the social reinforcement of cross-gender behavior but there is limited empirical evaluation. That said, generally, a number of authors from varied theoretical persuasions have found that clinic referred boys have either neutral or encouraging parents. Page 674.

37. **Answer: E.** Page 672.

38. **Answer: A.** Clomipramine's side effect profile and tolerance generally place it outside first-line consideration, but is worth trying if selective serotonin reuptake inhibitors fail. Page 559.

39. **Answer: B.** Permanency planning and placement, as mandated by law, includes (i) family reunification; (ii) child adoption; and (iii) long-term placement with kin or nonrelative foster caregivers who are granted legal guardianship. Page 698.

40. **Answer: A.** Page 567.

41. **Answer: A.** Pruning can lead to losses of up to 30,000 synapses per second, resulting in the loss of approximately half of cortical synaptic connections present before puberty. This is thought to affect preferentially excitatory synapses, accompanied by decreases in brain glucose metabolism, oxygen use, and blood flow. Page 281.

42. **Answer: C.** The ideographic approach rejects simple labels of classification and may be theory driven, as in psychoanalytic or behavioral theories, or may be used eclectically. Page 305.

43. **Answer: B.** Although attention deficit hyperactivity disorder (ADHD) pathology tends to take similar course regardless of the additional condition of Tourette's syndrome, there appears to be a distinction between tic-related obsessive–compulsive disorder and nontic-related obsessive–compulsive disorder. Pages 572–573.

44. **Answer: A.** Page 441.

45. **Answer: C.** However, dopaminergic circuits are influenced by inputs from multiple neurotransmitter systems including norepinephrine and serotonin. Page 436.

46. **Answer: E.** All are examples of policy, but what differentiates policies is the degree to which they have been formalized. Simply put, a policy is a set of principles used to guide decisions or procedures. Page 35.

47. **Answer: E.** The defendant psychiatrist is entitled to an appeal when sanctioned by the American Psychiatric Association. Page 21.

48. **Answer: A.** The other answers may be accurate but could be subsumed under the correct answer. Page 901.

49. **Answer: B.** Id encompasses the mental representations of the instinctual forces, whereas drive is applied to a stimulus arising from within the individual that arouses the mind and incites mental activity. Page 828.

50. **Answer: E.** Logical operations are crucial in mastering basic reading and mathematics skills, and they are also necessary for conducting social interactions, with its increasing complexity of groups, games, and rules. Page 270.

51. **Answer: A.** Although stuttering has at times been thought to be a learned behavior, most researchers today consider stuttering to have a biological component. All of the other statements are true. Page 424.

52. **Answer: B.** Provides a clinical working definition for infancy. Page 252.

53. **Answer: A.** However, the availability of so-called traditional services received by the children of military families in this study might have been greater than in other settings. Overall, the systems-of-care model appears to be beneficial in reducing the use of residential and out-of-home placements and achieving improvements in functional behavior in youth with severe emotional and behavioral disorders who are served in multiple systems. Page 894.

54. **Answer: B.** Page 240.

55. **Answer: A.** Page 151.

56. **Answer: B.** UGTs catalyze Phase II metabolic reactions. Page 747.

57. **Answer: B and D.** These two phases remove the active form of the drug from the body. Page 743.

58. **Answer: A.** Statutes immunize clinicians for making good faith reports about child abuse to child protective services. However, the advice to the mother falls outside the reporting requirements and could be grounds for a suit. Page 1024.

59. **Answer: E.** Describing psychosocial ills in detail, such as sexual abuse history details, also increases risk. It is fine to agree with trainees, but if you disagree with the trainee's findings and treatment plan you should specifically note that in the record and amend the diagnosis and plan accordingly. There are compliance guidelines for how to write a note when a trainee sees a patient with or without you. Page 1030.

60. **Answer: B and D.** Tremor and weight gain are also common, among other side effects. Page 769.

61. **Answer: A.** The 29-item measure is the Acute Stress Checklist for Children. Page 705.

62. **Answer: C.** The 1989 United States government's report of the Secretary's Task Force on Youth Suicide showed that suicide was the leading cause of death among sexual minority youth. In this report, about 30% of sexual minority youth commit suicide annually. Gay youth are two to three times more likely to commit suicide than other youth. Sexual orientation has an independent association with suicide attempts for males. For females, the association of sexual orientation with suicidality may be mediated by drug use and violence or victimization. Page 82.

63. **Answer: A.** Cochlear implants are most effective if present during the development of speech and language. Access to early language, whether signed or spoken is an important intervention. Page 72.

64. **Answer: B.** Low socioeconomic status (father unemployed or unskilled worker) is the strongest predictor of general mental health problems. Page 88.

65. **Answer: B.** In fact, the reverse is true; children with nonverbal learning disability appear to have deficits that are primarily nonverbal in nature. Page 369.

66. **Answer: E.** The shorter half-life of lithium in children is due to the faster glomerular filtration rates in the young and has practical implications in that reliable blood levels can be obtained after 4 days of dose initiation or adjustment (5 half-lives × 18 hours). Page 769.

67. **Answer: B.** Brain size in children ages 2 to 4 with autism has been observed to be 5% to 10% larger than typically developing counterparts. With further aging, however, brain growth decelerates, resulting in adult brain sizes equal to that which is typically expected or slightly larger. Pages 387 and 390.

68. **Answer: B.** Parents and the child should be told explicitly that confidentiality does not extend to situations that pose a clear danger to the child or others. Page 341.

69. **Answer: E.** This compares with 25% in the 1970s. Page 928.

70. **Answer: E.** Page 856.

71. **Answer: D.** For most children, physical aggression begins to subside around age 3 or 4. At the same time, verbal aggression increases between ages 2 and 4, as language skills increase. Overall, however, all kinds of aggression tend to diminish in frequency by age 5 or 6 years of age. Aggressive behavior in preschool children is generally focused around the assertion of physical needs and wants. Page 266.

72. **Answer: C.** Page 744.

73. **Answer: A.** A surprising statistic, but this question is meant to emphasize how the effect of fathers' influences on children is vastly underrepresented in the literature, despite their greater presence and engagement with their offspring. Page 4.

74. **Answer: D.** Given the high prevalence of abuse experiences in child psychiatric populations, maltreatment experiences should be screened routinely in all mental health evaluations. Page 693.

75. **Answer: E.** Bodily functions, lucky numbers, sexual or aggressive preoccupations, and fear of harm to oneself are less common. Page 550.

76. **Answer: B.** Freud's interest was not the treatment of children but confirming the centrality of childhood experience in shaping the adult psyche. With this motivation he supervised the analysis of Little Hans by his father. Page 826.

77. **Answer: B.** People can lose the capability of self-determination due to illness, mental disability, or due to the restriction of liberty, as upon incarceration. Page 141.

78. **Answer: B.** It is termed a mechanism of defense of which repression is one defense. Page 829.

79. **Answer: A.** Concrete services along with counseling that targets family communication, behavior management, and problem-solving skills typify a crisis intervention approach. Page 879.

80. **Answer: B.** Cultural formulation is a key concept in the biopsychosocial assessment. It serves as a sensitive instrument to address the requirements of a comprehensive assessment in culturally diverse or multicultural groups. The formulation has four main themes and includes (i) the cultural identity of the patient; (ii) cultural explanations of the patient's illness; (iii) cultural factors related to the psychosocial environment; and (iv) overall cultural assessment for diagnosis and treatment. Pages 61–62.

81. **Answer: B.** Oxcarbazepine's principal active metabolite is mostly glucuronidated (Phase II metabolism) and excreted in the urine. Page 772.

82. **Answer: E.** Page 2.

83. **Answer: A.** mRNA synthesized by the mother during oogenesis lies dormant within the egg until fertilization occurs. The embryo does not have the machinery for the proper transcription, translation, and processing of mature proteins and relies on the mother's mRNA. Page 184.

84. **Answer: D.** Infant intelligence quotient (IQ) tests were weak in predicting IQ in later development and are generally not administered presently. Page 310.

85. **Answer: A.** Page 41.

86. **Answer: C.** The number needed to treat (NNT) is the reciprocal of the absolute risk reduction (ARR) NNT = 1/ARR. Page 127.

87. **Answer: B.** Rather, pyromania is extremely rare in children. Page 488.

88. **Answer: A.** Page 365.

89. **Answer: C.** Page 160.

90. **Answer: E.** School reentry is highly stressful because of concerns about having fallen behind academically and the negative reactions of peers. The other options are not usually sources of pain, but support, although children may have worries about the others in their lives. Page 931.

91. **Answer: D.** It appears that improvement in ADHD symptoms is not as robust as with stimulants. There is also a delay to clinical effect, which requires more patience. Page 766.

92. **Answer: A.** This is an important point in pharmacokinetics due to the resulting increases in the volume of distribution (V_d), which consequently affects plasma concentration of a drug (C_p) relative to the amount of drug absorbed (D) as in the equation: $C_p = D/V_d$. Page 746.

93. **Answer: E.** Functional magnetic resonance imaging and positron emission tomography scan research in the field of autism has implicated differences in components of the limbic system, temporal lobe and frontal lobe. Page 388.

94. **Answer: A.** They occur during nonrapid eye movement stage 4 sleep and this stage occupies more time earlier in the night. Page 629.

95. **Answer: B.** On average, only about 50% of students ages 14 and older diagnosed with learning disabilities (LDs) graduate with regular high school diplomas. The employment prospect of these students is also troublesome—only about 60% of students ages 14 and older diagnosed with LDs have paid jobs outside the home. Thus, it is important to realize that the impact of LDs is not limited to any one academic domain; these are lifetime disorders with wide-ranging consequences. Page 416.

96. **Answer: A.** Page 634.

97. **Answer: C.** The usual dosage range is 50 to 200 mg daily. Page 763.

98. **Answer: B.** Neuropsychoanalysis seeks to achieve this aim by integrating the latest findings from cognitive neuroscience with psychoanalytic observations. Page 828.

99. **Answer: B.** A minor protective effect of breast-feeding has been observed repeatedly, which, according to some studies, is still detectable in adolescence. Page 608.

100. **Answer: D.** Page 972.

101. **Answer: C.** In practical terms this may mean diagnosing a patient based on a presentation that is reminiscent of another recent patient's presentation. Page 345.

102. **Answer: A.** Page 363.

103. **Answer: A.** Start at 25 mg nightly and titrate every 4 to 7 days. Most children respond in the 75 to 125 mg range. A baseline electrocardiogram should be obtained and monitoring is advised above 3.5 mg/kg after dose adjustments. Page 660.

104. **Answer: B.** Page 455.

105. **Answer: E.** These oppositional symptoms subsequently decrease in frequency. Page 457.

106. **Answer: C.** Each of these can increase vulnerability, but generally the parents' own traumatic experience with the event will influence a child's traumatic reactions. Page 940.

107. **Answer: D.** Approximately half of mental health disorders occur at or before age 14. Three-quarters occur by the age of 24. Page 921.

108. **Answer: B.** Over one-half was under the age of 18, and one-third was younger than age 15. Page 483.

109. **Answer: C.** Future suicidal tendencies were best predicted by anger or irritability, past history of suicidal thinking or behavior, and older age. Page 532.

110. **Answer: D.** The Stroop consists of naming the color of a flashed word. The other options represent bona fide neuropsychological tests. Having a basic knowledge of key neuropsychological tests is a reasonable expectation for a child psychiatrist. Page 545.

111. **Answer: C.** Those under 25 years of age account for 66%. Page 948.

112. **Answer: B.** To achieve these goals, the speech–language pathologist uses not only standardized tests but also criterion-referenced, observational, and dynamic assessments. Page 373.

113. **Answer: E.** A past medical and family history of syncope should also be investigated, as well as documentation of a normal physical examination within the past year. Page 764.

114. **Answer: D.** At birth, the brain is estimated to be about 10% of adult volume, then grows to 90% of adult volume by age 5. Boys' brains are typically about 10% larger than girls', and this difference persists into adulthood. Boys have greater growth in the amygdala, and girls have more growth in the hippocampus. In both boys and girls, information processing speed is parallel to synaptic pruning and myelinization, thus increasing between ages 6 and 12. Page 268.

115. **Answer: D.** An emerging body of empirical evidence indicates that risperidone is effective for serious behavior problems in children with autism, severe disruptive behavior and Tourette's syndrome. Page 774.

116. **Answer: B.** Page 975.

117. **Answer: B.** This is data from 2005. Page 946.

118. **Answer: D.** Page 1014.

119. **Answer: B.** Psychosocial dwarfism is not characterized by frontal bossing. Psychosocial dwarfism, also called deprivational dwarfism or hyperphagic short stature, is a syndrome of deceleration of linear growth combined with characteristic behavior disturbances (sleep disorder and bizarre eating habits), both of which are reversible by a change in the psychosocial environment. It differs from failure to thrive in that there is an absence of weight gain deceleration. Page 589.

120. **Answer: D.** Page 848.

121. **Answer: C.** This pattern is manifested in two or more areas: cognition, affectivity, interpersonal functioning, and impulse control. Page 680.

122. **Answer: A.** Two randomized controlled trials have demonstrated this. From a public policy perspective, adding a few additional family sessions to the standard treatment of adult patients in a clinical setting might be feasible. Page 175.

123. **Answer: D.** Page 843.

124. **Answer: C.** In other words, the intervention being studied is not successful. Page 115.

125. **Answer: A.** Cognitive changes seen in adolescence are accompanied by changes in social cognition and moral development. The development of formal operational thinking permits a growth in social perspective-taking and a decline in childhood egocentrism. It enables an adolescent to contemplate better what a social situation might look like from another person's point of view. Page 282.

126. **Answer: C.** Page 760.

127. **Answer: B.** The studies, which are of poor quality, show conflicting evidence. Page 463.

128. **Answer: B.** They were established through the Rockefeller Foundation at Massachusetts General, Colorado, and Duke. In the 1970s the National Institutes of Health began training grants to promote the growth of consultation–liaison psychiatry. In 2003, the field formally adopted the name of psychosomatic medicine and gained approval as a subspecialty by the American Board of Medical Specialties. Page 915.

129. **Answer: A.** Epilepsy is recurrent seizures without known stimuli. Page 958.

130. **Answer: E.** The Schedule for Affective Disorders and Schizophrenia for School-Aged Children or the Diagnostic Interview Schedule for Children are usually administered to children aged 5 and older and to their primary caregiver. Page 292.

131. **Answer: C.** You are permitted to observe the classroom and consult to staff about their questions on how to manage the student. Page 996.

132. **Answer: A.** Page 652.

133. **Answer: C.** The intraclass correlation coefficient is a test–retest reliability statistic used for continuous data such as scale scores. Page 351.

134. **Answer: E.** Physically aggressive behavior generally begins to subside by age 3, whereas verbal aggression increases between the ages of 2 and 4 (as language is developing). In general, both physical and verbal aggression diminish by age 5 or 6. In addition, although younger children focus aggression on assertion of their physical needs and wants, older children tend to focus aggression on social situations and needs. Page 266.

135. **Answer: B.** The multisystemic therapy condition was favorable at 4 months: they had fewer hospital days, fewer out-of-home placement days, fewer externalizing symptoms, better school attendance, and better family relations. By 16 months, however, there were few differences between the treatment conditions. Overall, this study supports the feasibility of in-home services as an alternative to inpatient care (less restrictive, similar results) and raises questions on how to best maintain and consolidate early gains. Page 883.

136. **Answer: D.** Trauma-focused cognitive-behavioral therapy has been used successfully with a wide age range of children with a variety of traumatic histories. A web-based training for trauma-focused cognitive-behavioral therapy is available as well. Page 707.

137–139. **Answers:** 137-C; 138-B; 139-A. Page 172.

140. **Answer: C.** Page 105.

141. **Answer: C.** Normative data should be reevaluated every 10 years as grossly outdated norms often yield inflated scores that may lead to falsely disqualifying infants in need of interventional services. Page 315.

142. **Answer: D.** In DSM-IV-TR, *mental retardation* is defined on the basis of three essential features: subnormal intellectual functioning, commensurate deficits in adaptive functioning, and onset before 18 years. Subnormal intellectual functioning is characterized by an IQ lower than 70, based in most cases on the administration of an appropriate standardized assessment of intelligence. Page 401.

143. **Answer: B.** School-aged children are more likely to witness catastrophic events and to understand better that death is irreversible. In order to master their fears, school-aged children's dreams often set themselves up as heroes. School-aged children can also experience anxiety, as they are better able to evaluate themselves as compared to others, and in so doing, perhaps feel inferior. Page 271.

144. **Answer: B.** Education of parents, patient, and teachers should be the initial treatment for tic disorders. Habit reversal training is a nonpharmacological approach for treatment. As tics tend to wax and wane, medications could be "chasing" the tics, although they are an option when tics cause functional impairment. Page 579.

145. **Answer: A.** The psychiatrist would try to address the patient's concerns to determine if they can be overcome, but her history of noncompliance and her inability to adhere to the recommendations of her physicians make her a poor transplant candidate. Page 941.

146. **Answer: B.** Page 619.

147. **Answer: C.** This capacity develops within the third stage of qualitative reorganization in an infant's life, according to Zeanah and colleagues. Page 257.

148. **Answer: C.** Page 107.

149. **Answer: A.** Because half the symptoms of oppositional defiant disorder describe hostility arising from negative affect, this finding is not entirely surprising. Page 472.

150. **Answer: A.** Whether the association is incidental, causal, or secondary is unclear. Psychodynamic generalizations about enuresis have been found to have little empiric support. Page 657.

151. **Answer: A.** Some argue that pathogenic care or maltreatment should not be a criterion for the diagnosis of reactive attachment disorder, as it is often difficult to obtain such a history at the time of presentation. However, possible support of the continued inclusion of this criterion is the report that children with excellent caregiving but a microdeletion in chromosome 7 typically show indiscriminate behavior, showing that other etiologies may play a role. Page 714.

152. **Answer: A.** Page 541.

153. **Answer: B.** Autism is a disorder with a spectrum of presentations. Although children share developmental delays in specific categories, syndrome expression varies widely. Page 384.

154. **Answer: C.** This speaks of several issues: the need to have systems in place that ensure follow-up with services; the potential mismatch between treatment recommendations and the patients' and families' wishes for treatment or ability to follow-up; the intense but transient nature of suicidal feelings and acts in youth. Rapid response teams, which provide vigorous clinical follow-up after discharge from the pediatric emergency department, have proved beneficial. Page 907.

155. **Answer: A.** This question refers to behavioral genetics and twin studies, which have demonstrated the equally influential effect of shared environment, at least for depressive disorders. Page 504.

156. **Answer: D.** This recommended upper limit is due to the seizure liability of bupropion. Page 766.

157. **Answer: B.** Selective mutism is most often seen in school settings, where the child refuses to speak despite being verbal at home. Cultural and linguistic differences can exacerbate the problem, especially when the child has limited English proficiency. Although most children eventually overcome their reluctance to talk in school, some, as well as up to 50% of monolingual English speakers, remain selectively mute for extended periods. The condition shows a 2:1 ratio in favor of girls. All other statements above are true. Page 421.

158. **Answer: B.** Group interventions with mothers facilitate indirect focusing on preschool children. Page 734.

159. **Answer: A.** A treating clinician should not switch to a forensic role, for a number of clinical and ethical reasons. If you are subpoenaed and compelled to testify in court, you can discuss the boy's care and treatment; however, you would not be able to comment on custody arrangements or the father's parenting ability, as you did not evaluate those aspects. Page 1002.

160. **Answer: C.** Individuals with tics may or may not have a premonitory urge or warning that a tic is about to occur. Coprolalia, obscene utterances, is rare in tic disorders. Page 570.

161. **Answer: B.** A large, tempting array of play materials is usually too stimulating for a group and leads to excessively active, disorganized interactions. A modest array of developmentally appropriate materials facilitates more productive group interaction. Page 845.

162. **Answer: C.** The ability to symbolize is the ability to let one thing stand for another, such as when a child "eats" from an empty toy spoon. Page 263.

163. **Answer: A.** Page 535.

164. **Answer: A.** Patients with bulimia nervosa should not be below 15% of the normal weight range. If they are, in most circumstances the correct diagnosis will be anorexia nervosa binge-purge subtype. Bulimia nervosa patients can be overweight. Page 593.

165. **Answer: A.** However, desipramine has generally not been used because of its association with a number of children who experienced cardiovascular events. Page 764.

166. **Answer: B.** Mendelian patterns of vertical transmission include, for example, Rett's and Fragile X syndromes. Height and intelligence are examples of nonmendelian polygenetic traits and it may be that some forms of childhood onset anxiety disorders and ADHD will also fall under this category (i.e., polygenetic transmission). Page 211.

167. **Answer: B.** Resilience does not preclude vulnerability. Although children of divorce can function just as well as their peers, the factors associated with the divorce, including age, gender, ethnicity and socioeconomic status can engender increased risk. Page 39.

168. **Answer: A.** The criteria for International Classification of Diseases (ICD)-10 hyperkinetic disorder are more restrictive than the DSM-IV criteria. Page 432.

169. **Answer: B.** Option A is displayed in reverse order of frequency; hypersexuality was the least common symptom. The others are in correct order but do not begin with the most common symptom. Page 515.

170. **Answer: D.** Theoretically, environmental factors could, in fact, be one of the explanations for allelic variation, but this would not capture the broader hypothesis. Page 190.

171. **Answer: C.** The second stage consists of massive changes in societal structure and function—establishment of evacuation centers and tent-cities, movement of refugees—which may lead to a breakdown of norms, structures, and functions. Page 728.

172. **Answer: B.** Page 224.

173. **Answer: B.** Fluvoxamine is given on a twice-daily schedule; and at low doses of sertraline (50 mg/day or less), children may require twice-daily dosing. Page 763.

174. **Answer: C.** The probability of making a type I error—of rejecting the null hypothesis, when in fact, it is true—decreases. Page 116.

175. **Answer: B.** Verbal skills are categorized under cognitive development, which also includes attentional skills. Page 326.

176. **Answer: D.** Mastery, autonomy, and independence are undervalued and disruption of the separation-individuation process occurs. Page 684.

177. **Answer: E.** Page 813.

178. **Answer: A.** This includes variables such as the child's attention, motivation, persistence, fatigue, rapport, and approach to questions. Page 359.

179. **Answer: B.** Relative to the general population, individuals with mental retardation are more likely to show psychosis, autism, and behavior disorders, and are less apt to be diagnosed with substance abuse and affective disorders. Page 404.

180. **Answer: D.** Selective serotonin reuptake inhibitors or bupropion should be added after mood stabilizers have shown nonresponse. (Whether the addition of antidepressants help depression in bipolar disorder has been raised.) For seasonal depression light therapy should be considered. Page 521.

181. **Answer: A.** Page 52.

182. **Answer: D.** The secure infant may protest and cry after a separation from a parent, but such a response will not be prolonged or excessive. Page 254.

183. **Answer: A.** This was found in a Finnish study at 21-year follow-up. This speaks to gene–environment interaction. The presumed genotype may be "sensitive" not only to dysfunction in the family environment but to protective environmental factors as well. Page 1015.

184. **Answer: D.** Psychological testing of a parent might be indicated if the mental health of the parent is an issue; however, the results should be used adjunctively and not serve as the sole basis for an opinion. A custody evaluation referral from all parties involved is preferred to avoid the appearance of bias and being a "hired gun." Page 1008.

185. **Answer: B.** Currently, the classification of child psychiatric disorders has a limited role in providing a prognosis and has a limited explanatory value. Page 302.

186. **Answer: D.** Rett's disorder is more common in females and usually lethal for males *in utero*, as it is associated with a genetic defect in MECP2, a regulator gene located on the X chromosome. It is not associated with peripheral ammonia levels as originally suspected by Rett. Medical conditions associated with Rett's disorder include seizures, and feeding, respiratory, movement, and orthopedic problems. Page 393.

187. **Answer: A.** Although confidentiality is often used interchangeably with privacy, there exists a distinction between the two terms. Confidentiality refers to a mode of management of private information. Page 146.

188. **Answer: C.** Page 372.

189. **Answer: B.** Page 756.

190. **Answer: C.** For alcohol, 80%. Page 616.

191. **Answer: B.** The typical starting dose of 0.5 mg is first given at bedtime with increases of 0.5 mg every 3 to 5 days to a total of 1.5 to 3 mg per day in two to three divided doses. Page 781.

192. **Answer: A.** Cohen's *d* is a common metric to assess the effect size of an intervention. This metric is calculated by taking the mean of the treated group on a measure of interest (e.g., Hamilton Depression rating scores), subtracting it from the mean of the control group, and then dividing this difference by the standard deviation of the control group. This calculation creates a score indicating the difference in outcomes between the intervention group and the controls. Page 790.

193. **Answer: C.** Page 806.

194. **Answer: A and C.** These two core constructs are interdependent: both high warmth with lax discipline and strict discipline without affection have been linked with poor adjustment. Page 294.

195. **Answer: D.** The term "double agentry" refers to serving two parties simultaneously and is a dilemma that can arise when the psychiatrist is not clear about his role. This term is more frequently used in the setting of a consultation in which a child psychiatrist has a duty to the school or consulting body and not necessarily to the patient or student. This dilemma in consultation can be minimized by informing the patient or student about the limits of confidentiality in this setting. However, as in the question, double agentry can also arise in pursuing the parents' agenda without regard to the child's best interests. Page 19.

196. **Answer: E.** When consulting to schools, one needs to be mindful of the impact of recommendations for the consultee and everyone else in the school system. Teachers are in the frontline and often ideally positioned to help a student, but have many other students under their instruction. Page 983.

197. **Answer: E.** Known as the four Ds. Page 1018.

198. **Answer: A, C, and D.** The interpersonal emphasis has its origin in the work of Meyer and Sullivan. Meyer theorized that mental illness was a result of poor environmental adaptation, including relationships. Sullivan postulated that mental illness was partly due to poor communication and a lack of understanding of one's behavior in relationships. Bowlby's attachment theory emphasized the importance of relational bonds between people. Page 820.

199. **Answer: D.** The Closeness Circle is a series of concentric circles with the adolescent's name in the center. The goal is to place significant relationships within the appropriate circles of closeness/importance in the adolescent's life and helps to identify the emotional valence of these relationships. Page 822.

200. **Answer: A.** This question is intended to emphasize the amount of information in multiple domains that observation of play can yield during an infant or toddler assessment. Page 313.

Test Three

Questions

1. In juvenile diabetes, depression is an independent risk factor for ALL of the following EXCEPT:
   A. Diabetic retinopathy
   B. Repeat hospitalization
   C. Adaptation to disease
   D. Prolactin elevation
   E. Metabolic control

2. Lithium levels above which point can affect multiple organs and be fatal?
   A. 4.0 mEq/L
   B. 3.2 mEq/L
   C. 2.5 mEq/L
   D. 1.6 mEq/L
   E. 1.2 mEq/L

3. True or False: The number needed to treat is always a whole number, rounded off to an integer.
   A. True
   B. False

4. In the biopsychosocial model of formulation, which of the following components belong in the biological realm?
   A. Inborn temperament
   B. Patterns of behavior
   C. Emotional development
   D. Family constellation
   E. Patterns of cognition

5. According to Kolvin, which of the following is FALSE for childhood onset schizophrenia?
   A. It is episodic in nature
   B. Children with this condition have poorer premorbid social functioning
   C. Children with this condition have poorer premorbid language functioning
   D. Transient autistic symptoms are commonly seen in toddler years
   E. All of the above

6. ALL of the following are examples of commonly used language test batteries EXCEPT:
   A. Clinical Evaluation of Language Fundamentals
   B. Oral and Written Language Scales
   C. Test of Early Language Development—4
   D. Vineland Adaptive Behavior Scales—2
   E. Preschool Language Scale—4

7. Classic characteristics of language in verbal children with autism spectrum disorders include ALL of the following EXCEPT:
   A. Echolalia
   B. Failure to use pronoun reversals
   C. Monotonous intonation
   D. Nonreciprocal speech
   E. Poor syntax

8. The Edinburgh High Risk Study has focused on the identification of a range of characteristics that identify individuals who are at increased risk for the development of schizophrenia. These characteristics include:
   A. Situational anxiety, depression, isolated hallucinations, social withdrawal, schizotypal features, and lower verbal intelligence quotient (IQ) scores
   B. Situational anxiety, depression, lower performance IQ scores, social withdrawal, schizotypal features, and isolated hallucinations
   C. Isolated hallucinations, mania, lower performance IQ scores, social withdrawal, and schizotypal features
   D. Chronic delusions, situational anxiety, isolated hallucinations, decreased verbal IQ, and social withdrawal

9. The most current consensus recommendations from experts in pediatric bipolar disorder suggest medication taper may be considered once remission has been maintained for:
   A. 6 months
   B. 12 to 24 months
   C. 24 to 36 months
   D. >36 months
   E. After adolescence

10. True or False: Although often described as involuntary, research suggests that tics are not analogous to other involuntary movements, such as choreas or dystonias.
    A. True
    B. False

11. Which of these patients could be diagnosed with pica?
    A. A toddler who eats his own hair
    B. A teenager with autism who eats raw potatoes
    C. A severely retarded adult who eats feces
    D. A normally developed adult who eats his own fingernails
    E. All of the above

12. Which of the following is true of hearing impairment in children under the age of 18 years in the United States?
    A. It affects 5% of children in this age group
    B. The most common form is the result of inner ear infection
    C. Acquired hearing loss is responsible for 60% of permanent hearing impairment
    D. Genetic defects are the most common cause of permanent sensorineural hearing loss
    E. All of the above

13. Relaxation training for children typically involves ALL of the following techniques EXCEPT:
    A. Progressive muscle relaxation
    B. Deep breathing
    C. Systematic desensitization
    D. Pleasant imagery

14. The most dramatic piece of legislation for children and families in recent years is the Personal Responsibility and Work Opportunity Reconciliation Act of 1996 in which government effectively reduced public entitlements to cash benefits resulting in ALL of the following EXCEPT:
    A. States are granted greater flexibility in the use of federal welfare funds
    B. States are obliged to impose work requirements for those receiving federal assistance
    C. States are obliged to provide a basic health care plan for children under the poverty line
    D. States are obliged to impose a 5-year lifetime limit for federal assistance

15. When a clinician interviews a child with severe visual impairment, and the child gazes in his or her direction, the clinician is more likely to ascribe which of the following to the child:
    A. Intelligence
    B. Developmental delay
    C. Anxiety
    D. Sexual reactivity
    E. A personality disorder

16. True or False: A recent pharmacokinetic study of paroxetine showed that children metabolize this selective serotonin reuptake inhibitor (SSRI) more slowly than adults do.
    A. True
    B. False

17. In a major study, Treatment for Adolescents with Depression Study, fluoxetine was found to be:
    A. Less efficacious than both placebo and cognitive-behavioral therapy (CBT)
    B. As efficacious as both placebo and CBT
    C. More efficacious than both placebo and CBT
    D. Unapprovable for the treatment of depression in children and adolescents

18. The Individual with Disabilities Education Act defines "emotional disturbance," previously known as "serious emotional disturbance," as:
    A. An inability to learn that cannot be explained by intellectual, sensory, or health factors
    B. An inability to build or maintain satisfactory interpersonal relationships with peers and teachers
    C. Inappropriate types of mood or behavior under normal circumstances
    D. A tendency to develop physical symptoms or fears associated with personal or school problems
    E. All of the above

19. Major changes in family, school, and neighborhoods, along with successes in preventive medicine, such as immunizations, accounted for the emergence of which field?
    A. Child and adolescent psychiatry
    B. Psychiatry
    C. Pediatrics
    D. Developmental behavioral pediatrics
    E. Internal medicine

20. True or False: Electroconvulsive therapy is the treatment of choice for catatonia if pharmacological management fails.
    A. True
    B. False

21. Preschool children often have fears and worries because:
    A. Their capacity for imagination is increasing
    B. There is little differentiation between fantasy and reality
    C. They are preoccupied with the constancy of important people in their lives
    D. They feel simultaneously powerful and helpless
    E. All of the above

22. True or False: The Diagnostic and Statistical Manual of Mental Disorders (DSM)-IV does not require evidence of conduct disorder prior to age 15 years for a diagnosis of antisocial personality disorder.
    A. True
    B. False

23. What is the treatment of night terrors?
    A. Reassure the child
    B. Wake the child
    C. Have the child sleep with the parents as needed
    D. Mirtazapine
    E. Hydroxyzine

24. According to Freud, development in the school-aged child is characterized by:
    A. A sexually dormant interlude
    B. An attempt to master the basics of the industry of society, by building on academic abilities
    C. An opportunity for society to correct the influence of the family
    D. Establishment of the superego
    E. None of the above

25. Meta-analysis is a research synthesis of a set of studies that uses what statistic to indicate the strength of relationship between a treatment (or other independent variable) and the dependent variables?
    A. Analysis of variance
    B. Multiple regression
    C. *T*-test
    D. Effect size
    E. None of the above

26. Morphometric magnetic resonance imaging studies of subjects with trichotillomania support findings for decreased volumes in the:
    A. Left frontal cortex
    B. Right frontal cortex
    C. Left parietal cortex
    D. Right parietal cortex

27. True or False: The electroencephalogram pattern during rapid eye movement sleep is low voltage, fast, and resembles the electroencephalogram of wakefulness.
    A. True
    B. False

28. Anna Freud's classic, *The Ego and the Mechanisms of Defense*, enumerated several patterns of defense already in the analytic literature, including repression and reaction formation, but which of the following mechanisms of defense did she discover?
    A. Identification with the aggressor
    B. Regression
    C. Projection
    D. Sublimation
    E. Undoing

29. What is the typical starting dose of paroxetine for children?
    A. 5 to 10 mg
    B. 25 to 50 mg
    C. 12.5 to 25 mg
    D. 10 to 20 mg
    E. 75 to 100 mg

30. At about 7 to 9 months, a shift of qualitative reorganization occurs in infants as they develop a sense of intersubjectivity, which consists of:
    A. The understanding that they are connected to, but not in complete union with, their caregivers
    B. The understanding that others can understand their thoughts, feelings, gestures, and sounds
    C. The understanding that others can see the things from their perspective
    D. The understanding that even when others cannot be seen or heard, they still exist

31. True or False: The first code of ethics of the American Medical Association was based upon Thomas Percival's *Code of Medical Ethics*.
    A. True
    B. False

32. Placebo-controlled studies have shown the efficacy of which tricyclic antidepressant in children and adolescents with obsessive–compulsive disorder (OCD)?
A. Desipramine
B. Clomipramine
C. Imipramine
D. Amitriptyline
E. Nortriptyline

33. At higher doses, venlafaxine selectively inhibits which of the following neuronal functions?
A. Serotonin reuptake
B. Dopamine reuptake
C. Norepinephrine reuptake
D. A and B
E. A and C

34. Attention deficit hyperactivity disorder (ADHD) is one of the most common childhood onset psychiatric disorders affecting approximately what percentage of children worldwide?
A. 0.5% to 1%
B. 1% to 2%
C. 3% to 5%
D. 5% to 6%
E. 5% to 12%

35. Two groups of subjects are initially free of disease. One group has experienced the exposure and the other group has not. What type of study is this?
A. Case–control
B. Cross-sectional
C. Ecological
D. Cohort

36. Which of the following statements is TRUE?
A. The negative outcome of abuse cannot be avoided
B. Psychotropic medications are more often prescribed for children in social service care than those in the community
C. Most children and adults involved in maltreatment receive mental health services
D. The Adoption and Safe Family Act of 1997 recommended that abused children who were removed from their homes be in permanent placement by the end of the first year
E. Parental substance abuse rarely affects the management of child maltreatment

37. Neuroanatomical structures that have been implicated in tic disorders include ALL of the following EXCEPT:
A. Corticostriatal thalamocortical circuit
B. Basal ganglia
C. Medulla oblongata
D. Cortex
E. Globus pallidus

38. Maternal smoking during pregnancy is associated with later behavioral problems in the child. Which of the following is a confounding factor?
A. Fetal development
B. Birth weight
C. Maternal antisocial behavior
D. The father
E. None of the above

39. Case reports identify which of the following as a comorbid occurrence with gender identity disorder, one that might conceivably be linked by traits of behavioral rigidity and obsessionality?
    A. Schizophrenia
    B. Bipolar disorder
    C. Parent–child relational problem
    D. Pervasive developmental disorder, not otherwise specified
    E. Psychological factors affecting medical condition

40. The DSM-III classified conduct disorder by dividing it into four subgroups according to whether children were socialized or undersocialized, and aggressive or nonaggressive, but how does DSM-IV classify conduct disorder?
    A. By degree of legal involvement
    B. By degree of antisocial behaviors
    C. By age of onset
    D. By lack of remorse
    E. By degree of externalizing behaviors

41. True or False: The system-of-care model places the child and family at the center of the clinical process and as full partners at all levels of system planning.
    A. True
    B. False

42. True or False: The course of borderline personality disorder (BPD) is highly stable with symptoms persistent.
    A. True
    B. False

43. ALL of the following psychotropic medications have narrow therapeutic indices for clinical effectiveness, but significant adverse effects with toxicity EXCEPT:
    A. Lithium
    B. Oxcarbazepine
    C. Valproate
    D. Carbamazepine
    E. Nortriptyline

44. True or False: A forensic evaluation affords the opportunity for therapeutic treatment for those clients who may not necessarily have access to psychiatric services.
    A. True
    B. False

45. A method of coping that uses strategies that avoid confronting pain, such as avoidance, denial, and wishful thinking is known as:
    A. Active coping
    B. Accommodative coping
    C. Inhibited coping
    D. Passive coping
    E. None of the above

46. The President's New Freedom Commission on Mental Health Report (2003) presented six major goals for a transformed mental health system, including which of the following:
    A. Elimination of disparities in mental health care
    B. Privatization of Medicaid mental health services
    C. Reduction of the intrusion of technology to access mental health care
    D. Screening of high school students' mental health
    E. Increasing Americans' understanding of mental health's limited impact on overall health

47. In studies of 3-year olds and preschool aggression, what percentage displays little or no aggression?
    A. 92%
    B. 76%
    C. 53%
    D. 38%
    E. 28%

48. Epidemiological studies suggest the percentage of children suffering "extreme functional impairments" from psychiatric disorders is in what range?
    A. 0.5% to 0.75%
    B. 1% to 2%
    C. 3% to 6%
    D. 5% to 9%
    E. 10% to 14%

49. Which of the following statements describing the psychoanalytic concept of resistance in the therapeutic process is FALSE? It is a defense against:
    A. Affects
    B. Repression
    C. Undesirable self-representations
    D. Unwanted drive derivatives

50. True or False: IQ scores are predictive of academic abilities in school-aged children.
    A. True
    B. False

51. The DSM-IV includes ALL of the following categories EXCEPT:
    A. Disorder of verbal expression
    B. Disorder of written expression
    C. Learning disorder, not otherwise specified
    D. Mathematics disorder
    E. Reading disorder

52. Which of the following is the statistic of choice to describe the center of a distribution if data are normally distributed?
    A. Mean
    B. Median
    C. Mode
    D. None of the above

53. True or False: IQ is stable from infancy.
    A. True
    B. False

54. Approximately what fraction of individuals with posttraumatic stress disorder (PTSD) experience one or more comorbid lifetime diagnoses?
    A. Three-fourths
    B. Two-thirds
    C. One-third
    D. One-half
    E. One-fourth

55. Which of the following is true of the genetics of homosexuality?
    A. Monozygotic male twins have concordance rates between 22% and 30%
    B. Monozygotic female twins have concordance rates of 48%
    C. Dizygotic male twins have concordance rates between 52% and 66%
    D. Dizygotic female twins have concordance rates of 48%
    E. All of the above

56. Compared to healthy controls, the rates of psychological disorders in children with chronic medical illness are:
   A. Lower than children without a chronic medical illness
   B. The same as children without a chronic medical illness
   C. Two to four times the rate of children without a chronic medical illness
   D. Four to six times the rate of children without a chronic medical illness

57. Which of the following is the normal milestone for a child's ability to eat solid food?
   A. 2 months
   B. 4 months
   C. 6 months
   D. 8 months
   E. 12 months

58. Psychometric tests are based on their reliability and validity. What is the least acceptable score of the reliability coefficient generally recommended for diagnostic tests?
   A. 0.40
   B. 0.60
   C. 0.80
   D. 0.90
   E. 5.0

59. Typically, impairment resulting from psychopathology is assessed in four domains and includes each of the following EXCEPT:
   A. Interpersonal relationships
   B. Academic/work performance
   C. Social and leisure activities
   D. Family relationships
   E. Ability to enjoy and obtain satisfaction from life

60. Which of the following statements about serving snacks in a group is FALSE?
   A. It is a nurturing, tangible support
   B. Promotes more intimate, relaxed interactions that often help task accomplishment
   C. The food should be voted on by the group, with the leaders retaining veto power
   D. Dietary restrictions should be accommodated by the entire group whenever possible
   E. Protests about the snack selection should be understood as part of the group attempting to establish and maintain its trust in the group leadership

61. Which of the following statements is NOT a DSM-IV criterion for Asperger's disorder?
   A. Impairment in social interaction
   B. Restricted, repetitive and stereotyped patterns of behavior, interests, and activities
   C. Clinically significant general delay in language
   D. Lack of clinically significant cognitive delay
   E. Does not meet criteria for another specific pervasive developmental disorder

62. Studies by Hetherington and colleagues found that the long-term effects of divorce and remarriage appear to be related to a number of factors including ALL of the following EXCEPT:
   A. Child's development status
   B. Child's sex
   C. Child's temperament
   D. The degree of amicability in the divorce proceedings
   E. The availability of support systems

63. The world's first statute regarding adoption was passed in:
   A. Massachusetts 1851
   B. California 1943
   C. New York 1789
   D. Virginia 1865
   E. Kansas 1918

64. True or False: A personality disorder cannot be diagnosed in a child.
    A. True
    B. False

65. The proton magnetic resonance spectroscopy study conducted by Thomas and colleagues in children with schizophrenia showed which one of the following?
    A. The ratio of N-acetylaspartate (NAA) to creatine was significantly lower in the frontal lobes of children with schizophrenia
    B. The ratio of NAA to creatine was significantly lower in the parietal lobes of children with schizophrenia
    C. The ratio of NAA to creatine was significantly lower in the occipital lobes of children with schizophrenia
    D. The ratio of NAA to creatine was significantly higher in the occipital lobes of children with schizophrenia
    E. The ratio of NAA to creatine was equivocal in the occipital lobes of children with schizophrenia

66. Besides psychosocial dwarfism, other disorders involving short stature, include ALL of the following EXCEPT:
    A. Intrauterine growth retardation
    B. Hypopituitarism
    C. Turner's syndrome
    D. Fragile X syndrome
    E. The osteochondrodystrophies

67. Which TWO of the following are risk factors for Stevens–Johnson syndrome while on lamotrigine therapy?
    A. Acute discontinuation
    B. Rapid dose escalation
    C. Fluoxetine cotreatment
    D. Carbamazepine cotreatment
    E. Valproate cotreatment

68. In resilience research, what is the conceptual definition of vulnerability factors?
    A. The factors that propagate or produce the risk condition
    B. The factors that exacerbate the negative effects of the risk condition
    C. The factors that indicate the inherent weaknesses in the individual
    D. The factors that hinder positive adaptation in spite of the risk condition
    E. All of the above

69. True or False: The proportion of adolescents in poor and near-poor families without insurance decreased between 1995 and 2002.
    A. True
    B. False

70. True or False: Less than half of the National Institute of Mental Health funded intervention proposals and programs include a family component.
    A. True
    B. False

71. In the field of infant assessments, one of the most commonly used instruments following the Piagetian model is the Infant Psychological Development Scale, which assesses an infant's ability to perform ALL of the following EXCEPT:
    A. Grasp object permanence
    B. Understand means-ends
    C. Respond to social cues
    D. Understand cause–effect relationships
    E. Imitate vocalizations and gestures

72. In the treatment of ADHD with atomoxetine, doses above which amount are not likely to produce additional benefit?
    A. 0.6 mg/kg
    B. 0.8 mg/kg
    C. 1.0 mg/kg
    D. 1.2 mg/kg
    E. 1.4 mg/kg

73. Higher rates of suicide are found in both children and adults with epilepsy. Which epilepsy in adults accounts for the highest rate?
    A. Parietal lobe
    B. Frontal lobe
    C. Absence
    D. Rolandic
    E. Temporal lobe

74. True or False: Children with less language ability may exhibit greater levels of physical aggression than their more verbal peers.
    A. True
    B. False

75. Which TWO of the following organizations were formed specifically for the mission of education and training?
    A. Association for Academic Psychiatry
    B. American Association of Psychiatric Clinics for Children
    C. American Association of Directors of Psychiatric Residency Training
    D. American Academy of Child & Adolescent Psychiatry
    E. American Academy of Psychiatrics

76. A study by Richard Green of 66 feminine boys and 56 control boys examined sexual orientation in fantasy and behavior, initially at 7 years of age and again at 19 years of age. Which statement(s) capture(s) the findings?
    A. 75% to 80% of the previously feminine boys were bisexual or homosexual at follow up
    B. 0% to 4% of the control boys were bisexual or homosexual
    C. Of those available at follow up, only one youth at the age of 18 years was gender dysphoric to the extent of considering sex reassignment surgery
    D. All of the above

77. What are the most common compulsions in adolescents?
    A. Cleaning rituals
    B. Repeating actions (doing and undoing)
    C. Checking rituals
    D. None of the above
    E. All of the above

78. Hermine von Hug-Hellmuth was credited as the first to undertake psychoanalytic therapy of children and adolescents. What was the most significant observation she made regarding the therapy and the expression of unconscious conflict in children as compared with adults?
    A. That regression was a common component of the therapy
    B. That children require therapeutic aids in expression of unconscious conflict
    C. That spontaneous play could stand in the place of verbal communications
    D. That a working alliance with parents was essential for child improvement
    E. That free association unfolds in similar ways

79. True or False: In interviewing adolescents, clinicians can decrease resistance by beginning the history taking by inquiring first about the adolescent's interests, strengths, and musical preferences.
    A. True
    B. False

80. Which of the following types of therapy groups requires substantial cognitive growth and ability in its members, especially regarding emotionally charged topics?
    A. Social skills group
    B. Support group
    C. Didactic group
    D. Goal-focused group
    E. All of the above

81. True or False: When genes are expressed, for example, as in the transcription of growth hormone, they are expressed in all cell lineages that have the gene.
    A. True
    B. False

82. Which professional organization established in 1924 attempted to unify the disciplines of psychiatric diagnosis and child treatment by bringing together psychiatrists, psychologists, social workers, and the judiciary interested in child guidance?
    A. American Academy of Child & Adolescent Psychiatry
    B. American Board of Psychiatry and Neurology
    C. American Association of Psychiatric Clinics for Children
    D. American Orthopsychiatric Association

83. Angelman and Prader-Willi syndromes, disorders of genomic imprinting, share ALL of the following features EXCEPT:
    A. Both are rare disorders with a prevalence of 1 in 10,000 births
    B. Both are the result of deletions from maternally derived chromosomes
    C. Individuals with both disorders are hypotonic as infants
    D. Individuals with both disorders have some degree of mental retardation (MR)
    E. Both disorders are caused by a deletion on chromosome 15 or by receiving two copies of chromosome 15 from one parent

84. True or False: A psychoanalytic finding indicates that parental harshness appears to weaken the superego functions of the child.
    A. True
    B. False

85. Symptoms frequently reported in children with conversion disorder include ALL of the following EXCEPT:
    A. Nonepileptic seizures
    B. Paralysis or paresis
    C. Sensory symptoms
    D. Gait disturbances
    E. Auras

86. The possibility of which adverse event cautions against the abrupt discontinuation of clonidine?
    A. Seizures
    B. Orthostatic hypotension
    C. Rebound hypertension
    D. Withdrawal dyskinesia
    E. None of the above

87. A living donor transplant is possible for which organs?
    A. Kidney
    B. Lung
    C. Liver
    D. Heart
    E. A, B, and C

88. For the treatment of anorexia nervosa, the following form of psychotherapy has been proven most effective:
    A. CBT
    B. Dialectical-behavior therapy
    C. Psychodynamic psychotherapy
    D. Interpersonal psychotherapy (IPT)
    E. No specific psychotherapy approach has proven most effective

89. During the middle phase of IPT for depressed adolescents, the therapist teaches the adolescent-specific strategies that can help with interpersonal difficulties. One strategy is to facilitate discussion of painful feelings and to help the adolescent use emotional experiences to better understand the link between mood and relationships. What is this technique called?
    A. Communication analysis
    B. Behavior change techniques
    C. Encouragement of affect
    D. Role playing
    E. Interpersonal experiments

90. Why should the long-term use (greater than a month) of anticholinergic medications be avoided if possible in children?
    A. The risk of extrapyramidal symptoms
    B. The risk of widespread cavities
    C. The risk of an acute dystonic reaction
    D. The risk of tardive dyskinesia
    E. The risk of parkinsonian symptoms

91. Approximately how many children are forced into prostitution worldwide each year?
    A. 50,000
    B. 100,000
    C. 200,000
    D. 500,000
    E. 1 million

92. A therapeutic dose of a benzodiazepine can be detected in the urine for how long?
    A. Less than 24 hours
    B. 24 to 48 hours
    C. 3 days
    D. 5 to 7 days
    E. 1 week

93. Which is the type of neuronal receptor at which a neurotransmitter binds to a receptor protein, resulting in a change in the permeability of the associated ion channel in milliseconds, and the influx of ions such as Ca^{2+}, Na^+, K^+, or Cl^-?
    A. Ionotropic
    B. G-protein-coupled
    C. Serotonergic
    D. Glutamatergic
    E. Dopaminergic

94. Which of the following medications can increase serum lithium levels?
    A. Nonsteroidal anti-inflammatory drugs
    B. Caffeine
    C. Theophylline
    D. Tetracyclines
    E. A and D

95. Child abuse and neglect are MOST LIKELY associated with which of the following?
    A. Chronic alcohol abuse among caretakers
    B. Poverty
    C. Mental illness of the guardians
    D. Single parent families
    E. Immigration

96. True or False: For all tricyclic antidepressants, vital signs and electrocardiograms should be obtained when the maintenance dose has been achieved.
    A. True
    B. False

97. True or False: Persons with Asperger's disorder tend to have better verbal IQ than performance IQ, and persons with classic autistic disorder tend to have better performance IQ than verbal IQ.
    A. True
    B. False

98. Stierlin proposed which of following concepts to describe ways in which families negotiate a pathological separation to overcome fear of prolonged fusion?
    A. Triangulation, projective identification, and parentification
    B. Binding, delegating, and expulsion
    C. Prescribing the symptom, exceptional solution, and paradoxical intervention
    D. All of the above
    E. None of the above

99. What is a potentially fatal complication from chronic ipecac abuse?
    A. Liver failure
    B. Renal failure
    C. Cardiac failure
    D. Emphysema
    E. Osteoporosis

100. Which antipsychotic is unlikely to produce neurological side effects even at high doses?
    A. Risperidone
    B. Quetiapine
    C. Olanzapine
    D. Haldol
    E. Fluphenazine

101. Insecure attachment behaviors include ALL of the following EXCEPT:
    A. Disrupted play
    B. Preoccupation with the parent's presence
    C. Difficulty being comforted
    D. Monitoring and seeking proximity to the parent

102. True or False: It is best to withhold from a child her health status if her illness is serious and life limiting.
    A. True
    B. False

103. Which of these is a federal law that had a major impact on the emergence of in-home, community-based care?
    A. Tax Equity and Fiscal Responsibility Act of 1982
    B. The Adoption Assistance and Child Welfare Act of 1980
    C. The Omnibus Budget Reconciliation Act of 1987
    D. Aid to Dependent Families with Dependent Children
    E. State Children's Health Initiative Program

104. The usual domains assessed by adaptive behavior scales include ALL of the following EXCEPT:
    A. Independent living skills
    B. Processing speed skills
    C. Functional communication and academic skills
    D. Fine and gross motor skills
    E. Social behaviors

105. What percentage of child custody cases result in the need for expert testimony?
    A. 4% to 5%
    B. 6% to 10%
    C. 11% to 15%
    D. 16% to 20%
    E. 21% to 25%

106. Some psychotropic medications follow first-order (or linear) kinetics best described by which of the following statements?
    A. The amount of drug eliminated is variable regardless of plasma level
    B. The amount of drug eliminated per unit of time is fixed regardless of the plasma level
    C. The amount of drug eliminated is proportional to the CYP 450 system being utilized
    D. The amount of drug eliminated is proportional to its amount circulating in the bloodstream

107. Routine use of laboratory testing yields findings that alter the working diagnosis in a psychiatric evaluation in which percentage of cases?
    A. 15%
    B. 12%
    C. 5%
    D. 1%
    E. 0.5%

108. Stimulants are used in the treatment of narcolepsy. What other class of medication can be useful?
    A. Antipsychotic
    B. Tricyclic antidepressant
    C. SSRI
    D. Orexin activating
    E. B and D

109. Interviewer-based interviews have ALL the following theoretical and practical advantages EXCEPT:
    A. The meaning of the ratings is precisely known
    B. Provide opportunities to cross-check discrepant information
    C. Enable the use of efficient open-ended questioning strategies
    D. The person being interviewed decides the presence or absence of psychopathology
    E. Less prone to overdiagnosis on the basis of symptom reports

110. Who is the most common abuser of a child in Munchhausen syndrome by proxy?
    A. Father
    B. Coach
    C. Older sibling
    D. Biological mother
    E. Adoptive mother

111. The most effective treatment for stuttering is:
    A. CBT
    B. Pharmacological intervention
    C. Psychodynamic therapy
    D. Reducing stressful environmental triggers
    E. Speech therapy

112. Which of the following statistics would most likely be used for descriptive research?
    A. *T*-test
    B. Analysis of variance
    C. Correlation
    D. Multiple regression
    E. Histogram

113. The central features of the Response to Intervention model include ALL of the following EXCEPT:
    A. Classroom performance measures
    B. High-quality classroom instruction
    C. Monitoring of IQ every 3 years
    D. Research-based instruction and intervention
    E. Universal screening

114. How long can alcohol be detected in the urine?
    A. Less than 24 hours
    B. 24 to 48 hours
    C. 3 to 5 days
    D. 1 week

115. Which of the following medications has been associated with the greatest amount of weight gain?
    A. Fluoxetine
    B. Lithium
    C. Valproate
    D. Quetiapine
    E. Olanzapine

116. In children, milder forms of delirium may be mistaken for:
    A. Depression
    B. Regression
    C. Provocative behavior
    D. Part of the illness
    E. All of the above

117. The transactional ecological framework of development asserts that a child's behavior is the product of three reciprocal transactions: those between the child's characteristics (his or her genetic, biological, cognitive, social, and emotional competencies) interacting with the broader ecological context (the multiple levels of social organization including family, neighborhood, and child care) AND:
    A. The caregiving environment
    B. The age of onset of early education
    C. The development of sense of transactional agency
    D. The exposure to multiple environments outside the home

118. Which TWO options delineate the two main goals of IPT?
    A. Decrease social anxiety
    B. Improve self-esteem
    C. Increase social supports
    D. Decrease depressive symptoms
    E. Improve social functioning with significant relationships

119. True or False: Neuropsychological studies of childhood onset schizophrenia have revealed deficits in attentional capacities and the processing of information.
    A. True
    B. False

120. The prevalence of intellectual disability in the general population is 1%. What percentage of individuals with intellectual disability have epilepsy?
    A. 3%
    B. 5%
    C. 10%
    D. 20% to 40%
    E. 50%

121. Which of the following questions might a child ask during a disaster, according to Vogel and Vernberg?
    A. "Is Earth a safe place?"
    B. "Is this happening to me?"
    C. "Is God upset at me?"
    D. "Is this grandma's fault?"
    E. "Is this real or a dream?"

122. Most persons with MR in childhood are those with
    A. Mild MR
    B. Moderate MR
    C. Severe MR
    D. Profound MR

123. Which of the following has a key role in the formation of memories?
   A. Extracellular-signal-related kinase
   B. Brain-derived neurotrophic factor
   C. Cyclic adenosine monophosphate
   D. Inositol

124. True or False: Soft neurological signs are nonfocal motor deficits.
   A. True
   B. False

125. Which of the following psychoanalytic concepts refers to the mental function that encompasses all the capacities of the mind to manage and channel the arousal and activity incited by the drives?
   A. Id
   B. Ego
   C. Superego
   D. Preconscious
   E. Censor

126. Which of the following is a manualized, cognitive-behavioral treatment for anxiety disorders in children and adolescents and has empirical support through randomized controlled trials?
   A. Kendall's the "Coping Cat"
   B. Frederick's the "Shy Lion"
   C. Johnson's "Captain Conquer"
   D. Thompson's "Where Did the Cowboys Go?"
   E. Tuttle's "C'mon, Get Over It"

127. True or False: If an adolescent has suicidal thinking and a plan, the indication is to admit him or her to an inpatient psychiatric unit.
   A. True
   B. False

128. True or False: Studies have unequivocally demonstrated that children with cancer suffer significantly from abnormal psychosocial functioning and emotional and behavioral problems.
   A. True
   B. False

129. Delayed onset PTSD can be diagnosed if symptoms emerge after what period from the traumatic event?
   A. 1 month
   B. 3 months
   C. 6 months
   D. 9 months
   E. 1 year

130. Research utilizing Mary Main's Adult Attachment Inventory has indicated how the father's role can have an effect on family formation in the setting of the mother's negative experience with her own parents. What is this effect?
   A. Destructive
   B. Ameliorative
   C. None
   D. Malign

131. Which of the following choices describes a major difference between DSM-IV and International Classification of Disease (ICD)-10?
   A. DSM-IV is intended to be useful for both clinical work and research, whereas ICD-10 provides separate clinical and research descriptions
   B. DSM-IV provides separate clinical and research descriptions, whereas ICD-10 is useful for both clinical work and research
   C. DSM-IV and ICD-10 are both intended for clinical purposes but have been co-opted for research
   D. DSM-IV and ICD-10 are both intended for research but have been co-opted for clinical purposes

132. What is a normative psychological task of adolescence?
   A. Identity consolidation
   B. Developing a satisfactory and realistic body image
   C. Developing increased independence from parents and adequate capacities for self-care
   D. Developing appropriate control and expression of increased sexual and aggressive drives
   E. All of the above

133. What percentage of children in the United States will grow up living with only one parent?
   A. 20%
   B. 33%
   C. 50%
   D. 75%
   E. 10%

For questions 134–136, match the type of preventive intervention with its proper description.

134. Indicated preventive intervention

135. Selective preventive intervention

136. Universal preventive intervention
   A. Targeted to individuals whose risk of developing mental disorders are significantly higher than average
   B. Targeted to individuals who are identified as having minimal but detectable signs or symptoms foreshadowing mental disorder, but who do not meet standard diagnostic criteria that define a mental disorder
   C. Targeted to the general public or a whole population group that has not been identified on the basis of individual risk

137. Enuretic events occur during which part of the night or sleep cycle?
   A. During deep sleep (stages 3 or 4)
   B. The first third of the night
   C. The last third of the night
   D. During rapid eye movement sleep
   E. In each stage of sleep

138. True or False: Children under 10 years of age require larger, weight-adjusted doses of most hepatically metabolized medications than do adults to achieve comparable blood levels and therapeutic effects.
   A. True
   B. False

139. Which of the following statements about autistic disorder is TRUE?
   A. Children with autism are overly concerned with the nonsocial environment
   B. Children with autistic disorder enjoy being social
   C. Parents of children with autism have unusually high levels of education
   D. Autistic disorder does not have any associated medical disorders
   E. Children with autism have average intelligence

140. When was the *International Classification of Causes of Death*, the publication presently known as the ICD, adopted by the International Statistical Institute?
   A. 1649
   B. 1764
   C. 1811
   D. 1893
   E. 1930

141. The term *non nil null hypothesis* is best described by what statement?
   A. The mean of the population of those who receive the intervention is equal to the mean of the population of those who do not
   B. To reject the null hypothesis, the treatment group would have to exceed the control group by an amount necessary to make a functional difference
   C. The mean of the population of those who receive the intervention is less than the mean of the population of those who do not
   D. To accept the null hypothesis, the treatment group would have to *not* significantly differ from the control group
   E. None of the above

142. Diffusion tensor imaging tractography allows the study of which of the following?
   A. The degree of directional dependence of water diffusion in the brain
   B. Ellipsoid geometrical representations of the diffusional properties of water at a given voxel in the brain
   C. The orientation of an ellipsoid's longest axis representing the local orientation of brain fibers
   D. The connectivity of white matter in the brain by reconstructing the pathways of nerve fiber bundles based on the principal direction of water diffusion
   E. None of the above

143. Cohen's *d* is a common metric used to assess the effect size of clinical intervention studies that indicates the difference in outcome between the control and intervention samples. Conventionally, which two numbers indicate a small and large effect size, or *d*?
   A. 1.2 and 0.6
   B. 0.6 and 1.2
   C. 50 and 100
   D. 0 and 1
   E. 0.2 and 0.8

144. Which of the following parenting styles leads to the best outcome in children's academic and social performance?
   A. Low responsivity and low demandingness
   B. High responsivity and low demandingness
   C. High responsivity and high demandingness
   D. Low responsivity and high demandingness

145. In the Four Ps model of psychiatric formulation, which domain of factors is concerned with the features that identify current symptoms, the diagnostic reasoning about the role of inciting events, and possible concurrent illness?
   A. Predisposing
   B. Precipitating
   C. Perpetuating
   D. Protective

146. Cytogenetic methods for gene studies include ALL of the following, EXCEPT:
   A. Karyotyping
   B. Linkage analysis
   C. Fluorescence *in situ* hybridization
   D. Microarray comparative genomic hybridization

147. Children with which disorder are thought to be at increased risk for having epilepsy?
   A. ADHD
   B. Anorexia nervosa
   C. Oppositional defiant disorder
   D. Generalized anxiety disorder

148. Which of the following large studies showed the superiority of CBT over SSRI alone for the treatment of pediatric OCD?
    A. Pediatric Obsessive–Compulsive Disorder Treatment Study
    B. Multimodal Treatment Study of Children with ADHD
    C. Treatment for Adolescents with Depression Study
    D. Child/Anxiety Multimodal Treatment Study
    E. Research Unit on Pediatric Psychopharmacology

149. The early embryonic development of the nervous system is characterized, in part, by the migration of populations of neurons. In the case of corticogenesis, development depends in part on:
    A. Radial glial cells
    B. Astrocytes
    C. Ependymal cells
    D. Oligodendrocytes
    E. Schwann cells

150. In a natural history study by Skoog and Skoog of 251 adult patients with OCD followed over 30 years, what was the most common course of the disorder?
    A. Episodic course (one episode lasting less than 5 years)
    B. Chronic illness (continuous, unremitting severity lasting over 5 years)
    C. Intermittent illness (periods of OCD interspersed with completely symptom-free periods)
    D. Deteriorating course

151. Which of the following is the best description of the psychodynamic concept of internalization?
    A. The process by which experiences with the external world, primarily in relationships, form stable intrapsychic structures or capacities
    B. The attribution of internal conflicts to the external environment and a search for external solutions
    C. The ability to take account of one's own and others' mental states in understanding why people behave in specific ways
    D. The unconscious displacement onto the therapist of patterns of feelings, thoughts, and behaviors originally experienced in relation to significant figures during childhood

152. What are the major concepts of death as viewed from a child developmental perspective?
    A. Irreversibility, finality, causality, and inevitability
    B. Beginnings, transitions, and endings
    C. Denial, bargaining, anger, guilt, and acceptance
    D. Corporeality, ethereality, and transcendence

153. Which of the following is the most well validated and widely disseminated treatment for childhood PTSD?
    A. Dialectical-behavior therapy
    B. Mentalization-based treatment
    C. Parent–child therapy
    D. Trauma-focused CBT
    E. Habit reversal training

154. The blockade of which part of the dopaminergic neuron is a significant mechanism of action of stimulant drugs, such as amphetamine and cocaine?
    A. D1 receptor
    B. D2 receptor
    C. Dopamine transporter
    D. Monoamine oxidase
    E. D3 receptor

155. True or False: Stimulants have no impact on aggressive symptoms in youth with ADHD.
    A. True
    B. False

156. When is the peak time for violence, crime, and sexual activity for adolescents?
    A. Midnight to 1 a.m.
    B. 10 p.m. to midnight
    C. 7 p.m. to 10 p.m.
    D. 3 p.m. to 6 p.m.

157. What are two clinician-based rating scales for the assessment of manic symptoms and their severity in youth?
    A. Young Mania Rating Scale
    B. The Mood Disorder Questionnaire
    C. Kiddie-Schedule for Affective Disorders and Schizophrenia Mania Rating Scale
    D. A and B
    E. A and C

158. The International Algorithm Project put forth a simple method for ranking available treatments according to their level of empirical support. Medications with good empirical support, based on consistently positive results in randomized control trials would receive what classification?
    A. Class A
    B. Class B
    C. Class C
    D. None of the above

159. A presenting complaint and reason for referral may be described quite differently, depending on the informant. These discrepancies are referred to as:
    A. Parental discordance
    B. Informant variance
    C. Splitting
    D. Projection
    E. Wishful thinking

160. True or False: Principle I of the Nuremberg Code contains the definition of consent from which the medical definition of informed consent is derived.
    A. True
    B. False

161. All of the following statements are accurate regarding automatic thoughts EXCEPT:
    A. They are defined as cognitions that stream rapidly through an individual's mind
    B. Individuals typically do not question them for believability
    C. They are typically delusional
    D. They may be valid worries
    E. They occur with increased intensity and frequency in disorders such as anxiety, depression, and OCD

162. Which of the following developments contributed to the increased interest in social policy among mental health professionals?
    A. Implementation of federally sponsored social programs such as Project Head Start
    B. The inception of an additional postgraduate year in many residency programs devoted to the study of mental health and social policy
    C. Securing funding for research often requires the demonstration of the practical application of findings and their potential to address societal needs
    D. The greater reimbursement provided for psychiatrists with social policy credentials
    E. A and C

163. True or False: Girls' levels of satisfaction with their body and physical appearance increase as they pass through adolescence.
    A. True
    B. False

164. Which of the following is CORRECT regarding medicines that could be used to address specific symptoms secondary to a disaster?
    A. SSRIs–PTSD
    B. Atypical antipsychotics—aggression
    C. Mood stabilizers —affective dysregulation
    D. Alpha adrenergic agents—impulsivity
    E. All of the above

165. True or False: The newly emerging literature on Pediatric Autoimmune Neuropsychiatric Disorders Associated with Streptococcal Infections (PANDAS) has been increasingly supportive of the association between streptococcal infection and OCD.
    A. True
    B. False

166. The modern era of community-based systems of care for children was ushered in by the publication of:
    A. George W. Bush's Executive Order for Faith-Based and Community Initiatives
    B. Jane Knitzer's "Unclaimed Children"
    C. The National Institute of Mental Health's statistics on the lack of such services
    D. George Orwell's "Animal Farm"

167. True or False: The majority of children with cancer want to know everything about their disease.
    A. True
    B. False

168. Statistics from community samples reveal roughly what percentage of male children interested in playing with fire?
    A. 5%
    B. 15%
    C. 25%
    D. 60%
    E. 80%

In the following questions, match the appropriate phrase to the neuroimaging term.

169. Pixel

170. Voxel

171. Resolution

172. Signal-to-noise ratio

173. Partial volume effect

174. Tesla (T)

175. Field of view

176. Contrast
    A. The height and width of the two-dimensional slice of brain tissue being imaged
    B. A useful index of image quality
    C. A basic unit of a two-dimensional digital image called a picture element
    D. The size of the voxels from which a radio signal is being measured
    E. The difference in the strength of signal acquired from adjacent tissues
    F. A three-dimensional cube of tissue in the brain called a volume element
    G. A unit of measurement that represents the number of magnetized water molecules within a specific volume of tissue
    H. When a signal from two differing structures included in the same voxel are averaged into a single signal

177. True or False: Language acquisition, including vocabulary and the fundamentals of linguistic semantics, occurs even with very little environmental support.
    A. True
    B. False

178. Clinicians are susceptible to a number of collection biases in the process of interviewing and diagnosing a patient. Which of the following biases is the definition of an illusory correlation?
    A. Arriving at a diagnostic determination before collecting all the relevant information
    B. Focusing on collecting information to confirm a diagnosis
    C. Making judgments based on the most readily available cognitive patterns
    D. Seeing correlations where none exist
    E. Ignoring disconfirming information

179. Which of the following terms best refers to the consistency of measurement of a test, or the degree to which test scores are free from random fluctuations of measurement?
    A. Validity
    B. Correlation
    C. Regression
    D. Standardization
    E. Reliability

180. Siblings of persons with autism:
    A. Are more likely to be affected with autism themselves
    B. Are less likely to have offspring who have autism
    C. Are at lower risk for cognitive problems
    D. Are at lower risk for language problems
    E. Are likely to have Asperger's disorder at twice the rate of the general population

181. In addition to the core constructs of warmth and control that are integral to "good parenting," which TWO other constructs are critical for resilient adaptation?
    A. Attachment
    B. Limit setting
    C. Communication
    D. Monitoring
    E. Consequences

182. Approximately what percentage of child patients newly diagnosed with epilepsy will go on to have intractable epilepsy?
    A. 1%
    B. 5%
    C. 10%
    D. 15%
    E. 20%

183. ALL of the following seems to distinguish those youths with major depressive disorder who have suicidal behavior from those with major depressive disorder alone, EXCEPT:
    A. Severity of depressed mood
    B. Intensity of negative self-evaluation
    C. Increased levels of hopelessness
    D. IQ
    E. Anhedonia

184. True or False: A mental health professional should know how to diagnose reactive attachment disorder based on the Strange Situation paradigm.
    A. True
    B. False

185. Studies have shown an inverse relationship between adult borderline personality disorder and:
    A. Education
    B. Income
    C. Bipolar disorder
    D. Security of attachment
    E. Cyclothymia

186. A shared criterion for all tic disorders, with the exception of tic disorder not otherwise specified, per DSM-IV classification is:
    A. Onset before age 18 years
    B. Multiple motor and vocal tics have been present during the illness
    C. Tics occur multiple times a day for at least 4 weeks but less than 12 months
    D. The first tics appeared before the age of 7
    E. Only motor or vocal tics have been present but not both

187. At a nascent cognitive level what is the definition of gender identity?
    A. A child's recognition that he or she is a member of one sex but not the other
    B. A child's awareness that he or she has genitalia
    C. A child's awareness that, generally, mothers and fathers behave differently
    D. A child's awareness that there is the "other sex"

188. The effects of parental conflict on the psychological well-being of children are mediated by what factor more than the parental conflict itself?
    A. The witnessing of reconciliation after the conflict
    B. The overall quality of the parent–child relationship
    C. The presence of a strong extrafamilial support network
    D. The practice of parents sharing the reasons for the conflict

189. It appears that depression and which other disorder are influenced by the same genetic factor?
    A. Social anxiety disorder
    B. Borderline personality disorder
    C. Generalized anxiety disorder
    D. Schizophreniform disorder
    E. None of the above

190. ALL of the following traits in patients with ADHD predict a greater probability of failure to diagnose and treat the disorder EXCEPT:
    A. Minority status
    B. Legal difficulties
    C. Female sex
    D. Low income

191. Which of the following models of classification views disorders as either present or absent?
    A. Dimensional
    B. Categorical
    C. Ideographic
    D. Archetypal

192. True or False: In the clinical assessment of infants, it is sufficient to provide results in the dichotomous categories of developmental delay or adequate age.
    A. True
    B. False

193. Heightened psychopathology in persons with MR has been linked to ALL of the following biological problems EXCEPT:
    A. Abnormal neurological functioning
    B. Biochemical anomalies associated with unusual behaviors such as self-injury
    C. High rates of sensory or motor impairments
    D. Increased rates of seizure disorder
    E. Increased susceptibility of addiction to substances

194. Which of the following is FALSE regarding MR and epilepsy in children in poor countries?
    A. Prevalence rates in developing countries is estimated to be in the range of 8 to 12 per 1,000 for children ages 3 to 10 years
    B. MR and epilepsy are the most common mental disorders in India
    C. Cerebral palsy and postnatal causes of MR are more common in developing countries than in developed countries
    D. The cost of medication to treat epilepsy is relatively low but access to care is limited
    E. The death rates for children in the community with mild MR is higher than the general population

195. Researchers and clinicians use which of the following tests to assess children's overall symptom levels on different maladjustment domains?
    A. Kiddie-Schedule for Affective Disorders and Schizophrenia
    B. Child Behavior Checklist
    C. Diagnostic Interview Schedule for Children—IV
    D. Behavior Assessment System for Children
    E. B and D

196. In transdisciplinary teams, where team members engage in a collaborative approach to assessments, what is the name of the term that describes the sharing of information and team members helping each other perform activities traditionally reserved within disciplines?
    A. Autonomy
    B. Role release
    C. Collaborative problem solving
    D. Cognitive collaborating
    E. Multidisciplinary collaborations

197. True or False: Lithium can be expected to have a lower plasma concentration in a child compared with an equivalent mg/kg dose in adults.
    A. True
    B. False

198. Over the last decade, which of the following has seen increased use by adolescents?
    A. Marijuana
    B. Steroids
    C. Prescription opiates
    D. Gamma-hydroxybutyrate
    E. Ecstasy

199. What is a side effect with desmopressin acetate?
    A. Mania
    B. Hyponatremia
    C. Gastrointestinal bleeding
    D. Enuresis
    E. Constipation

200. Gender identity is primarily determined through which of the following?
    A. Protein expression
    B. Heredity
    C. Sex hormones
    D. Socialization
    E. None of the above

Test Three

Answers

1. **Answer: D.** Prolactin elevation is not found. The other answers have been associated to varying degrees. Page 922.

2. **Answer: C.** However, signs of lithium toxicity can also occur at normal serum levels. Page 769.

3. **Answer: A.** This practice occurs by convention. Page 128.

4. **Answer: A.** Refer to Table 4.2.6.2. Page 378.

5. **Answer: A.** Childhood onset schizophrenia is a severe and pervasive condition with a nonepisodic and unremitting course. Page 494.

6. **Answer: D.** The Vineland is an example of a parent report questionnaire. This question's primary purpose is to make the reader aware of the variety of commonly used language test batteries that assess a child's communication abilities. Page 374.

7. **Answer: E.** When children with autism spectrum disorders begin talking, aspects of language form, including phonology, syntax, and morphology are relatively spared. These children generally show skills in language form that are at or close to those of mental-age mates. The other answers reflect common characteristics of language in autism. Page 422.

8. **Answer: A.** Such characteristics could help identify those individuals who would most likely benefit from selective preventive interventions. Page 175.

9. **Answer: B.** Page 522.

10. **Answer: A.** Page 815.

11. **Answer: E.** The definition of pica is the persistent eating of nonnutritive substances for at least a month in a manner that such eating is inappropriate to the developmental level and is not part of culturally sanctioned practice, so all of the answer options could be included. Page 584.

12. **Answer: D.** Genetic defects are the most common causes of permanent sensorineural hearing loss followed by complications of severe prematurity and intrauterine and postnatal infection. Pages 66–67.

13. **Answer: C.** Page 806.

14. **Answer: C.** This act replaced Aid to Families with Dependent Children with Temporary Assistance to Needy Families. Page 37.

15. **Answer: A.** A more favorable assessment of cognitive and social capacities occurs when the child uses gaze direction. Page 76.

16. **Answer: B.** Despite the shorter half-life of paroxetine in children, the investigators of the study still recommended once-daily dosing of the medication. Page 763.

17. **Answer: C.** This answer was one of the notable findings of the Treatment for Adolescents with Depression Study. Page 505.

18. **Answer: E.** A general mood of unhappiness or depression is also included. One or more of the conditions should be present to a marked degree for a long time and adversely affect educational performance. Page 987.

19. **Answer: D.** The field of developmental behavioral pediatrics emerged as the needs of pediatric patients changed. It is intended to enhance the capacity of pediatricians to identify, manage, and when necessary, refer children with behavioral and developmental concerns. Developmental behavioral pediatrics fellowships after pediatric residency are of 3 years' duration. Page 922.

20. **Answer: A.** Page 654.

21. **Answer: E.** Preschool children depend on routine and ritual to soothe their worries and to make the world seem less scary. At the same time, their imaginations are growing, and scary thoughts are often much scarier than reality. Because preschoolers have a simultaneous sense of power and helplessness, with the concurrent difficulty in distinguishing between fantasy and reality, they often have the concern that by thinking a scary thought, the thought will come true. Page 265.

22. **Answer: B.** Page 457.

23. **Answer: A.** The problem is transient and not serious. A benzodiazepine can be tried if a child is too embarrassed to sleep at a friend's house or becomes inhibited by usual daytime activities. If the problem persists into adolescence, a neurological evaluation is warranted to rule out sleep-related seizures. Page 629.

24. **Answer: A.** Freud described middle childhood as a period of latency, or sexual dormancy, although later theorists determined that school-aged children are not, actually, sexually "dormant." The superego develops before middle childhood, during the oedipal phase. Erikson's stage of industry versus inferiority also describes middle childhood. Page 267.

25. **Answer: D.** There are many types of effect size indices, including *d* effect size, *r*, the odds ratio, risk ratio, and number needed to treat. Page 118.

26. **Answer: A.** Page 567.

27. **Answer: A.** Neuronal firing, neurotransmitter release and uptake, and metabolic rates also resemble patterns of waking. Page 625.

28. **Answer: A.** She also discovered turning passive to active, denial, intellectualization, displacement, and altruistic surrender. Page 829.

29. **Answer: A.** The usual dosage range is 10 to 40 mg daily. Please note that paroxetine is not the preferred first line agent in children and adolescents, because it seems to have a higher rate for the emergence of suicidal thinking than other agents. Page 763.

30. **Answer: B.** This qualitative shift has profound impact on reciprocal communication and familial belonging. Page 257.

31. **Answer: A.** A historical fact that warrants mentioning. Page 147.

32. **Answer: B.** Page 764.

33. **Answer: E.** At lower doses (less than 150 mg daily), venlafaxine inhibits only serotonin reuptake. Page 766.

34. **Answer: E.** Page 432.

35. **Answer: D.** At times single cohorts are available, but the measurement of the exposure of each subject will allow the construction of two or several cohorts according to exposure levels. Page 152.

36. **Answer: B.** Children involved in the child protective service are two to three times more likely to be prescribed psychotropic medication than children in the community. Page 698.

37. **Answer: C.** Areas of the cortex, especially the motor strip have been implicated in connection with the corticostriatal thalamocortical track, which includes the basal ganglia as a way station. The globus pallidus is part of the basal ganglia. Page 574.

38. **Answer: C.** Maternal antisocial behavior is associated with smoking during pregnancy and, quite separately, with risk of child behavioral problems. Thus, the association between prenatal maternal smoking and later child behavioral problems could be accounted for entirely by the confounding effects of maternal antisocial behavior. Page 155.

39. **Answer: D.** Page 673.

40. **Answer: C.** By childhood or adolescent type, depending on whether there were symptoms prior to the age of 10 years. Page 455.

41. **Answer: A.** Family driven care is a cornerstone of the system-of-care approach. Page 891.

42. **Answer: B.** Findings are inconsistent, although, overall, the course of borderline personality disorder is considered less entrenched than it was historically. Page 687.

43. **Answer: B.** Page 744.

44. **Answer: B.** Forensic evaluations are only intended to help the court find the truth in a given situation and to address the legal question at hand. Whenever possible, forensic evaluations should be separated from treatment. Page 20.

45. **Answer: D.** Accommodative coping—accepting and adjusting to pain by regulating attention and thought patterns—is associated with lower levels of pain, somatic complaints, and emotional distress for those with chronic pain. Passive coping is associated with more distress. Page 638.

46. **Answer: A.** Page 895

47. **Answer: E.** This question is meant to highlight how normative physical aggression among 3-year olds is, but that this behavior diminishes upon school entry and through the elementary school years. Page 468.

48. **Answer: D.** Moreover, up to 10% to 20% have diagnosable disorders. Page 23.

49. **Answer: B.** Page 831.

50. **Answer: A.** Page 363.

51. **Answer: A.** The Diagnostic and Statistical Manual of Mental Disorders (DSM-IV) classifies types of learning disorders by referencing the primary academic areas of difficulty. The classification includes reading disorder, mathematics disorder, disorder of written expression, and learning disorder not otherwise specified. Page 411.

52. **Answer: A.** Page 106.

53. **Answer: B.** Although this belief was well rooted during the earlier decades of the 20th century, it has been discredited and infant intelligence quotient (IQ) tests are presently not used. Page 310.

54. **Answer: A.** Page 705.

55. **Answer: B.** Several studies have shown monozygotic male twins to have concordance rates between 52% and 66% and female twins 48%. For dizygotic male twins the concordance rates have been shown to be 22% to 30% and for female twins it is 16%. Page 83.

56. **Answer: C.** It varies by chronic medical illness. Page 912.

57. **Answer: C.** Page 371.

58. **Answer: D.** For screening tests, the reliability coefficient should be at least 0.80. Page 315.

59. **Answer: D.** The importance of including impairment in case definition has been well presented, because the prevalence of psychiatric disorders on the basis of symptoms alone reaches 50% but is under 20% if impairment is included in case definition. (Conversely, however, there are a number of impaired children who fall below specified cutoffs for diagnosis.) Page 162.

60. **Answer: C.** Page 845.

61. **Answer: C.** Page 394.

62. **Answer: D.** The quality of the home environment also plays a factor, but the amicability of the divorce is not specifically included in the study's findings. Page 39.

63. **Answer: A.** Page 1013.

64. **Answer: B.** However, the pattern of a personality disorder should be stable and of long duration. This criterion, along with the fluid developmental processes of children, makes the diagnosis difficult. Some authors argue that the diagnosis is warranted regardless of a child's age when patterns of perceiving reality and thinking about oneself and the environment become inflexible, maladaptive, chronic, cause subjective distress, and cause significant impairment. A diagnosis also allows for early intervention. Page 681.

65. **Answer: A.** Thomas and colleagues conducted a proton magnetic resonance spectroscopy study of children with schizophrenia and healthy children in which they found that the ratio of N-acetylaspartate to creatine was significantly lower in the frontal lobes of children with schizophrenia. Page 499.

66. **Answer: D.** Other disorders involving short stature include primary dwarfism, intra-uterine growth retardation with persistent small size, hypopituitarism from a variety of etiologies, Turner's syndrome (XO chromosomal pattern), osteochondrodystrophies, constitutionally delayed growth, and growth stunting secondary to chronic malnutrition with or without chronic disease. Fragile X is not associated with short stature. Page 590.

67. **Answer: B and E.** These risk factors are especially true for children. Page 772.

68. **Answer: B.** Vulnerability and protective factors modify the negative effects of adverse life events; the former factor worsens those effects. Page 293.

69. **Answer: A.** Page 52.

70. **Answer: B.** As parent involvement has been shown to enhance engagement in treatment, retention, and treatment outcome, the National Institute of Mental Health has encouraged the use of family interventions in investigative projects; more than half of National Institute of Mental Health funded intervention proposals and programs include a family component. Page 854.

71. **Answer: C.** Another ability the scale assesses is the manipulation of objects in space. The Brazelton Neonatal Behavioral Assessment Scale assesses social responsiveness. Page 318.

72. **Answer: D.** The total daily dose of atomoxetine usually falls between 0.8 and 1.2 mg/kg. Page 766.

73. **Answer: E.** In one retrospective chart review of children with suicide attempts, those with epilepsy had a rate 15 times that of the general population. Page 967.

74. **Answer: A.** Children with fewer words may have no other means to express their needs and frustrations. Page 265.

75. **Answer: A and C.** The American Association of Psychiatric Clinics for Children was formed in 1946 but not solely for education and training. Rather, the recently formed organizations of the American Association of Directors of Psychiatric Residency Training and the Association for Academic Psychiatry have this specific purview. Page 23.

76. **Answer: D.** Note that gender identity disorder was not assessed in this study. Page 676.

77. **Answer: E.** The answer options are listed in descending order of frequency from A to D. In adults, the most common compulsions are checking and cleaning. Page 550.

78. **Answer: C.** Furthermore, von Hug-Hellmuth observed that fully conscious analytic understanding of unconscious conflicts was not a prerequisite for therapeutic effect in children. Pages 826–827.

79. **Answer: A.** This is an important clinical point worth knowing, as adolescents are sensitive to feeling judged as vulnerable, "weird" or "different" which can occur with an exclusive focus on "problems." At the same time, the adolescent knows they are there for "a problem" and not mentioning the purpose can appear odd. Introducing the purpose of the visit, but focusing on more neutral, pleasant topics at first may be the right balance. Page 338.

80. **Answer: C.** Page 843.

81. **Answer: B.** Genes remain quiescent in some cell lineages or are repressed after a period of activity. This repression occurs via several mechanisms. Page 180.

82. **Answer: D.** The American Association of Psychiatric Clinics for Children grew out of the American Orthopsychiatric Association and was established in 1945, eventually issuing guidelines for training in child psychiatry. The American Academy of Child Psychiatry was founded in 1953 and was the first group to limit its membership to child psychiatrists only. Page 12.

83. **Answer: B.** The deletion on chromosome 15 (15q11-15q13) derives from the father in most cases of Prader-Willi syndrome and from the mother in most individuals with Angelman syndrome. This phenomenon is a classic example of genomic imprinting. Pages 205–206.

84. **Answer: A.** When a parent inflicts punishment that hurts the child, the child's focus is promoted on the external struggle with the parent and the child is distracted from the internal struggle with shame, guilt, or remorse. Page 830.

85. **Answer: E.** Page 634.

86. **Answer: C.** Page 781.

87. **Answer: E.** Lung transplant is unique in that two donors are necessary. Living donors may be biologically related, emotionally connected but not related, or unrelated and anonymous. Potential donors undergo a comprehensive psychological evaluation to ensure full autonomy, informed consent, and the absence of coercion. Page 943.

88. **Answer: E.** The Cochrane review of six small outpatient psychotherapy trials concluded that no specific psychotherapy approach can be recommended. Page 598.

89. **Answer: C.** All the choices listed are various therapeutic strategies employed in interpersonal psychotherapy for depressed adolescents. Page 823.

90. **Answer: B.** Anticholinergic medications decrease secretions, which can cause a Sjogren-like iatrogenic syndrome, which can lead to widespread cavities. Page 779.

91. **Answer: E.** Approximately 1 million children are forced into prostitution worldwide each year. Page 89.

92. **Answer: C.** Page 619.

93. **Answer: A.** These are also called class I receptors. Page 236.

94. **Answer: E.** Nonsteroidal anti-inflammatory drugs and tetracyclines can decrease urinary clearance of lithium. Page 769.

95. **Answer: B.** Child abuse can and does occur across all socioeconomic classes, but is most prevalent among the poor. Families earning $15,000 or less per year are 22 times more likely to abuse or neglect their children than families with annual incomes of $30,000 or more. Page 693.

96. **Answer: A.** Vital signs and electrocardiograms should be obtained prior to treatment and after dose adjustments. Page 764.

97. **Answer: A.** Page 389.

98. **Answer: B.** In the binding mode, the excessive binding of the family to the adolescent can force the growing adolescent into psychotic or suicidal behavior to free himself or herself from the family unit. In the delegating mode, the family allows the adolescent to depart from the family unit with attenuated supervision and connection to return periodically to share the tales of his or her exploits to compensate for the restricted life of the parents. In the expulsion mode, the adolescent is rejected by and extruded from the family to free him or her from the family unit. Page 858.

99. **Answer: C.** Cardiac failure may be caused by cardiomyopathy from ipecac abuse. Page 595.

100. **Answer: B.** Due to quetiapine's relatively low affinity for D2 receptors, it does not show the dose threshold effect resulting in neurological side effects observed with risperidone, olanzapine, and the first-generation agents. Page 774.

101. **Answer: D.** The answer is characteristic of a secure attachment. Page 254.

102. **Answer: B.** It is best to inform children honestly about their health status, doing so in a conversation over time, initially being sure to convey that they have a serious illness. Adults may initially voice discomfort when children acknowledge awareness of their own illness. Children perceive this discomfort and in turn join in a mutual pretense that they are unaware of the seriousness of their condition, often in an attempt to provide support to their parents. Children may fear the process of dying as much as death itself. Without the possibility of communicating their worries, they are left without possible supports. Younger children fear separation from parents rather than death per se. Page 976.

103. **Answer: B.** The rising number of children without permanent placement in foster care led to Public Law 96-272 and brought new focus and resources to home- and family-based intervention programs. The other answer options are real but do not apply. Page 880.

104. **Answer: B.** Page 367.

105. **Answer: A.** The majority of child custody cases do not reach the trial stage requiring expert testimony. Page 1008.

106. **Answer: D.** Page 743.

107. **Answer: D.** This question emphasizes the low yield of routine laboratory testing; however, laboratory evaluation is warranted when the history or physical findings suggest a particular medical diagnosis or as part of medication monitoring. Page 341.

108. **Answer: E.** Tricyclics, such as clomipramine, can be used to treat the cataplexy of narcolepsy. Modafinil, which activates orexin-containing neurons, can be used in lieu of stimulants. Monoamine oxidase inhibitors have also been used. Page 630.

109. **Answer: D.** The excepted option is the primary tenet of the respondent-based interview. Page 352.

110. **Answer: D.** In one review, the perpetrator was the mother in every case (98% biological mother and 2% adoptive mother). In another review, fathers were the perpetrators in 6.7% of cases. Page 720.

111. **Answer: E.** In general, speech therapy is used both to shape fluent speech and help the patient to stutter with less tension, avoidance, and interruption of the flow of communication. Stress or anxiety is not thought to play a role in the etiology. Neither anti-anxiety medication nor psychotherapy has been shown to be an effective treatment for stuttering. Page 424.

112. **Answer: E.** Descriptive research uses only descriptive statistics such as averages, percentages, histograms, and frequency distributions. Page 109.

113. **Answer: C.** Among the central features of all forms of the Response to Intervention model are (i) high-quality classroom instruction, (ii) research-based instruction, (iii) classroom performance measures, (iv) universal screening, (v) continuous progress monitoring, (vi) research-based interventions, (vii) progress monitoring during intervention, and (viii) fidelity measures. Page 416.

114. **Answer: A.** Detecting alcohol by urine is not very efficient or effective. A breathalyzer should be used. Page 619.

115. **Answer: E.** Olanzapine has been associated with the greatest amount of weight gain, but this side effect is particularly common and potentially prominent with all atypical antipsychotics as well as lithium and valproate. Aripiprazole and ziprasidone have been found to be more weight neutral, but can also cause weight gain in some patients. Page 609.

116. **Answer: E.** Page 649.

117. **Answer: A.** The triad consists of characteristics in the child, caregivers, and social environment; the caregiving environment refers to the dyadic relationship between caregiver and child and how the caregiver responds to the child's behavior. Page 252.

118. **Answer: D and E.** Interpersonal psychotherapy assumes that if one improves the relationships in the patient's life, one can change the course of the depressive episode. Page 820.

119. **Answer: A.** Page 369.

120. **Answer: D.** The more severe the intellectual compromise, the more likelihood epilepsy is present and emerges at an early age. Severe epilepsy itself, if it develops early in infancy and is intractable, can lead to significant impact on neuropsychological development. Page 963.

121. **Answer: A.** Vogel and Vernberg claimed that disasters challenge children's basic assumption that the world is a secure place, leaving them helplessly vulnerable. Page 729.

122. **Answer: A.** Most persons with an intellectual disability in childhood have mild mental retardation (MR) (about 85% of cases); the remainder of cases comprise those with moderate (about 10%), severe (about 4%), and profound (1%–2%). Page 401.

123. **Answer: A.** Extracellular-signal-related kinase is a member of the mitogen-activated protein kinase family of proteins. The extracellular-signal-related kinase pathway is necessary for the formation of new long-term memories. Page 200.

124. **Answer: A.** Page 439.

125. **Answer: B.** Page 828.

126. **Answer: A.** Page 545.

127. **Answer: B.** That is one option, but the goal is to provide the appropriate care in the least restrictive setting; without more information the right disposition here is unclear. Page 534.

128. **Answer: B.** Studies have been mixed. Several cross-sectional and comparative studies indicate that for the most part, aggregate scores on measures of depression, distress, or anxiety for children and adolescents with cancer fall within the normal range or are no different from their peers; some studies have reported lower levels of psychosocial problems when compared with healthy controls. In addition, younger children may be more adaptable than older children. Page 930.

129. **Answer: C.** Page 702.

130. **Answer: B.** The author indicates how the choice of a mate can be the product of a strong unconscious motivation to acquire a longed-for or unfinished aspect of oneself, which can contribute to stability in a marriage and the formation of a family. According to C. Eichberg's research, a husband can be positively ameliorative of a mother's negative upbringing experiences. Page 6.

131. **Answer: A.** Page 303.

132. **Answer: E.** Adolescent tasks include all of the above, as well as the development of satisfying relationships outside the family. Page 282.

133. **Answer: B.** Up to one-half of marriages end in divorce and the majority of women under the age of 30 who have children are unmarried. One-third of children grow up with only one parent. Page 1006.

134–136. **Answers:** 134-B; 135-A; 136-C. Page 173, Table 2.2.2.1.

137. **Answer: E.** Earlier studies suggested deep sleep. Page 657.

138. **Answer: A.** The reason for this is not obvious as it does not appear related to the greater liver-to-body mass ratio or the efficiency of CYPs in children. Page 749.

139. **Answer: A.** Children with autistic disorder are delayed in social development and their ability to relate to others, but do become preoccupied with nonsocial aspects of the environment. Page 384.

140. **Answer: D.** Page 306.

141. **Answer: B.** This distinction is especially important in practical applications of an intervention or exposure. Page 115.

142. **Answer: D.** This information is derived from diffusion tensors that are ellipsoid geometrical representations of the diffusional properties of water. Page 224.

143. **Answer: E.** Cohen's d is commonly used in meta-analytic studies assessing clinical efficacy of therapeutic interventions. This metric is calculated by taking the mean of the treated group on a measure of interest (e.g., Hamilton Depression Rating scores) subtracting it from the mean of the control group, and then dividing this difference by the standard deviation of the control group. Traditionally, a d of 0.2 is considered a small effect size, whereas a d of 0.8 is a large effect. Page 790.

144. **Answer: C.** Parents with high responsivity and high demandingness ("authoritative" style) tend to have the best outcome. Low responsivity and low demandingness describes a neglectful or uninvolved parent. High responsivity and low demandingness describes a permissive parent. Low responsivity and high demandingness describes an authoritarian style parent. Page 272.

145. **Answer: B.** Page 379.

146. **Answer: B.** Linkage analysis is not a cytogenetic method. Page 192.

147. **Answer: A.** Children with anorexia nervosa might be at increased risk for metabolic reasons, but this would represent provoking stimuli and therefore not epilepsy. Page 958.

148. **Answer: A.** The Pediatric Obsessive-Compulsive Disorder Treatment Study showed a 46% symptom improvement for cognitive-behavioral therapy (CBT) alone compared with 30% for sertraline. Although combined treatment showed a 53% improvement, the results suggest that CBT is the preferred first treatment for obsessive–compulsive disorder. Page 760.

149. **Answer: A.** Newly formed glutamatergic projection neurons migrate along radial glial guides that stretch between the ventricular surface and outer cortical surface. Note that all of the options represent central nervous system cells except E. A second type of migration independent of radial cell guides involves tangential movement of GABAergic neurons. Page 184.

150. **Answer: C.** In this study, 83% improved overall, with 20% recovering completely. Page 560.

151. **Answer: A.** Page 828.

152. **Answer: A.** Option C refers to Kubler—Ross's model for grief. Finality is also known as nonfunctionality and inevitability is also known as universality. Page 972.

153. **Answer: D.** Trauma-focused CBT has been used successfully with a wide age range of children with a variety of traumatic histories. A web-based training for trauma-focused CBT is available. Page 707.

154. **Answer: C.** The stimulants methylphenidate and amphetamine also facilitate the release of dopamine into the synapse from vesicles. Page 240.

155. **Answer: B.** Page 475.

156. **Answer: D.** The peak time for these behaviors is after school hours when many adolescents are unsupervised by an adult. Page 42.

157. **Answer: E.** Further studies to evaluate the validity of these rating scales are necessary. The Mood Disorder Questionnaire screens for bipolar spectrum disorders. Page 517.

158. **Answer: A.** Page 756.

159. **Answer: B.** At the very least, this points to troublesome lacks of continuity in the child's holding environment and a lack of a shared consensus between the child and important adults. Page 902.

160. **Answer: A.** Page 141.

161. **Answer: C.** Page 802.

162. **Answer: E.** The proliferation of programs such as Head Start, and the support of government funds enabled researchers and clinicians to apply their expertise to areas such as program development and evaluation, which had previously received scant attention. Page 36.

163. **Answer: B.** Girls' levels of satisfaction with their bodies and physical appearance decline as they pass through adolescence. Page 283.

164. **Answer: E.** In a comprehensive review, Donnelly proposes that broad-spectrum agents such as selective serotonin reuptake inhibitors are a good first choice because they are effective in treating core symptoms of posttraumatic stress disorder and comorbid symptoms (depression, anxiety). In addition, Donnelly suggests that adrenergic agents may be useful in alleviating symptoms of hyperarousal and impulsivity; mood stabilizers may be necessary in severe affective dyscontrol; and atypical neuroleptics may be required in cases of acute self-injurious behavior, dissociation, and aggression. Page 737.

165. **Answer: B.** This is a controversial diagnosis and some initial findings have not been replicated. It appears that considering an autoimmune mechanism is relevant only when the highly specific pattern of acute onset and associated symptoms are observed (not just obsessive–compulsive disorder with more distal infection). Page 555.

166. **Answer: B.** Published by the Children's Defense Fund in 1982, it exposed the lack of services for children with significant mental health needs. Knitzer's advocacy and those of others led to the development of the Child and Adolescent Service System Program, discussed in another question. Page 888.

167. **Answer: A.** A study of 8- to 16-year olds, showed that two-thirds wanted to know everything and one-third wanted to know as little as possible. Those who received information were significantly less anxious and depressed. Page 934.

168. **Answer: E.** Over 80% of boys were interested in fire play. Page 483.

169–176. Answers: 169-C; 170-F; 171-D; 172-B; 173-H; 174-G; 175-A; 176-E. Pages 215–216.

177. **Answer: A.** Language acquisition, including vocabulary and the fundamentals of linguistic semantics, occurs by age 4 or 5, even with very little environmental support. This is exemplified by deaf children's early communication even without language input. Page 262.

178. **Answer: D.** Page 345.

179. **Answer: E.** Page 360.

180. **Answer: A.** Siblings of persons with autism are at higher risk of having cognitive and language problems and have a 22-fold or greater risk of being affected with autism than the general population. Page 388.

181. **Answer: B and D.** Parental monitoring is defined as a "set of correlated parenting behaviors involving attention to and tracking of the child's whereabouts, activities, and adaptations." It has emerged as a powerful construct in resilience research. Page 294.

182. **Answer: C.** Approximately 70% of people with epilepsy will go into remission, defined as 5 or more years free of seizures (off or on medications). Childhood onset epilepsy without developmental or neurological disabilities has a better prognosis. Only 35% of those with mental retardation, cerebral palsy, or other neurological conditions will enter remission. Page 959.

183. **Answer: D.** IQ per se is not a predictor. Page 532.

184. **Answer: B.** The strange situation, which introduces stranger and caregiver–child separations, is a research method designed to assess the attachment classification of the relationship. The strange situation is not intended to provide a clinical diagnosis and should not be substituted for clinical observation. Page 715.

185. **Answer: D.** Insecure or disorganized attachment and borderline personality disorder have been associated in the attachment studies examining this issue. Page 684.

186. **Answer: A.** Option B is a criterion for Tourette's disorder only. Option C is a criterion for transient tic disorder only. Option D is not listed in any DSM criteria for tic disorders. Option E is a criterion for chronic motor or vocal tic disorder. Page 570.

187. **Answer: A.** Page 669.

188. **Answer: B.** This research study showed how the quality of parent–child relationships has greater influence than the presence of parental conflict. Page 9.

189. **Answer: C.** Page 540.

190. **Answer: B.** Page 441.

191. **Answer: B.** The categorical approach is sometimes referred to as the medical model of classification. Page 305.

192. **Answer: B.** In early child evaluations, assessing development involves an understanding of the child and his environment, as well as descriptions of infant behavior including qualitative aspects of behavior in the structured assessment setting. Page 313.

193. **Answer: E.** Heightened psychopathology in persons with MR has been linked to specific biopsychosocial problems. Biologically, these include increased rates of seizure disorders, abnormal neurological functioning, which in most cases is undetected, high rates of sensory or motor impairments, biochemical or neurological anomalies associated with unusual behavior such as severe self-injury, and genetic causes that carry higher than usual risks of certain maladaptive or psychiatric vulnerabilities. There is no evidence to support statement E. Page 404.

194. **Answer: E.** Premature deaths are more common in children, who are in institutions, with moderate and severe retardation. Page 94.

195. **Answer: E.** These two assessments capture a wide range of child functioning and are well normed. They include a list of symptoms from diverse maladjustment domains, which collectively yield scores on discrete subscales such as attention, conduct, or depressive problems; they also include composite scores, which indicate aspects of overall maladjustment. Page 292.

196. **Answer: B.** Page 372.

197. **Answer: A.** Drugs primarily distributed in body water will have a lower plasma concentration in children compared with adults because the volume of distribution (V_d) is higher in children and adolescents. The volume of distribution (V_d) affects plasma concentration of a drug (C_p) relative to the amount of drug absorbed (D), as in the equation: $C_p = D/V_d$. Page 746.

198. **Answer: C.** Marijuana use and alcohol use has been on the decline over the last decade. Page 617.

199. **Answer: B.** Hyponatremic seizures have been reported with intranasal desmopressin acetate. Page 661.

200. **Answer: D.** Studies of infants with ambiguous genitalia established that gender identity is primarily determined through socialization. Page 270.

Test Four

Questions

1. In interpersonal psychotherapy, clinical depression is conceptualized with which of the following THREE components?
   A. Symptom formation
   B. Gradual exposure
   C. Transference
   D. Social functioning
   E. Personality

2. Which of the following is the principal metabolite of dopamine?
   A. Vanillylmandelic acid
   B. 3-Methoxy-4-hydroxy-phenyl glycol
   C. Homovanillic acid
   D. Monoamine oxidase (MAO)
   E. L-Dopa

3. When is sexual preference established typically?
   A. At birth
   B. During middle childhood
   C. In adolescence
   D. In college
   E. By age 3

4. Which of the following treatment programs has significant empirical support for adolescents with depression?
   A. Multisystemic therapy
   B. Dialectical-behavior therapy
   C. Interpersonal psychotherapy (IPT)
   D. Electroconvulsive therapy
   E. Mentalization-based treatment

5. True or False: In preschool children with attention deficit hyperactivity disorder (ADHD), the inattentive subtype is more common.
   A. True
   B. False

6. What proportion of children in sub-Saharan Africa are infected with HIV?
   A. One-half
   B. One-third
   C. Three-fourths
   D. One-quarter
   E. One-fifth

7. Which of the following statements is true?
   A. The mean length of sleep for high school students is approximately 12.3 hours a night
   B. Adolescents experience an increase in appetite, referred to as developmental hyperphagia, which is seen across species
   C. The sleep phase shift seen in adolescence occurs due to earlier night-onset and earlier morning-termination of melatonin secretion
   D. Adolescents with sleep problems are less likely to develop learning difficulties or have impaired academic performance

8. What is the range suggested by epidemiological studies for the percentage of children with diagnosable psychiatric disorders?
   A. 1% to 2%
   B. 3% to 5%
   C. 5% to 10%
   D. 10% to 20%
   E. 20% to 30%

9. In assessing a child who presents with somatic symptoms it is important to:
   A. Enlist the patient's view by making a statement such as "nothing is wrong, so what do you think is wrong?"
   B. Refrain from asking about prior treatment experiences, which have likely been alienating or discouraging
   C. Try to convey over time how the symptoms are purely psychological
   D. Explore timing, context, and social reinforcement of any symptoms
   E. See the child before the parents

10. True or False: More than 50% of children who experiment with drugs go on to become regular users.
    A. True
    B. False

11. Which of the following statements reflects the result of epidemiological findings?
    A. Children are more accurate reporters of their externalizing symptoms and parents more accurate reporters of their child's internalizing symptoms
    B. Children are more accurate reporters of their internalizing symptoms and parents more accurate reporters of their child's externalizing symptoms
    C. Children and parents are more accurate reporters of the child's internalizing symptoms and other adults are better reporters of externalizing symptoms
    D. Children and parents are more accurate reporters of the child's externalizing symptoms and other adults are better reporters of internalizing symptoms
    E. None of the above

12. In the multisite study, Treatment of ADHD in Children with Tourette's syndrome (TACT), 136 children (ages 7–14) with ADHD and a chronic tic disorder were randomized to one of four treatments: clonidine, methylphenidate, clonidine and methylphenidate, or placebo. What was the major result of the study?
    A. Clonidine treatment was superior to placebo on teacher and parent measures of ADHD
    B. Methylphenidate treatment was superior to placebo on teacher and parent measures of ADHD
    C. Combined treatment with clonidine and methylphenidate was superior to placebo on teacher and parent measures of ADHD
    D. All three active treatments were superior to placebo on teacher and parent measures of ADHD
    E. None of the above

13. True or False: There is a higher rate of psychosis among patients with epilepsy.
    A. True
    B. False

14. ALL of the following are reasons why scores among tests assessing psychological functioning may vary EXCEPT:
    A. The scores on the tests are reported in different units of measurement
    B. The tests lack enough easy items to discriminate between low scorers and enough hard items to assess upper levels of ability
    C. The tests may not be correlated or only moderately related
    D. Scores may improve because of familiarity with the test or test items or prior exposure
    E. The tests may have the same content despite differing in their name

15. Speece and Brent concluded that most studies found the age of acquisition of the three concepts of death they reviewed—irreversibility, nonfunctionality, and universality—to occur between:
    A. Ages 3 and 5
    B. Ages 5 and 7
    C. Ages 8 and 10
    D. Ages 10 and above

16. What is the minimum acceptable level of reliability for a neuropsychological or psychological test?
    A. 95%
    B. 85%
    C. 80%
    D. 75%
    E. 60%

17. Which of the following is true of acute otitis media and its sequelae?
    A. It affects about 10% of children ages 6 to 24 months
    B. It is very uncommon after age 6 years
    C. About 10% of children with acute otitis media have a middle ear effusion 1 month after an episode of infection
    D. Surgical insertion of primary ear care tubes is indicated when middle ear effusion associated hearing loss is greater than 5 dB
    E. All of the above

18. ALL of the following represent the community-based system-of-care principles outlined by the Child and Adolescent Service System Program initiative, EXCEPT:
    A. Treatment of children who are seriously emotionally disturbed, as exhibited by the presence of an Axis I diagnosis under the Diagnostic and Statistical Manual of Mental Disorders (DSM)
    B. Treatment of children who are seriously emotionally disturbed, as exhibited by the child's inability to function in at least one of his or her life domains (school, home, society)
    C. Access to a comprehensive array of services
    D. Treatment in the least restrictive environment possible
    E. Focus on access to mental health expertise rather than reliance on community resources

19. In the 1980s, which federal program assisted all 50 states in the development of an infrastructure for publicly funded community-based services?
    A. The Community Health Act
    B. The Help, Not Hate, Your Neighbor Act
    C. The Homer Simpson Donut Act
    D. The Child and Adolescent Service System Program
    E. The Child and Adolescent Mental Health Act

20. Which of the following terms defines the patterns of behaviors, acquired and transferred over time, which prescribe the norms, customs, roles, and values inherent in political, economic, religious, and social aspects of family life?
    A. Culture
    B. Ethnicity
    C. Cultural context
    D. Cultural identity
    E. Cultural mask

21. The diagnosis of which of the following was the first major clinical application of diffusion tensor imaging, a relatively new neuroimaging modality?
    A. Bipolar disorder
    B. Glial brain tumors
    C. Childhood autism
    D. Temporal lobe seizures
    E. Ischemic stroke

22. True or False: When a child learns two languages, each language is represented in its own language center.
    A. True
    B. False

23. According to DSM-IV-TR, a person with a diagnosis of moderate mental retardation would have which of the following.
    A. An IQ of 90
    B. An IQ of 75
    C. An IQ of 60
    D. An IQ of 45
    E. An IQ of 30

24. True or False: An estimate for the prevalence of a condition can be obtained by the proportion of subjects who score significantly above the cutoff on a screening phase instrument.
    A. True
    B. False

25. Each of the following has randomized controlled trials supporting its efficacy for anxiety disorders in children EXCEPT:
    A. Fluvoxamine
    B. Clonazepam
    C. Fluoxetine
    D. Sertraline
    E. Paroxetine

26. The Pediatric OCD (Obsessive–Compulsive Disorder) Treatment Study (POTS), the largest pediatric trial of cognitive-behavioral therapy (CBT) for OCD to date, found which of the following results with regard to efficacy?
    A. CBT + SSRI > CBT alone > SSRI alone
    B. CBT + SSRI > SSRI alone > CBT alone
    C. CBT + SSRI > CBT alone = SSRI alone
    D. CBT + SSRI = SSRI alone > CBT alone
    E. CBT alone > CBT + SSRI > SSRI alone

27. In a review of 22 studies on fire behavior in children and adolescents, researchers found that 82% of identified firesetters were male, and the average age of these children was:
    A. 5 years
    B. 10 years
    C. 13 years
    D. 16 years
    E. 18 years

28. In infant and toddler assessments, the TWO most common types of scoring used to provide a representation of the child's performance relative to other children are:
    A. Standard scores
    B. t-scores
    C. Age equivalent scores
    D. Deviation scores
    E. z-scores

29. An assessment of the adaptive behavior of a child or adolescent patient provides information about which of the following?
    A. What potential of doing the child has in day-to-day life
    B. What the child is capable of doing in day-to-day life
    C. What the child actually does in day-to-day life
    D. How adaptive the child can be in the face of adverse circumstances
    E. How resilient the child can be in the face of adverse circumstances

30. Which of the following accounts for most in the success of solid organ transplantations?
    A. Increased health insurance coverage for transplantations
    B. Increased psychosocial supports for parents allowing for better management
    C. The introduction of cyclosporine in 1980
    D. The improvement of sutures
    E. More pleasant healthcare staff

31. True or False: Linkage analysis assesses the probability that a given phenotype and a particular genetic marker (or series of markers) are transmitted together from one generation to another.
    A. True
    B. False

32. A number of practical behavioral treatments can be implemented for patients with ADHD even upon first contact, which include ALL of the following EXCEPT:
    A. Star charts for target behaviors
    B. Clearly established house rules
    C. Written or pictorial instructions
    D. Gradual exposure to the offending stimulus
    E. Contingent rewards for accomplishing tasks

33. Which of the following best characterizes the epidemiology of suicide among males 15 to 24 years old?
    A. A rapid rise began in the 1960s, peaked in 1977, and has declined since
    B. A rapid rise began in the 1980s and continues
    C. A decline since the 1950s
    D. Intermittent peaks every 10 to 20 years corresponding with economic recessions over the past five decades
    E. None of the above

34. ALL of the following are true of a child by age 5 EXCEPT:
    A. Interested in sexual differences
    B. Enjoys the company of other children
    C. Engages in interactional play with rules
    D. Names and copies a triangle
    E. Judges peers by their qualities

35. Which of the following statistics would most likely be used in associational research?
    A. Histogram
    B. Correlation
    C. *t*-test
    D. Analysis of variance
    E. Frequency distribution

36. Regarding the etiology of Asperger's disorder, which of the following statements is TRUE?
    A. In some cases, up to one-third of immediate family members have significant social difficulties
    B. There is no associated familial relationship
    C. There is a decreased risk for depression and anxiety in family members
    D. Autism and Asperger's disorder are not etiologically related
    E. Females are more affected than males

37. Which of the following is the appropriate measure of central tendency for ordinal-level data (i.e., ordered data but not normally distributed)?
    A. Mean
    B. Median
    C. Mode
    D. None of the above

38. Which of the following is the most compelling theory for enuresis?
  A. Children with enuresis have difficulty concentrating the urine that they produce at night
  B. Children with enuresis are scared of their caregivers
  C. Children with enuresis do not like waking up to go to the bathroom
  D. Children with enuresis have the regressive desire to be in diapers
  E. None of the above

39. Around what age does pretend play begin?
  A. 18 months
  B. 24 months
  C. 4 years
  D. 5 years
  E. 6 years

40. What type of variable interacts with an independent variable to cause the change in the dependent variable?
  A. Active independent variable
  B. Moderator variable
  C. Extraneous variable
  D. Attribute independent variable
  E. Mediator variable

41. True or False: A semistructured clinical interview gives the interviewer latitude in the specific form of questions used.
  A. True
  B. False

42. Some studies document that ALL of the following factors are predictive of chronic delinquency in youth EXCEPT:
  A. Low socioeconomic status
  B. Poor academic performance
  C. Convicted parents
  D. Low intelligence
  E. Poor parental childrearing

43. True or False: A therapeutic group should avoid containing only one representative of any critical attribute or category, including race, religion, ethnicity, gender, or level of diagnostic severity.
  A. True
  B. False

44. The most frequent comorbidities with oppositional defiant disorder and conduct disorder are ALL of the following EXCEPT:
  A. ADHD
  B. Major depressive disorder
  C. Substance abuse
  D. Psychotic disorder, not otherwise specified

45. Which of the following medications has the single highest association with incidental suicidal ideation?
  A. Paroxetine
  B. Fluoxetine
  C. Bupropion
  D. Imipramine
  E. Venlafaxine

46. What is the prevalence of anxiety disorders in children and adolescents?
  A. 4% to 20%
  B. 1% to 10%
  C. 5% to 50%
  D. Less than 3%

47. When a clinician interviews a child with deafness, what is a common response on the clinician's part?
    A. Exaggeration of positive affect to engage child
    B. Feelings of dominance
    C. Intellectualization of affect
    D. Rationalization
    E. Speaking in a soft voice

48. What percentage of affected individuals with neurofibromatosis have an intellectual disability?
    A. 15%
    B. 33%
    C. 50%
    D. 66%
    E. 90%

49. True or False: One historical development that fueled mental health professionals' interest in social policy was the recognition that children develop within the social context.
    A. True
    B. False

50. Child psychiatric epidemiology started in the mid-1960s with:
    A. Dutch population surveys
    B. Scandinavian school surveys
    C. The Danish juvenile delinquency registry
    D. British Isle of Wight surveys
    E. None of the above

51. For very young children showing some early symptoms of a disorder, which diagnostic system is considered by some to be more appropriate than the DSM?
    A. Diagnostic System Zero to Three, Revised
    B. Diagnostic System for Infants and Toddlers
    C. Diagnostic and Statistical Manual for Mental Disorders, which begin in infancy
    D. Diagnostic and Statistical Manual for Emotional or Behavioral Impairments, which begin in infancy
    E. International Classification of Diseases

52. In psychoanalytic thought, object relations theories use a metapsychology organized around the concept of which of the following?
    A. Mechanisms of defense
    B. The tripartite model
    C. Freud's dual drive theory
    D. Internal representational world
    E. Erikson's stages of development

53. True or False: The incidence of seizure disorders in children with autism increases through adolescence.
    A. True
    B. False

54. True or False: The best predictor of longer term consequences for the psychosocial adjustment of children of divorce is their initial response to the divorce.
    A. True
    B. False

55. Which of the following is the most widely used measure of the development of infants and toddlers in both clinical and research settings?
    A. Bayley Scales of Infant Development—II
    B. Mullen Scales of Early Learning
    C. Battelle Developmental Inventory
    D. Brigance Diagnostic Inventory of Early Development—Revised
    E. Early Learning Accomplishment Profile for Infants

56. What did both of the Surgeon General's Conference on Children's Mental Health in 2000 and the President's New Freedom Commission on Mental Health in 2003 acknowledge regarding child and adolescent psychiatry?
    A. The workforce of child psychiatrists requires more training
    B. The shortage of child psychiatrists is a national crisis
    C. Child psychiatrists should adhere to a multisystemic model
    D. The workforce of child psychiatrists is overworked and underpaid
    E. Child psychiatry should be included in mental health parity for insurance reimbursement

57. Taking information out of context and ignoring relevant details describes which of the following cognitive errors?
    A. Arbitrary inference
    B. Selective abstraction
    C. Ignoring evidence
    D. Overgeneralization
    E. Absolutism

58. ALL of the following symptoms are common presentations of Munchhausen syndrome by proxy in Rosenberg and Sheridan's reviews EXCEPT:
    A. Diarrhea
    B. Fracture
    C. Fever
    D. Seizure
    E. Apnea

59. Which of the following is true in providing child psychiatric services as part of a consultative service to early care and education programs?
    A. The child can be observed in a natural setting, which includes peer interactions
    B. The clinician must focus solely on classroom-specific reduction of particular behaviors
    C. The clinician can observe the child without the need for collateral information from parents or other caregivers
    D. Children generally behave similarly at home and in child care programs

60. Which of the following best characterizes the prognosis in pediatric OCD?
    A. 60% of children with OCD will improve such that they no longer meet criteria
    B. 40% of children with OCD will recover
    C. 60% of children with OCD will continue to meet criteria for the disorder or have subthreshold symptoms
    D. None of the above
    E. A, B, and C

61. In the biopsychosocial model of formulation, which of the following components belong in the psychological realm?
    A. Inborn temperament
    B. Constitution
    C. Emotional development
    D. Family constellation
    E. Intelligence

62. Some psychotropic medications follow zero-order (or nonlinear) kinetics, best described by which of the following statements?
    A. The amount of drug eliminated is variable regardless of plasma level
    B. The amount of drug eliminated per unit of time is fixed regardless of the plasma level
    C. The amount of drug eliminated is proportional to the CYP 450 system being utilized
    D. The amount of drug eliminated is proportional to its amount circulating in the bloodstream

63. The following examples would lead you to consider which diagnosis? Running for class president, despite having no friends; early-afternoon anxiety attached with persecutory delusions, followed by successful participation in a soccer game in the afternoon; chronic complaints of boredom; describing teacher as "girlfriend."
    A. ADHD
    B. Somatization disorder
    C. Borderline personality disorder
    D. Phase of life problem
    E. No diagnosis

64. True or False: In psychoanalytic thought, ego functions conceptualize the inner voice of conscience, which maintains ideals and values, observing and criticizing any shortfall of the self.
    A. True
    B. False

65. Although ethical codes in medicine date back to the fifth century BC, they received scant attention in the modern medical literature until the 1990s. Greater awareness and interest in medical ethics can be attributed to ALL of the following EXCEPT:
    A. An increasingly consumer-centered approach to medicine with its emphasis on patient rights
    B. High-technology medical developments that offer a multitude of choices yet also introduce the need for health care rationing and decisions about prolonging life
    C. An increasingly diverse populace with multiple moral codes in the postmodern era
    D. Changes in the delivery of health care that has altered the autonomy of the physician and challenges traditional ethical codes

66. The five AREST principles followed by mental health professionals to help children and families who are victims of a catastrophe include ALL of the following EXCEPT:
    A. Anticipate
    B. Redifferentiate
    C. Empower
    D. Supervise and assess
    E. Terminate
    F. Treat

67. ALL of the following are Phase I metabolic reactions involved in the biotransformation of drugs EXCEPT:
    A. Hydroxylation
    B. Conjugation
    C. Reduction
    D. Hydrolysis

68. Heavy use of cannabis can be detected in the urine for how long?
    A. 1 day
    B. 3 days
    C. 5 days
    D. 7 days
    E. 10 days

69. True or False: Paroxetine can cause birth defects.
    A. True
    B. False

70. What is likely the most common preoccupation in adolescents with body dysmorphic disorder?
    A. Hair
    B. Teeth
    C. Legs
    D. Skin
    E. Eyes

71. ALL of the following statements about the diagnosis of reactive attachment disorder (RAD) are true EXCEPT:
    A. The identified patient must have a developmental age of at least 9 months
    B. Pervasive development disorder is an exclusion criterion according to DSM
    C. Hypervigilance is a common symptom for both posttraumatic stress disorder (PTSD) and RAD
    D. Large head circumference may be conducive to the diagnosis of RAD with autistic-like features
    E. Failure to thrive is not a criterion in the diagnosis of RAD

72. Which of the following is the normal milestone for a child's ability to use a cup to drink?
    A. 18 months
    B. 15 months
    C. 12 months
    D. 10 months
    E. 6 months

73. Reassessment and contemporaneous documentation of the need for continuation of restraints must be done how often for children ages 9 to 17?
    A. Every half hour
    B. Every hour
    C. Every one and a half hours
    D. Every two hours
    E. Whenever the child is calm enough for a reassessment

74. A landmark study by Avshalom Caspi and colleagues showed reduced likelihood of antisocial behavior in maltreated children with the presence of a genotype conferring what?
    A. High levels of a serotonin transporter
    B. Low levels of a serotonin transporter
    C. High levels of prefrontal dopamine receptors
    D. High levels of MAO A enzyme
    E. Low levels of MAO A enzyme

75. ADHD has a high rate of comorbid psychiatric disorders including ALL of the following EXCEPT:
    A. Oppositional defiant disorder
    B. Conduct disorder
    C. Anxiety disorder
    D. Learning disorder
    E. Dysthymic disorder

76. The incidence of maternal depression can lead to disengaged parenting practices resulting in poor development. In one study, what was the incidence of depression in single mothers with young children?
    A. Twice the national average
    B. Three times the national average
    C. Equal to the national average
    D. Less than the national average

77. Atomoxetine has ALL of the following black box warnings EXCEPT:
    A. Hepatitis
    B. Increased aggression
    C. Increased hostility
    D. Increased suicidal thinking
    E. Seizures

78. Zucker and Bradley summarized data from six follow-up reports on 55 boys with gender identity disorder. Which of the following conclusions from this study is accurate?
    A. 90% were classified as homosexual
    B. 30% were classified as heterosexual
    C. 80% were classified as homosexual
    D. 50% were classified as heterosexual
    E. None of the above

79. Each of the following answer options are intellectual considerations associated with cancer, using Chesler and Barbarin's model of stress and coping, EXCEPT:
    A. How do children become aware that they have a serious situation and that they have a condition about which they ought to worry?
    B. What conclusions do children draw from the many verbal and nonverbal cues displayed by parents, relatives, and medical staff?
    C. What do children make of the rapidity with which family members will come from afar to visit?
    D. How are siblings provided information so that they are not left to imagining the worst?
    E. How will children with cancer do their schoolwork?

80. True or False: In official diagnostic systems such as the DSM-IV, etiological factors are included in classification.
    A. True
    B. False

81. True or False: A stepparent can obtain custody in place of a natural parent.
    A. True
    B. False

82. True or False: Boys with gender identity disorder have more externalizing than internalizing symptoms.
    A. True
    B. False

83. Which of the following large studies evaluated the long-term treatment with methylphenidate (and other medications to a lesser degree) on 576 children with ADHD?
    A. Pediatric OCD Treatment Study
    B. Multimodal Treatment Study of Children with ADHD (MTA) Study
    C. Treatment for Adolescents with Depression Study (TADS)
    D. Children and Adolescents Anxiety Multimodal Treatment Study
    E. Research Units on Pediatric Psychopharmacology

84. True or False: In forensic evaluations, the practice of accepting retainer fees or contingency fees is equally ethical.
    A. True
    B. False

85. What is a common sleep disorder in adolescence?
    A. Circadian rhythm sleep disorder
    B. Narcolepsy
    C. Somnambulism
    D. Night terrors

86. Fonagy and colleagues assert that security of attachment is linked to what?
    A. The caregiver's soothing statements
    B. The caregiver's affective attunement
    C. The caregiver's mental health
    D. The caregiver's mentalizing capacity
    E. The caregiver's affective stability

87. Rather than viewing obsessions and compulsions as separate entities, several investigators consider that OCD might be better viewed as consisting of four or more subtypes. In one model, the four subtypes are ALL of the following EXCEPT:
    A. Aggressive, sexual, religious, and somatic obsessions with checking compulsions
    B. Obsessions with themes of death with undoing compulsions
    C. Symmetry obsessions with counting, arranging, ordering, and repeating compulsions
    D. Contamination obsessions with cleaning and washing
    E. Hoarding obsessions with hoarding and collecting compulsions

88. Which of these is NOT a setting in which pediatric psychology services for medically ill children is commonly provided?
    A. Summer camps
    B. Outpatient medical clinics
    C. Specialty facilities
    D. Outpatient clinics for children with psychiatric problems
    E. Schools

89. The bioavailability of a medication in the systemic circulation is determined in part by its presystemic clearance, which is also called:
    A. First-pass effect
    B. Second-pass effect
    C. Third-pass effect
    D. Conjugation
    E. Metabolism

90. Which condition is characterized by an acquired aphasia secondary to a seizure disorder?
    A. Broca's aphasia
    B. Gerstmann syndrome
    C. Landau-Kleffner syndrome
    D. Pragmatic learning impairment
    E. Wernicke's aphasia

91. True or False: When you receive a subpoena, it means you are alleged to have done something wrong.
    A. True
    B. False

92. What are the barriers to diagnosing and providing mental health treatment in the primary care setting?
    A. Insufficient training of pediatricians to recognize and treat mental health problems
    B. Inadequate outpatient mental health resources
    C. Time
    D. Reimbursement
    E. All of the above

93. Regarding meeting length, which of the following represents the optimal amount of time for a group therapy meeting?
    A. 20 to 30 minutes
    B. 45 to 50 minutes
    C. 45 to 75 minutes
    D. 60 to 90 minutes
    E. Duration increases linearly with age range

94. During the middle phase of IPT for depressed adolescents, the therapist teaches the adolescent specific strategies that can help with interpersonal difficulties. One strategy is to act out the skills that the adolescent is learning in the treatment, such as affective expression, effective communication, and decision-making strategies. What is this technique called?
    A. Communication analysis
    B. Behavior change techniques
    C. Encouragement of affect
    D. Role playing
    E. Interpersonal experiments

95. Each of the following is an element in Chesler and Barbarin's stress coping model EXCEPT:
    A. Cognitive-behavioral
    B. Intellectual
    C. Emotional
    D. Existential
    E. Practical
    F. Interpersonal

96. The onset of symptoms in autism appears to occur typically:
    A. Within the first 2 months of life
    B. Within the first or second year of life
    C. Between ages 5 and 7 years
    D. After the onset of puberty
    E. After age 18 years

97. ALL of the following should be part of a pretransplant psychiatric evaluation, EXCEPT:
    A. Screening of potential recipients for the presence of significant Axis I diagnoses
    B. Assessment of a child's relationship with caregivers
    C. Determination of the child and family's motivation for transplant
    D. Evaluation of the child and family's ability to comply with treatment recommendations
    E. Administration of the Millon Preadolescent or Adolescent Personality Clinical Inventory

98. Preschoolers struggle to deal with separations because:
    A. Their repertoire of coping abilities is still developing
    B. They have increased cognitive abilities
    C. They are able to reassure themselves easily
    D. They have never experienced a successful separation
    E. They are emotionally stable

99. True or False: In psychoanalytic thought, the concept of identification is one mechanism of internalization.
    A. True
    B. False

100. Habit reversal is used to treat stuttering when relaxation training is paired with:
    A. Awareness training and psychoeducation about the nature of the disorder
    B. Awareness training and contingency management
    C. Distraction and psychoeducation about the nature of the disorder
    D. Contingency management and distraction
    E. Contingency management and psychoeducation about the disorder

101. Which of the following is an example of indirect prevention-minded treatment and has empirical evidence demonstrating positive outcome?
    A. Consulting with a school social worker to help him with at risk teenagers
    B. Treatment of a mother with major depressive disorder who has a young child and counseling her about the child's increased anxiety
    C. Couples therapy for a couple on the verge of divorce for which you bring the children in as part of your treatment
    D. Family therapy

102. True or False: Children are more likely to develop PTSD symptoms if they display dissociative symptoms following the trauma.
    A. True
    B. False

103. A number of epilepsies can result in significant mental retardation, which includes ALL of the following EXCEPT:
    A. Infantile spasms or West syndrome
    B. Lennox-Gastaut
    C. Epileptic encephalopathies
    D. Landau-Kleffner Syndrome
    E. Childhood absence

104. Which of the following describes the type of neuronal receptor at which the binding of the neurotransmitter to the receptor protein leads to a change in the protein conformation?
    A. Ionotropic
    B. G-protein-coupled
    C. Serotonergic
    D. Glutamatergic
    E. Dopaminergic

105. Which of the following is a side effect of cyclosporine, an immunosuppressant?
    A. Delirium
    B. Somatization disorder
    C. Hypochondriasis
    D. Adjustment disorder
    E. Schizophreniform disorder

106. In resilience research, what is the BEST conceptual definition of a protective factor?
    A. Factors that inoculate the individual from significant adverse circumstances
    B. Factors that serve to offset the negative effect of vulnerability factors
    C. Factors that strengthen the core structures of the individual and personality
    D. Factors that modify the effects of risk in a positive direction
    E. All of the above

107. True or False: Crisis-intervention and family-preservation services in child welfare have proved to be more effective than treatment as usual.
    A. True
    B. False

108. In the 18th century, John Locke put forth the argument that the human mind at birth was:
    A. Bestowed by divine right
    B. A blank slate
    C. Equal among all other minds
    D. Influenced by hereditary factors

109. Children who make "mastery-oriented attributions"
    A. Give credit to their ability when they succeed
    B. Attribute failures to their lack of innate ability
    C. Display learned helplessness
    D. Are unable to determine if their performance is due to luck, ability, or effort
    E. Compare their abilities with those of their peers

110. Parents of a seriously ill, dying child may find themselves wishing that the child would finally die to relieve everyone of the emotional and financial burden and suffering. This unacceptable wish is transformed through which defense mechanism?
    A. Reaction formation
    B. Altruism
    C. Suppression
    D. Humor
    E. Projection

111. The diagnostic criteria for anorexia nervosa include ALL of the following EXCEPT:
    A. Refusal to maintain body weight at or above a minimally normal weight for age and height
    B. Intense fear of gaining weight or becoming obese
    C. Disturbance in the way in which one's body weight or shape is experienced
    D. A pattern of bingeing or purging
    E. The absence of at least three consecutive menstrual cycles (amenorrhea), in women who have had their first menstrual period

112. Which of the following is the most frequently encountered problem in the treatment of childhood cancer?
  A. Death
  B. An angry parent
  C. The pursuit of unorthodox therapies
  D. Nonadherence to treatment
  E. Diversion of opiates to another adult or adolescent sibling in the child's family

113. Which of the following statements is TRUE?
  A. Parent–child conflict appears to decrease in mid-adolescence
  B. Most parent–child relationships are not able to weather the stresses of parent–child conflict in adolescence
  C. Authoritarian parents have the most success in raising adolescents who are socially competent and academically successful
  D. None of the above

114. What is the percentage occurrence of rashes in adults on lamotrigine treatment?
  A. 0.5%
  B. 1%
  C. 2%
  D. 5%
  E. 10%

115. A potential physiological factor that could reinforce weight loss is:
  A. Increased pH in the stomach
  B. Increased corticotrophin releasing hormone after fasting
  C. Decreased levels of serotonin in the brain
  D. Decreased absorption in the intestines over time

116. Among the tricyclic antidepressants, which one is most selective in its capacity to block norepinephrine uptake?
  A. Desipramine
  B. Clomipramine
  C. Imipramine
  D. Amitriptyline
  E. Nortriptyline

117. True or False: One strategy in using desmopressin acetate is to rapidly titrate the initial dosage (to max 50 µg) until dryness is achieved; maintain this dosage for 4 to 6 weeks; then decrease the dosage by 10 µg every 4 weeks.
  A. True
  B. False

In the following questions, match each of the following imaging modalities to the phrase that best describes it.

118. Computed tomography

119. Positron emission tomography

120. Single photon emission computed tomography

121. Magnetic resonance imaging (MRI)

122. Anatomical MRI

123. Functional MRI

124. Diffusion tensor imaging

125. Magnetic Resonance Spectroscopy

126. Multimodal MRI

127. Electroencephalography

128. Magnetoencephalography
    A. Provides information concerning the volumes and occasionally the shapes of particular brain regions
    B. Uses radiotracers to track and then produce images of various *in vivo* biochemical and neurophysiological processes by the measurement and detection of gamma-ray emissions
    C. Provides information about the direction and integrity of neural fiber tracks in the brain *in vivo*
    D. Measures the extracranial magnetic field produced by the intraneuronal ionic current flow within appropriately oriented cortical pyramidal cells
    E. Uses the changes in the deoxyhemoglobin concentration within a corresponding voxel in the brain as an indirect measure of the change in local neuronal activity associated with the performance of a task
    F. Uses an array of detectors placed around the subject to measure the attenuation of multiple x-ray beams passing through the same body region from many different angles
    G. Measures brain electrical activity directly, and consequently neuronal activity, by the use of scalp electrodes
    H. Uses single-proton nuclei to generate a radio signal from the brain that carries information about the microscopic environment in which the hydrogen nucleus finds itself
    I. Provides biochemical information of the brain in the form of a series of spectral peaks of differing intensities at differing radiofrequencies in the MRI signal that originate from various nuclei
    J. Measures minute amounts of radioactively labeled molecules in the subject that emit photons whose spatial orientation and time of emission is independent of any other photon released, and is detected and measured by collimators
    K. Incorporates data for individual subjects from two or more MRI modalities

129. The voluntary consent of a human subject involves four essential attributes according to the Nuremberg Code, which include ALL of the following EXCEPT:
    A. The person should have access to an attorney
    B. The person should have legal capacity to give consent
    C. The person should have free power of choice
    D. The person should have sufficient knowledge of the subject for which he consents
    E. The person should comprehend the subject for which he consents

130. A child with snoring and mouth breathing is found to have obstructive sleep apnea. Which of the following hormones may be affected?
    A. Prolactin
    B. Thyroid-stimulating hormone
    C. Oxytocin
    D. Adrenocorticotropin hormone
    E. Growth hormone

131. Residential care of a child with borderline personality disorder has what purpose?
    A. Help the parents regain control
    B. Help the child function in school
    C. Interrupt coercive cycles of interaction between parent and child
    D. Interrupt addictive patterns involving drugs, food, promiscuity, or self-injury
    E. C and D

132. The diagnostic criteria for PTSD and Major Depressive Disorder share how many symptoms in common?
    A. One
    B. Two
    C. Three
    D. Four
    E. Five

133. For a pediatric residency program to be accredited, it must have how many months of child and adolescent psychiatry exposure?
    A. 0 months
    B. 1 month
    C. 2 months
    D. 3 months
    E. 6 months

134. The basic flow of biological information is from DNA to RNA (transcription) and from RNA to protein (translation). Transcribed RNA typically undergoes a number of modifications before it is ready for export from the nucleus as mRNA, including excision of intervening regions of the RNA that do not encode for proteins. The active regions (exons) are then spliced together. A single gene may contain a number of splice sites that allows for different exons of the gene to be brought together. As a result, a single gene may produce nearly identical proteins. This alternative splicing regulatory mechanism permits:
    A. Proteins to be expressed
    B. Proteins to be eliminated
    C. Proteins to be expressed in different forms, within differing tissues, or at varying developmental periods
    D. Genes to be eliminated
    E. Genes to be acid washed

135. Each of the following is a specific phobia, EXCEPT:
    A. Animal type
    B. Natural-environment type
    C. Blood-injection type
    D. Situational type
    E. Other type

136. Attachment theory originated with the work of:
    A. Mary Ainsworth
    B. Mary Main
    C. John Bowlby
    D. Margaret Mahler
    E. Melanie Klein

137. The recommended pharmacological intervention for obesity in adolescents is:
    A. Sibutramine
    B. Orlistat
    C. Dextroamphetamine
    D. Fen-phen (fenfluramine/phentermine)
    E. None of the above

138. How is developmental psychopathology characterized?
    A. Domain-specific weakness in a child's development
    B. Static or cross-sectional disturbances in a child's development
    C. Patterns of a child's behavioral maladaptation over time
    D. Isolated lacunae in a child's development

139. Randomized control trials looking at the efficacy of multisystemic therapy in the treatment of violent and chronic juvenile offenders have demonstrated ALL of the following findings EXCEPT:
    A. Reduction in long-term rate of criminal offences
    B. Reduction in rate of drug use and drug-related offences
    C. Improvement in family functioning
    D. Reduction in rate of sex offender recidivism
    E. Reduction in rate of other mental health problems

140. In one study of 180 youths, what percentage discharged from an inpatient psychiatric hospital attempted suicide within 5 years of discharge?
    A. 5%
    B. 15%
    C. 25%
    D. 50%
    E. 70%

141. What percentage of male U.S. high school students report having used steroids in the past year?
    A. 1%
    B. 3%
    C. 5%
    D. 10%
    E. 15%

142. True or False: Measures of infant information processing have been shown to be related significantly to IQ scores later in development.
    A. True
    B. False

143. Two groups of subjects are selected according to health status, with and without the disease of interest. What type of study is this?
    A. Case–control
    B. Cohort
    C. Ecological
    D. Cross-sectional

144. What is a potential concern of informed consent when working with parents of children who are dying of a serious illness in the hospital?
    A. Parents cannot make rational decisions in such circumstances
    B. The outcome is unpredictable and as such informed consent is meaningless
    C. Informed consent is complicated by the parents' disagreement about care
    D. The healthcare team risks using this as an excuse to avoid the difficult responsibility of formulating treatment recommendations
    E. Informed consent is not required at the terminal stages of treatment

145. Which of the following is true regarding genetic factors in tic disorders?
    A. The concordance rate for Tourette's syndrome (TS) in monozygotic twins is 90%
    B. The risk of an offspring of a parent with TS developing TS is 10% to 15%
    C. Offspring of a parent with TS have no increased risk of developing OCD
    D. There has been little research done in the search for genes related to TS
    E. It is likely that one gene is responsible for the phenotype of TS

146. Aripiprazole is classified as which of the following?
    A. D2 receptor blocker
    B. Partial dopamine agonist
    C. Partial dopamine antagonist
    D. Dopamine agonist
    E. Dopamine antagonist

147. True or False: The well-known Apgar screening test has been shown in studies to be a consistent predictor of subsequent infant development.
    A. True
    B. False

148. Valproate has multiple pharmacological effects on the brain including ALL of the following EXCEPT:
    A. Decreased dopamine turnover
    B. Increased serotonin antagonism
    C. Decreased release of aspartate
    D. Enhanced GABAergic inhibition
    E. Increased potassium influx

149. Which of the following is the most comprehensive epidemiological survey of psychiatric disorders in the United States?
    A. Framingham Study
    B. Clinical Antipsychotic Trials of Invention Effectives
    C. TADS
    D. National Comorbidity Survey
    E. MTA Study

150. The inheritance of pica occurs by which pattern?
    A. Autosomal dominant
    B. Autosomal recessive
    C. X-linked dominant
    D. No known inheritance pattern

151. What is the most salient feature observed in children and adolescents who meet DSM-IV-TR criteria for gender identity disorder?
    A. Dysphoria that he or she identifies with and prefers the gender role or characteristics of the other sex
    B. Depressive symptoms
    C. Posttraumatic stress symptoms
    D. Strong identification with and preference for one parent over another
    E. Strong identification with and preference for the gender role characteristics of the other sex

152. The most prevalent type of communication problems in children are:
    A. Aphasias due to focal lesions
    B. Childhood apraxia of speech
    C. Phonological disorders
    D. Specific language impairments
    E. Stuttering disorders

153. True or False: Less than 5% of children with a tic disorder have an isolated motor tic disorder.
    A. True
    B. False

154. Seizure disorder is common in ALL of the following pervasive developmental disorders, as described in DSM-IV or the literature, EXCEPT:
    A. Autistic disorder
    B. Asperger's disorder
    C. Rett's disorder
    D. Childhood disintegrative disorder
    E. Heller's syndrome

155. True or False: Individual psychodynamic therapy is most clearly indicated in cases where the patient's difficulties are the product of intrapsychic conflicts and the patient adheres to object representations that are developmentally regressive.
    A. True
    B. False

156. Which of the following models of classification assesses for disorders by way of continuous measurable characteristics of function or dysfunction?
    A. Dimensional
    B. Categorical
    C. Ideographic
    D. Archetypal

157. At what level do most researchers set the probability value (alpha) to reject the null hypothesis?
    A. 0.80
    B. 0
    C. -1 to 1
    D. 0.6 to 0.8
    E. 0.05

158. There is evidence that adolescents metabolize ALL of the following SSRIs faster than do adults EXCEPT:
     A. Fluvoxamine
     B. Sertraline
     C. Citalopram
     D. Paroxetine

159. Qualified speech–language pathologists are certified by which of the following organizations?
     A. American Psychiatric Association
     B. American Speech–Language Hearing Association
     C. American Academy of Child and Adolescent Psychiatry
     D. National Cued Speech Association
     E. National Autism Association

160. True or False: Prospective naturalistic studies of pediatric bipolar disorder have shown that 70% to 90% of youth will eventually recover (e.g., no significant symptoms for 2 months) from their index mood episode.
     A. True
     B. False

161. True or False: Section 504 refers to a section of the Individuals with Disabilities Education Act.
     A. True
     B. False

162. Which assessment instrument for delirium has been evaluated in children?
     A. Cognitive Test for Delirium
     B. Confusion Assessment Method
     C. Delirium Rating Scale
     D. Intensive Care Delirium Screening Checklist
     E. Delirium Detection Score

163. What is an assessment of a child's communication abilities in a natural setting by observing the child's spontaneous language use and understanding in familiar contexts called?
     A. Norm-referenced assessment
     B. Assessment of baseline function
     C. Authentic assessment
     D. Dynamic assessment
     E. Criterion-referenced assessment

164. True or False: Violence among youth is more likely to be a group phenomenon than the violence perpetrated by adults.
     A. True
     B. False

165. Randomized, controlled studies have shown the following medication to be effective in anorexia nervosa:
     A. Chlorpromazine
     B. Olanzapine
     C. Fluoxetine
     D. Cyproheptadine

166. True or False: All genes are active at the same time.
     A. True
     B. False

167. By 14 years of age, what percent of boys are enuretic at least once a week?
     A. 1%
     B. 5%
     C. 10%
     D. 15%
     E. 20%

168. Which TWO of the following people are considered the founders of child psycho-analysis?
  A. Donald Winnicott
  B. Melanie Klein
  C. Margaret Mahler
  D. Anna Freud
  E. Benjamin Spock

169. Which of the following large studies indicated that combined treatment of adolescent depression with fluoxetine and CBT had the highest rate of positive response (71%) compared with placebo or either treatment alone?
  A. POTS
  B. MTA Study
  C. TADS
  D. Children and Adolescents Anxiety Multimodal Treatment Study
  E. Research Units on Pediatric Psychopharmacology

170. According to the National Institute of Mental Health data which of the following is true of multidimensionally impaired children?
  A. Brief, transient episodes of psychosis and perceptual disturbance, typically in response to stress
  B. Nearly daily periods of emotional lability disproportionate to precipitants
  C. Impaired interpersonal skills despite desire to initiate social interactions
  D. Cognitive deficits, indicated by multiple deficits in information processing
  E. All of the above

171. True or False: A full diagnostic interview battery is difficult to complete when administered to an individual with an IQ much below 70.
  A. True
  B. False

172. According to the Structural School of Family Therapy the term psychosomatic families refers to families of patients with _____ and other psychosomatic disorders.
  A. Dysthymic disorder
  B. Childhood schizophrenia
  C. Anorexia nervosa
  D. Munchhausen syndrome by proxy
  E. Conduct disorder

173. True or False: Autism occurs more frequently in males than females, but females are more likely to show intellectual disability.
  A. True
  B. False

174. ALL of the following are components of McHugh and Slavney's four perspectives in psychiatric assessment and are used as an alternative to the biopsychosocial model for formulation EXCEPT:
  A. Disease
  B. Dimension
  C. Behavior
  D. Life story
  E. Social issues

175. Secure attachment has been associated longitudinally with ALL of the following attributes in the child EXCEPT:
  A. Development of social and emotional competence
  B. A sense of confidence and efficacy in novel or challenging situations
  C. A preoccupation with memories of parental treatment of the child
  D. Ability to manage stress

176. The Individuals with Disabilities Education Act recognizes ALL of the following categories under which a child can be identified as having a disability EXCEPT:
  A. Autism
  B. Emotional disturbance
  C. Inadequate educational experience
  D. Orthopedic impairment
  E. Visual impairment

177. True or False: Compared with adults, adolescents have a lower risk of dystonic reactions to conventional antipsychotic agents.
  A. True
  B. False

178. What treatment modality is an empirically supported treatment for procedure-related pain in pediatric patients?
  A. IPT
  B. Psychodynamic therapy
  C. CBT
  D. Reiki
  E. Meditation

179. Four categories of techniques are generally employed in the child psychiatric interview, which include engagement, projective, direct questioning, and interactive techniques. Which of the following describes the technique of engagement?
  A. Techniques to put the child at ease so that the child will provide accurate and meaningful clinical information
  B. Techniques to allow the child to reveal underlying themes or issues that the child may be unable to verbalize directly
  C. Techniques required to clarify particular points or to elicit specific information
  D. Techniques needed to clarify how the child relates to, as well as accepts or integrates, input from others

180. Estimates suggest that approximately what percentage of people with mental retardation have known "organic" causes, with known prenatal, perinatal, and postnatal insults?
  A. 10%
  B. 25%
  C. 50%
  D. 70%
  E. 85%

181. Which of the following SSRIs has the longest half-life?
  A. Sertraline
  B. Fluvoxamine
  C. Fluoxetine
  D. Citalopram
  E. Paroxetine

182. ALL of the following biological risk factors are associated with the development of disruptive behavior disorders EXCEPT?
  A. Male sex
  B. Parent–child conflict
  C. Low birth weight
  D. Antenatal and perinatal complications
  E. Brain injury

183. Which of the following statements is TRUE?
  A. For infants, sleep begins with an initial REM period
  B. In adults, REM sleep occupies about 20% of total sleep time
  C. In adults, sleep typically begins with nonrapid eye movement stage 4 sleep
  D. None of the above
  E. All of the above

184. Which of the following medications can decrease serum lithium levels?
A. Nonsteroidal anti-inflammatory drugs
B. Caffeine
C. Theophylline
D. Tetracyclines
E. B and C

185. Which of the following psychiatric disorders among maltreated children was found to be elevated in comparison to the general child psychiatric population?
A. Eating disorder
B. Substance abuse
C. Conduct disorder
D. Reactive attachment disorder
E. PTSD

186. Which TWO of the following factors result in greater clearance and shorter elimination half-life of lithium in children from 9 to 12 years of age?
A. Greater liver-to-body mass ratio
B. Increased glomerular filtration
C. More efficient CYP enzymes
D. Increased volume of distribution

187. True or False: Following the publication of Anna Freud's classic *The Ego and the Mechanisms of Defense*, a devoted effort to develop a comprehensive catalog of defensive mechanisms was begun but was never completed.
A. True
B. False

188. Which of the following is true of treatment studies of childhood onset schizophrenia?
A. There are no trials comparing atypical antipsychotics in this population
B. Two randomized controlled trials showed the superiority of atypical antipsychotics over placebo
C. Randomized controlled trials have shown the superiority of atypical antipsychotics over typical antipsychotics
D. A single trial in a small group of treatment refractory childhood onset schizophrenia patients demonstrated the efficacy of clozapine over risperidone
E. All of the above

189. What is the estimate for the prevalence of language difficulties in preschool children?
A. 1% to 6%
B. 7% to 15%
C. 16% to 23%
D. 24% to 31%
E. 32% to 42%

190. Beginning at about 4 months, an infant's responsive cooing, her growing repertoire of emotional responses, and her proclivity toward direct imitation of others' behaviors serve to facilitate what?
A. An increased attachment to her caregiver
B. A greater sense of her separation and individuality
C. Reciprocal and contingent social interactions
D. A greater awareness of her vocal, emotional, and social skills

191. A. Damien Martin has written that homosexuality is a normal variation in sexual orientation and behavior and that the prejudice faced by sexual minority is similar to prejudice faced by other minority groups, but it differs in a significant way:
A. Sexual minority youth are older when they first face prejudice
B. Sexual minority youth are younger when they first face prejudice
C. Sexual minority youth often have a different sexual orientation then their parents
D. Sexual minority youth are more successful in school than their peers
E. Sexual minority youth enter the work force at an earlier age

192. Which of the following terms describes the proportion of patients with an undesired consequence in the intervention group in comparison with the control group?
    A. Absolute risk reduction
    B. Number needed to treat
    C. Correlation, *r*
    D. Cohen's *d*
    E. Number needed to harm

193. True or False: The course of trichotillomania appears to be chronic.
    A. True
    B. False

194. Which of the following mood stabilizers has shown marked effects in reducing aggression and self-reported irritable mood in medication trials?
    A. Divalproex
    B. Lithium
    C. Carbamazepine
    D. Oxcarbazepine
    E. Lamotrigine

195. True or False: In their influential works regarding the best interests of the child in custody cases, Goldstein, Freud, and Solnit recommend that judges award shared custody to the divorcing parents.
    A. True
    B. False

196. When a patient is prescribed tricyclic antidepressants, a corrected QT interval (QTc) on electrocardiogram greater than which of the following would warrant a dose reduction followed by a repeat electrocardiogram?
    A. 150 ms
    B. 320 ms
    C. 420 ms
    D. 450 ms
    E. 500 ms

197. True or False: Fathers who are present at the birth of their child are more verbal about their babies and more intimately attached to them at follow-up.
    A. True
    B. False

198. Which of the following is FALSE regarding Williams syndrome?
    A. The disorder is characterized by distinct facial features
    B. Affected children have significant visual–spatial deficits
    C. Children with both Williams and Down syndrome share similar cognitive profiles
    D. The disorder is a result of the deletion of genes on chromosome 7
    E. Affected children demonstrate unusual musical abilities

199. Which of the following proposed brain circuit models accounts for OCD?
    A. Cortico-striato-thalamo-cortical circuit
    B. Cortico-nigro-striato-cortical circuit
    C. Mesocortico-limbic-mesocortical circuit
    D. Cortico-amygdalo-caudal-cortical circuit

200. The California Supreme Court case of *Tarasoff v. Board of Regents* ruled that a psychiatrist has a duty to protect an intended victim of a patient's threat of violence, if it is likely that such a threat would be carried out. This ruling occurred in which year?
    A. 1864
    B. 1915
    C. 1974
    D. 1983
    E. 1992

1. **Answer: A, D, and E.** Interpersonal psychotherapy was originally conceptualized as intervening in symptom formation and social functioning; it influences personality less because of its short duration. Page 820.

2. **Answer: C.** Page 241.

3. **Answer: B.** Gender identity is established by age 3. Sexual preference, however, is typically established during middle childhood. Page 268.

4. **Answer: C.** Interpersonal therapy has received empirical support of efficacy for depressed adolescents. Page 790.

5. **Answer: B.** The hyperactive subtype is more common; however, the symptoms related to hyperactivity tend to decrease with age. Page 433.

6. **Answer: D.** Approximately one-fourth of the young population in sub-Saharan Africa is infected. Page 89.

7. **Answer: B.** The mean length of sleep for high school students is 7.5 hours per night, much less than the 9.3 hours mean for children between the ages of 10 and 12. This reduced length of sleep time is accompanied by a sleep phase delay, with a tendency to fall asleep later and wake up later. The delay occurs due, in part, to later night-onset and later morning-termination of melatonin secretion. Page 282.

8. **Answer: D.** Up to 9% suffer from "extreme functional impairments" from psychiatric disorders. Page 23.

9. **Answer: D.** Remember also, many patients—or anyone, for that matter—know a friend or relative who was reassured about a symptom and later found to have serious physical disease. Page 639.

10. **Answer: B.** Page 617.

11. **Answer: B.** Behaviors resulting from attention deficit hyperactivity disorder (ADHD), conduct disorder, and oppositional defiant disorder, for example, represent externalizing symptoms; whereas anxiety and depression, for example, represent internalizing symptoms. Page 902.

12. **Answer: D.** The combined treatment group showed the most improvement at 59%. Page 779.

13. **Answer: A.** The sum of the data suggests this is true and seems to be associated most strongly with temporal lobe epilepsy. Early onset psychosis and lower intelligence quotient (IQ) is also associated with epilepsy. The concept of forced normalization was introduced by Landolt in the 1950s: patients with abnormal electroencephalographies (EEGs) who had their EEGs normalized with treatment were observed to develop psychopathology. Page 967.

14. **Answer: E.** This question emphasizes the critical analysis of test scores by listing pitfalls in comparing test scores: a full list with associated terms is found in a table in the Lewis textbook. Page 364.

15. **Answer: B.** Most children acquire the concepts of death between ages 5 and 7. Earlier studies that cited an older age had methodological limitations. Page 972.

16. **Answer: C.** Reliability is represented by the reliability coefficient, symbolized by the letter r with two identical subscripts and range from 0.00 (no association between scores) to 1.00 (perfect reliability). Page 360.

17. **Answer: B.** Acute otitis media (AOM) affects about two-thirds of the children in the age range of 6 to 24 months. AOM is very uncommon after the age of 6 years. About 45% of children with AOM have a middle ear effusion (MEE) 1 month after an episode of AOM and about 10% have MEE 3 months after an episode of AOM. When the MEE associated hearing loss is greater than 20 dB loss, the surgical insertion of pressure-equalization tubes is indicated. Page 67.

18. **Answer: E.** Page 891.

19. **Answer: D.** The Child and Adolescent Service System Program. The other answers are inventions, except for the donut. In 1984, the Child and Adolescent Service System Program was transformed into the Child and Adolescent Branch of the Center for Mental Health Services of the Substance Abuse and Mental Health Services Administration, which established the Comprehensive Community Mental Health Services for Children and Their Families Program. Got all that? This program has funded over 80 systems of care throughout the nation. Page 888.

20. **Answer: A.** Culture is the correct term. Pages 57–58.

21. **Answer: E.** Diffusion tensor imaging can demonstrate changes in contrast between tissues within minutes following an ischemic insult in comparison with conventional imaging, which shows changes only after many hours. Page 224.

22. **Answer: B.** This is true for adults learning a second language. If a child learns two languages, both will be represented in the same language center. This is an example of activity-dependent plasticity, where connections are shaped according to external input. Another example is the visual cortex, which requires visual stimuli for its proper development. Page 186.

23. **Answer: D.** Various levels of mental retardation (MR) are specified in the Diagnostic and Statistical Manual of Mental Disorders (DSM)-IV-TR: mild (IQ 50–70), moderate (IQ 35–49), severe (IQ 20–34), and profound (IQ < 20). Page 401.

24. **Answer: B.** This approach is wrong as the proportion of screened positives in a survey is made up of the sum of true positives and false positives, which is very different from the prevalence rate, which corresponds to the sum of true positives and false negatives. Pan laboratory screening and other testing approaches (e.g., electrocardiographies) that do not take into consideration factors such as sensitivity, specificity, positive predictive value, negative predictive value, rate of false negatives, rate of false positives, and other parameters can be problematic for the patient and leads to a poor allocation of resources. Page 163.

25. **Answer: B.** Page 545.

26. **Answer: A.** Page 807.

27. **Answer: B.** Page 483.

28. **Answer: A and C.** The other choices are common forms of standard scores. Page 314.

29. **Answer: C.** Adaptive behavior scales measure what the child actually does as opposed to what he or she is capable of doing in home, school, or the community. Page 367.

30. **Answer: C.** The first attempts at solid organ transplantation in children involved cardiac transplants for infants in the 1960s. The children died within a few days. Cyclosporine made possible the resistance to graft rejection. Page 939.

31. **Answer: A.** Page 192.

32. **Answer: D.** Page 443.

33. **Answer: A.** Page 529.

34. **Answer: E.** Children entering first grade (age 5–6) generally judge their peers by whether they are nice. Not until age 10 or 11 will a child judge peers on their qualities. Page 269.

35. **Answer: B.** Associational inferential statistics such as correlation and multiple regression are most likely used in associational research compared with the other statistics listed. Page 109.

36. **Answer: A.** Asperger's disorder is more common in males. Immediate family members have increased risk for depression and anxiety as well as significant social difficulties. Page 395.

37. **Answer: B.** Page 106.

38. **Answer: A.** The other options are inventions. Whether they have been considered is unknown. Genetic linkages, given enuresis can run in families, have been examined, as has urine osmolality, arginine vasopressin, circadian rhythms, arginine vasopressin at the receptor level, and sodium and potassium excretion. Page 657.

39. **Answer: B.** Pretend play begins around age 2. Page 263.

40. **Answer: B.** Page 119.

41. **Answer: A.** Page 345.

42. **Answer: B.** Conduct disorders are also a predictive factor. Page 44.

43. **Answer: A.** Page 844.

44. **Answer: D.** ADHD comorbidity is about ten times more common than expected; major depression comorbidity is about seven times more; and substance abuse comorbidity in adolescents is about four times more than expected. Page 456.

45. **Answer: E.** This observation along with its lack of significant results in pediatric depression provides strong caution against its routine use in pediatric psychopharmacology. Page 766.

46. **Answer: A.** Page 538.

47. **Answer: A.** The interviewer is likely to exaggerate positive affect. She may also feel disempowered and helpless, especially if the child is a user of sign language. Page 76.

48. **Answer: C.** Approximately half of affected individuals with neurofibromatosis also have an intellectual disability. The region of the gene that is mutated determines if the child develops cognitive deficits in addition to other clinical features (i.e., benign tumors). Page 202.

49. **Answer: A.** As there was greater understanding of the influence of the immediate environment and social institutions such as school, the parents' workplace, and mass media on the physical and mental health of children, this realization promoted a number of ecological studies assessing the effect of these environmental influences. Page 36.

50. **Answer: D.** The Isle of Wright surveys had key design characteristics that provided a model for surveys in the years following. Page 157.

51. **Answer: A.** Some states allow for billing under the DC:0-3R. Page 896.

52. **Answer: D.** Page 830.

53. **Answer: A.** Page 341.

54. **Answer: B.** Page 1007.

55. **Answer: A.** The choices are all bona fide infant/toddler assessments. Page 318.

56. **Answer: B.** There are approximately 7,000 child and adolescent psychiatrists, well below the estimated need of 20,000. Page 24.

57. **Answer: B.** Page 803.

58. **Answer: B.** The four presentations that were common in both Rosenberg's and Sheridan's reviews were seizures, apnea, diarrhea, and fevers, with apnea the most common presentation. Page 720.

59. **Answer: A.** Consultative delivery models afford the clinician an opportunity to observe the patient in a natural setting (e.g., the child care program), observe interactions with several peers, obtain information about the child's functioning from other adults in addition to the parents, and enlist the assistance of many adults in supporting treatment recommendations. Additionally, children often behave very differently at home versus their child care programs, where the degree of structure and behavioral expectations may vary considerably. Page 266.

60. **Answer: E.** Two-thirds of the 60% who no longer meet criteria recover, hence the 40% figure for recovery. Option C is a restatement of the first two options. Page 560.

61. **Answer: C.** Refer to Table 4.2.6.2. Page 378.

62. **Answer: B.** Zero-order kinetics occurs when metabolizing or eliminating mechanisms are exceeded or saturated. Paroxetine demonstrates zero-order kinetics at clinically relevant doses. Page 743.

63. **Answer: C.** The description in the question reflects a number of characteristics found in borderline personality disorder, including disturbance in self-perception, affective instability, chronic feelings of emptiness, and unstable intense personal relationships. Page 682.

64. **Answer: B.** This is the function of the superego. Page 828.

65. **Answer: C.** Although we may live in the postmodern age, the other answers are more specific to the challenges of the present-day physician, which has brought about renewed interest in medical ethics. Page 17.

66. **Answer: E.** Mental health interventions for children and families exposed to mass disaster should follow the five AREST principles, for which specific interventions will differ according to the particular characteristics of each country. AREST is Anticipate, Redifferentiate, Empower, Supervise and Assess, Treat and Follow-up. Page 731.

67. **Answer: B.** Conjugation is a Phase II reaction. Page 747.

68. **Answer: E.** Single use of cannabis can be detected for 1 to 3 days; moderate use for 3 to 5 days; and heavy use for 10 days or more. Page 619.

69. **Answer: A.** Exposure to paroxetine during the first trimester of pregnancy may increase the risk for congenital malformations, especially cardiac malformations. Page 763.

70. **Answer: D.** Page 635.

71. **Answer: D.** Children with reactive attachment disorder and autistic-like features have normal or small (not large) head circumference. Page 715.

72. **Answer: A.** Page 371.

73. **Answer: D.** Somewhat germane: Yale's inpatient unit for children under 16 years of age was able to reduce dramatically the use of restraints by adapting the Collaborative Problem Solving approach to care. Page 906.

74. **Answer: D.** This study by Caspi and colleagues was published in *Science* in 2002, titled, "Role of genotype in the cycle of violence in maltreated children." Page 294.

75. **Answer: E.** Page 439.

76. **Answer: B.** This Kagan and Fuller study observed the finding in a sample of 948 single mothers with young children. Page 38.

77. **Answer: E.** Page 768.

78. **Answer: B.** Sixty-two percent were homosexual, the rest were not rated or other; 12% showed persistent gender identity disorder. Page 677.

79. **Answer: E.** The model proposed by Chesler and Barbarin helps to organize issues across five domains of stress and coping (intellectual, practical, interpersonal, emotional, and existential). The examples above fit under intellectual considerations, except E, which refers to a practical consideration, another domain. Page 929.

80. **Answer: B.** Different etiological factors may result in similar conditions and the same etiological factor may be associated with a range of clinical conditions. Etiological factors are not generally included in diagnostic systems such as the DSM-IV. Page 303.

81. **Answer: A.** Children are generally placed with natural parents; however, this presumption is overcome by "clear and convincing evidence" that the best interests of the child require placement with a nonbiological parent. Page 1009.

82. **Answer: B.** Page 673.

83. **Answer: B.** The Multimodal Treatment Study of Children with ADHD provided convincing evidence of the long-term benefits of methylphenidate. Children were assigned to one of four treatment groups: medication management, behavioral treatment, combined medication and behavioral treatment, and community care. The combined treatment and medication management group did significantly better than the other two groups. Page 757.

84. **Answer: B.** It is preferable for the psychiatrist to accept a retainer, that is, payment up front, instead of a contingency fee, as the latter is an unethical practice. A retainer fee lessens the possibility of bias, whereas a contingency fee creates a vested financial interest in the outcome of the evaluation. Page 20.

85. **Answer: A.** A sleep debt develops as the adolescent stays up late each night then arises early for school, which leads to increased late morning awakenings and a shift in the body's timing mechanisms. Sufficient sleep, at least 9 to 10 hours each night in adolescence, is particularly important. Page 631.

86. **Answer: B.** Mentalization is the biologically prepared capacity to interpret the mental states that give behavior meaning and intentionality. Page 684.

87. **Answer: B.** There is evidence that these subtypes correlate with treatment response, neuroimaging results, neuropsychological function, and genetics. Page 550.

88. **Answer: E.** Page 915.

89. **Answer: A.** Presystemic clearance, or the first-pass effect, occurs in the intestinal and hepatic transporters through metabolism and conjugation. Page 745.

90. **Answer: C.** Some children go through a period of normal development, and then suddenly or gradually lose language skills in association with a seizure disorder. The affected child usually stops paying attention to speech, although audiological testing shows normal hearing; the child may stop talking, or regress in language ability, although nonverbal skills are preserved. The seizure disorder itself is often of unknown origin. This condition is known as Landau-Kleffner syndrome (LKS). Page 423.

91. **Answer: B.** A subpoena is a legal document that in most cases compels you to appear at a specified proceeding, produce documents, or both. It generally means that the recipient, you, has information that is relevant to a legal dispute involving other parties. Page 999.

92. **Answer: E.** Some of the factors are interrelated. There is a disincentive to recognize and treat mental health disorders when diagnosis and treatment are time consuming and tax one's skills, when reimbursement is low, and when there is a dearth of mental health clinicians for referrals. Page 924.

93. **Answer: D.** Page 845.

94. **Answer: D.** All the choices listed are various therapeutic strategies employed in interpersonal psychotherapy for depressed adolescents. Page 823.

95. **Answer: A.** Page 929.

96. **Answer: B.** Signs and symptoms of concern in autism, including language delay, social unrelatedness, or unusual environmental sensitivities, are typically observed within the first or second year of life. Page 388.

97. **Answer: E.** Elements of an evaluation include understanding the social supports available to the family; assessment of psychosocial stressors in the family, such as financial pressures or marital discord; and assessment of the family's understanding of the risks and benefits of the transplant. A developmental, social, educational, family, and past psychiatric history is indicated. Page 941.

98. **Answer: A.** Preschoolers often struggle to deal with separations because they are still learning coping skills. Older children have increased cognitive skills, more experience, and the ability to reassure themselves. Page 264.

99. **Answer: A.** Identification is the psychological process by which one individual becomes like another. Page 828.

100. **Answer: A.** Page 816.

101. **Answer: B.** The child is less likely to have internalizing or externalizing behaviors if the mother receives effective treatment. In prevention-minded treatment, traditional treatment is delivered to a patient but includes strategies that are designed to indirectly benefit other family members. Each of the answers reflects approaches that could be preventive. The correct answer has evidence behind it. Page 173.

102. **Answer: A.** Page 701.

103. **Answer: E.** All of the above except absence can be associated with severe MR. LKS represents language loss in children who were previously normally developing correlated with paroxysmal EEG changes in the speech centers. Behavioral and psychomotor disturbances can be present in the condition, and word deafness is a first sign. Audiograms, however, are normal. LKS can be mistaken for autism. Pages 963–964.

104. **Answer: B.** These are also called class II receptors, and the conformational change in the receptor is relayed to an associated G-protein that, in turn, regulates two major classes of molecules: ion channels and second messenger generating enzymes. Page 236.

105. **Answer: A.** Cyclosporine can cause frank psychotic symptoms, especially in high doses. Patients who undergo bone marrow transplants may be particularly susceptible. Cyclosporine is metabolized by the P450 system. Page 944.

106. **Answer: D.** Vulnerability and protective factors modify the negative effects of adverse life events; the latter modifies them in a positive direction. Page 293.

107. **Answer: B.** Several large, methodologically sound studies in aggregate have led to the conclusion that such an approach has no superior benefit. The reasons are thought to be several. In general, children and families served by the child welfare system have needs that outstrip those provided by intensive home-based family preservation programs that employ the crisis intervention model. Page 880.

108. **Answer: B.** John Locke's argument had far-reaching social and political influence, refuted notions of royal heredity, and influenced the political founders of the United States, who wrote in the Declaration of Independence that "all men are created equal." This argument emphasizes the influence of environment above that of heredity, and is an important example of the centuries old "nature versus nurture" debate. Page 11.

109. **Answer: A.** Children who make mastery-oriented attributions give credit to their own abilities when they succeed ("I'm great at math") but attribute failure to factors that are controllable ("I need to study harder."). Children with learned helplessness tend to attribute their failure to an innate lack of ability. Page 273.

110. **Answer: A.** Such thoughts horrify parents and may lead them to become extra protective in their caring. Page 976.

111. **Answer: D.** A pattern of bingeing or purging is not a diagnostic criterion for anorexia nervosa. Page 593.

112. **Answer: D.** Surviving childhood cancer is more likely than death. Angry parents and diversion of opiates can happen; however, the pursuit of alternative treatments falls under the category of nonadherence (if it is an alternative treatment that is harmful or replaces, rather than supports, best evidence care), which is the most common problem listed. Rapport and cultural understanding are keys to increasing adherence. Page 930.

113. **Answer: A.** The apparent decrease in parent–child conflict in middle adolescence coincides with decreased time spent with parents and a turn toward greater involvement with, and reliance on, peers. Despite the mutual stresses of increased conflict during adolescence, most parent–child relationships remain solid. Page 284.

114. **Answer: E.** Lamotrigine is well documented to cause skin rashes that are usually mild and seen within the first few months of treatment, but the risk for potentially fatal Stevens–Johnson syndrome is also present. Page 772.

115. **Answer: B.** After only 8 hours of fasting, there is an increased secretion of corticotropin-releasing hormone, which is a potent anorectic agent. This may be effective in assisting some with anorexia to continue their decreased calorie intake. Page 595.

116. **Answer: A.** This highly selective property of desipramine probably plays a role in its effectiveness in children with ADHD. This agent is not used often in children with ADHD because of its association with cardiovascular events in children and sudden death. Page 764.

117. **Answer: A.** Seventy-one percent achieve complete dryness without relapse. Page 661.

118–128. **Answers:** 118-F (Pages 216–217); 119-B (Page 217); 120-J (Page 217); 121-H (Page 218); 122-A (Page 219); 123-E (Page 221); 124-C (Page 223); 125-I (Page 225); 126-K (Page 227); 127-G (Page 228); 128-D (Page 229).

129. **Answer: A.** Page 141.

130. **Answer: E.** The secretion of growth hormone, which normally occurs during stage 4 nonrapid eye movement sleep, may be affected by multiple awakenings. Page 629.

131. **Answer: E.** Residential care for children with borderline personality disorder has little empirical support but can accomplish the aforementioned goals. Page 688.

132. **Answer: E.** This question points out the challenge in determining the presence of posttraumatic stress disorder (PTSD) among the differential of comorbid diagnoses. Page 705.

133. **Answer: A.** Child and adolescent psychiatry experience is not required. Pediatric residency programs must have 1 month, as well as other integrated training experiences, in developmental–behavioral pediatrics. Page 924.

134. **Answer: C.** Long question meant to convey information about basic, posttranscriptional, and regulatory mechanisms for RNA. Another regulatory mechanism involves the addition of long stretches of adenine nucleotides, the poly(A) tail, to the mRNA messenger prior to being shuttled out of the nucleus. Page 181.

135. **Answer: C.** Blood injection. The options are listed to help you remember the five types. Evolutionary theorists speculate that the five types correspond to evolutionary dangers and have become embedded in the genetic code, hence their irrationality. Page 541.

136. **Answer: C.** Attachment theory was developed by John Bowlby and refined in collaboration with Mary Ainsworth and others. Page 711.

137. **Answer: E.** For the time being, drug treatment for adolescent obesity is at an experimental stage and only off-label prescribing of the currently available antiobesity drugs (sibutramine and orlistat) is possible. Page 611.

138. **Answer: C.** When the environment cannot sufficiently compensate or cannot nurture a child with his or her unique needs or difficulties, these factors can combine to produce a pattern of maladjustment that over time can lead to psychopathology. Page 252.

139. **Answer: D.** Page 860.

140. **Answer: C.** The greatest risk is 6 months to 1 year after discharge. Page 532.

141. **Answer: B.** Page 620.

142. **Answer: A.** Studies have indicated information processing theories of human intelligence may play a role in the next generation of developmental assessment instruments; however, at present they are difficult to administer under normal clinical conditions. Page 311.

143. **Answer: A.** Case–control studies are particularly indicated for rare diseases. Page 153.

144. **Answer: D.** A or C may be accurate at times, but the correct answer is D. For example, if a child is on life support, the team should inform the parents the child has died and invite input from the family members about whether they would like to be present when life support is removed and their preferences on timing. One must avoid leading the family to think they are being asked whether they think treatment is likely to be effective or whether or not they "wish to allow their child to die." Page 977.

145. **Answer: B.** Several approaches in the genetic study of Tourette's syndrome (TS) have indicated that one single gene is not responsible for the phenotype of TS. The concordance rate for TS in monozygotic twins is closer to 50% and increases to 77% if chronic motor tic disorders are included. Page 573.

146. **Answer: B.** Aripiprazole binds with presynaptic dopamine receptors, which is purported to turn down the dopamine system in brain regions with increased dopaminergic tone. Page 776.

147. **Answer: B.** Studies have shown that the Apgar test is an inconsistent predictor of subsequent infant development. Page 316.

148. **Answer: B.** Valproate also decreases N-methyl-D-aspartate induced currents and inhibits sodium influx in neurons. Page 771.

149. **Answer: D.** The study compromised just fewer than 6,000 individuals ages 15 to 54. Page 702.

150. **Answer: D.** Except as mediated by MR, there are no known genetic factors in the etiology of pica. Page 584

151. **Answer: E.** Page 669.

152. **Answer: C.** Phonological disorders are the most prevalent type of communication problem. Six percent of school age children have phonological disorders, and the prevalence is higher for preschoolers, with estimates ranging from 10% to 15%. Page 424.

153. **Answer: B.** Most children with a tic disorder have only motor tics. Less than 5% of children with a tic disorder have isolated phonic tic disorder. Page 571.

154. **Answer: B.** Seizure disorder is common in all pervasive developmental disorders except Asperger's disorder and pervasive developmental disorder, not otherwise specified. Heller first described Childhood Disintegrative Disorder. Page 391.

155. **Answer: A.** Page 832.

156. **Answer: A.** Unlike the categorical classification which views disorders as dichotomous, the dimensional approach to classification relies on the assessment of dimensions of function or dysfunction by reducing phenomena to various dimensions along which a child can be placed. For example, consider Axis V, the Global Assessment of Functioning. Page 305.

157. **Answer: E.** Page 115.

158. **Answer: A.** What this finding means is that adolescents (as a general demographic) need higher doses than typical adult doses for sertraline, citalopram, and paroxetine because they can metabolize these medications faster. Page 506.

159. **Answer: B.** Speech–language pathologists are usually licensed by their state as well. Page 371.

160. **Answer: A.** For patients who have recovered, 80% will experience one or more recurrences in a period of 2 to 5 years. Page 518.

161. **Answer: B.** Section 504 of the Rehabilitation Act, which ensures that all children receive a free and appropriate public education, is more closely related to the American Disabilities Act. The American Disabilities Act prohibits the denial of educational services to students with disabilities. Schools can generate an accommodation plan for such a student called a 504 Plan. Students with more severe disorders have safeguards under the Individuals with Disabilities Education Act (IDEA). Roughly, 504 Plans allow accommodations so that students with disabilities can access their education, whereas IDEA mandates specialized instruction and related services if necessary to meet students' unique needs. Each child under IDEA has an IEP (Individualized Education Plan) with parental input and consent and due process guarantees. Page 984.

162. **Answer: C.** It is composed of 10 items. Page 649.

163. **Answer: C.** Page 374.

164. **Answer: A.** When compared to adult crime, crimes committed by juveniles are more likely to involve more than one assailant. Page 468.

165. **Answer: D.** Cyproheptadine. Although there have been studies that suggest the efficacy of all these medications in anorexia nervosa, only cyproheptadine has had several double-blind studies that show it to be effective, especially in high doses, up to 24 mg per day, in facilitating weight gain and reducing depressive symptomatology. Page 598.

166. **Answer: B.** Differences in the pattern of expression of genes over the life span are responsible for the physical and cognitive functioning of individual organisms from Drosophila to humans. For example, the hemoglobin genes active during fetal life are different from those that are active in adulthood. Page 178.

167. **Answer.** A. Page 655.

168. **Answer: B and D.** Klein coined the term "play analysis," and Anna Freud studied the ego mechanisms of defense. Page 827.

169. **Answer: C.** The Treatment for Adolescents with Depression Study randomly assigned 439 adolescents, ages 12 to 17, in four groups: fluoxetine alone, cognitive-behavioral therapy alone, combination treatment, or pill placebo. However, combined treatment was not significantly better than medication only, and cognitive-behavioral therapy alone was not superior to placebo. Page 757.

170. **Answer: E.** All of the above statements are true. Page 494.

171. **Answer: A.** Page 353.

172. **Answer: C.** Page 855.

173. **Answer: A.** Gender ratio in a review by Fombonne was 4.3:1, male to female; however, the ratio is variable with associated cognitive disability, which occurs more frequently in females with autism. Page 386.

174. **Answer: E.** Table 4.2.6.4 is particularly helpful in understanding the four perspectives. Page 380.

175. **Answer: C.** Preoccupation over memories of the parent, specifically negative ones, is not indicative of a secure attachment. Page 254.

176. **Answer: C.** As per these exclusionary criteria, a child cannot be diagnosed with a learning disability unless other factors such as other disorders or lack of exposure to high quality and age, language, and culture appropriate educational environments have been ruled out. All of the other categories are recognized by IDEA under which a child can be identified as having a disability. Page 411.

177. **Answer: B.** Page 742.

178. **Answer: C.** Page 916.

179. **Answer: A.** Page 338.

180. **Answer: C.** Estimates suggest that approximately one-half of people with MR have known organic causes. Page 405.

181. **Answer: C.** Fluoxetine's half-life is estimated at 48 to 72 hours. In addition, fluoxetine has an active metabolite, norfluoxetine, with an elimination half-life of 7 to 14 days. Citalopram has the second longest half-life at 33 hours. Page 763.

182. **Answer: B.** Although parent–child conflict is a family risk factor that is related to disruptive behavior disorders, it is not a biological risk factor. Page 459.

183. **Answer: E.** By 6 months of age, the specific EEG waveforms that are used to subclassify the four stages of nonrapid eye movement sleep have emerged. Page 625.

184. **Answer: E.** Caffeine and theophylline promote lithium excretion via the kidneys. Page 769.

185. **Answer: E.** Compared with community controls, maltreated children have elevated externalizing and internalizing behavior problems according to parent and teacher report. They also have increased rates of PTSD; depression diagnoses; reactive attachment disorder; dissociative symptoms; self-destructive behavior and borderline traits; sexually inappropriate behaviors; drug- and alcohol-related problems; eating disorders; oppositional defiant disorder, and conduct disorder. When compared with psychiatric controls, however, elevated rates of externalizing and internalizing problems and most psychiatric disorders, with the exception of PTSD, have not been found. Page 694.

186. **Answer: B and D.** Increased body water in children results in an increased volume of distribution (V_d). Changes in tubular reabsorption also appear to be a factor. Page 749.

187. **Answer: A.** After pursuing the goal of an exhaustive list of defenses, the conclusion was reached via clinical observation that any aspect of ego functioning may be used in the service of defense so the attempt to delineate a comprehensive list of specific mechanisms was impossible and too reductionistic. Page 829.

188. **Answer: A.** There is only a narrow evidence base to guide treatment for childhood onset schizophrenia (COS). There are no trials comparing atypical antipsychotics in this population. Two randomized controlled trials have established the superiority of typical antipsychotics over placebo in COS. A single trial in a small group of treatment refractory COS patients demonstrated the efficacy of clozapine over haloperidol. Page 500.

189. **Answer: B.** Page 419.

190. **Answer: C.** The period between 2 and 7 months is marked by an increase in social reciprocity between infant and caregiver, which follows from an increased awareness of the world and motor development. Page 257.

191. **Answer: C.** Sexual minority youth are not able to use positive identification with their parents' sexual orientation to help them navigate this issue for themselves. Page 83.

192. **Answer: E.** The number needed to harm is a useful measure of the frequency of undesired consequences resulting from a treatment. Page 128.

193. **Answer: A.** Page 567.

194. **Answer: A.** Lithium, on the contrary, has shown mixed results. Page 476.

195. **Answer: B.** They recommend awarding full custody to the "psychological parent." However, there is controversy regarding this recommendation. Page 40.

196. **Answer: D.** Also, a QRS complex longer than 120 ms or a PR interval greater than 200 ms warrants a dose reduction followed by a repeat ECG. Page 764.

197. **Answer: A.** This question touches on the powerful and long-term impact of the father's experience of witnessing his child's birth. Page 7.

198. **Answer: C.** Williams syndrome is a rare genetic disorder (1 per 20,000 live births) caused by a deletion on chromosome 7. The disorder is characterized by distinct facial features, a variable degree of MR, cardiovascular disease, and a very distinct cognitive profile (with prominent visual–spatial deficits). Affected children are unable to integrate the parts of a picture into a whole pattern. They do, however, exhibit strengths in other cognitive areas such as verbal skills (normal quality of vocabulary, auditory memory, and social use of language). Many patients also have talent for singing or playing musical instruments. Pages 207–208.

199. **Answer: A.** It posits the existence of somatotopically organized connections between distant brain structures arranged into cortico-striato-thalamo-cortical circuits that subserve planning, execution, and termination of voluntary movements. Page 556.

200. **Answer: C.** Page 147.

Questions

1. The kappa statistic is commonly used to assess agreement across raters. Values above what number are considered to represent high levels of agreement?
   A. 0.005
   B. 0.60
   C. 0.01
   D. 0.75
   E. 1.0

2. Four categories of techniques are generally employed in the child psychiatric interview, which include engagement, projective, direct questioning, and interactive techniques. Which of the following describes projective techniques?
   A. Techniques to put the child at ease so that the child will provide accurate and meaningful clinical information
   B. Techniques to allow the child to reveal underlying themes or issues that the child may be unable to verbalize directly
   C. Techniques to clarify particular points or to elicit specific information
   D. Techniques to clarify how the child relates to as well as accepts or integrates input from others

3. A 4-year-old boy displays extreme sadness and distress when he must say good-bye to his preschool teacher at the end of the school year. Which of the following would be most helpful in the transition?
   A. Introducing the boy to his next, new teacher right away
   B. Visiting with the preschool teacher after the farewell
   C. Preventing any further contact between the boy and his teacher in the future
   D. Telling the boy that his teacher left because of his bad behavior
   E. Reassuring the boy that he will have many teachers in the future

4. True or False: Psychiatric disorders such as schizophrenia, bipolar disorder and Tourette's syndrome (TS) appear to exhibit mendelian patterns of inheritance.
   A. True
   B. False

5. Which of the following is NOT one of the diagnostic criteria for gender identity disorder (GID)?
   A. A strong and persistent cross-gender identification
   B. Persistent discomfort with his or her sex preference
   C. The disturbance is not concurrent with a physical intersex condition
   D. The disturbance causes clinically significant distress and impairment in social, occupational, or other important areas of functioning

6. In the treatment of selective mutism, introducing the child gradually and systematically into situations in which the child already speaks is an example of:
   A. Prompting
   B. Shaping
   C. Situational fading
   D. Individual fading
   E. Backwards chaining

7. In which part of the brain are about half of all noradrenergic neurons located?
   A. Substantia nigra
   B. Locus coeruleus
   C. Hippocampus
   D. Amygdala
   E. Thalamus

8. A developmental pediatrician is asked to evaluate a 24-month-old girl referred for regression in development. Her parents describe normal prenatal and perinatal development before recent loss of purposeful hand movements. DNA analysis is likely to reveal?
   A. Deletion on chromosome 15
   B. Disruption at the "fragile" site on the X chromosome
   C. Mutation in the LIS-1 gene
   D. Deletion on chromosome 7
   E. MeCP2 gene mutation

9. The 5-year training program in pediatrics, general psychiatry, and child and adolescent psychiatry, better known as the "Triple Board" began as a pilot training experiment in which year?
   A. 1946
   B. 1964
   C. 1985
   D. 1992
   E. 2000

10. Which of the following marks the start of adolescence?
    A. Gonadarche
    B. Adrenarche
    C. High school
    D. Breast development

11. Which of the following statements is TRUE?
    A. By age 2, many children with autism show clear repetitive behaviors
    B. By school age, many children with autism become more socially responsive
    C. Language skills of children with autism never improve
    D. Early intervention studies show no improvement in independent functioning
    E. Two-thirds of adults with autism achieve independence

12. In a survey of 785 adolescent and adult females, which ethnic group had the highest rate of anorexia nervosa?
    A. Asian-Americans
    B. African-Americans
    C. European-Americans
    D. Latino-Americans
    E. None, they were all found to be within the mean

13. What is the lifetime prevalence of bipolar disorder in the offspring of parents with bipolar disorder?
    A. 5% to 15%
    B. 15% to 25%
    C. 20% to 35%
    D. 35% to 50%
    E. Over 50%

14. In McHugh and Slavney's four perspectives in psychiatric assessment that serves as an alternative to the biopsychosocial approach to formulation, which component addresses "what a patient is"?
    A. Disease
    B. Dimension
    C. Behavior
    D. Life story

15. In the study of sexual orientation, what part of the brain, in both animals and humans, has received particular interest?
    A. Hypothalamus
    B. Caudate nucleus
    C. Medulla
    D. Mamillary bodies
    E. Hippocampus

16. Which of the following elements compose psychic reality?
    A. Thoughts
    B. Feelings
    C. Fantasies
    D. Perceptions of the external world
    E. All of the above

17. Each of these is a model for psychiatric consultation to pediatrics EXCEPT:
    A. Resource consultation
    B. Process-educative consultation
    C. Collaborative team
    D. Family systems consultation
    E. Administrative

18. True or False: Video surveillance of the mother and the child in the hospital has proved to be helpful in diagnosing Munchhausen syndrome by proxy.
    A. True
    B. False

19. True or False: According to International Classification of Diseases (ICD)-10, conduct disorder is not diagnosed if attention deficit hyperactivity disorder (ADHD) symptoms are present.
    A. True
    B. False

20. ALL of the following may be a medical consequence of taking anabolic steroids EXCEPT:
    A. Premature growth stoppage
    B. Mood swings
    C. Psychosis
    D. Development of male sexual characteristics in women
    E. Enlarged testicles

21. When is the best time to begin discussing with a child that he or she was adopted?
    A. When they are in late elementary school
    B. When they are preadolescent
    C. When they are adolescent
    D. When they ask whether they are adopted
    E. Early in life

22. True or False: It is not unethical to use human subjects as a means to accomplish goals of research.
    A. True
    B. False

23. Posttraumatic stress disorder (PTSD) symptoms in children are more likely to occur when there are additional stressors after the traumatic event including ALL of the following EXCEPT:
    A. Dislocation
    B. Reexperiencing
    C. Loss
    D. Separation from significant caregivers

24. In interpersonal psychotherapy for depressed adolescents (IPT-A), just as in the adult version (IPT), there are four identified problem areas upon which the therapy can focus. These four areas include ALL of the following EXCEPT:
    A. Conduct issues
    B. Grief
    C. Interpersonal disputes
    D. Role transitions
    E. Interpersonal deficits

25. In any given year, how many children under 15 will have epilepsy?
    A. One in 100
    B. One in 200
    C. One in 300
    D. One in 500
    E. One in 1,000

26. Which of the following sources is the BEST option for a forensic psychiatrist seeking ethical guidelines for a forensic evaluation?
    A. American Academy of Child & Adolescent Psychiatry
    B. American Academy of Psychiatry and the Law
    C. American Psychiatric Association
    D. Local and state statutes
    E. None of the above

27. Which of the following is NOT TRUE of children with childhood onset schizophrenia?
    A. Higher rates of early language impairment
    B. Higher rates of early social abnormalities
    C. Higher rates of early motor abnormalities
    D. Higher rates of cardiac abnormalities
    E. All of the above

28. At higher doses, venlafaxine can be associated with the risk of which side effect in a dose-dependent relationship?
    A. Urinary retention
    B. QTc lengthening
    C. Seizures
    D. Diastolic hypertension
    E. Systolic hypertension

29. Acute depression, intense anger, anxiety about future relationships, and social withdrawal can be characteristic of which group experiencing parental divorce?
    A. Preschool children
    B. Middle-school children
    C. Adolescents
    D. Boys
    E. Girls

30. Children acquire skills best when:
    A. They are under stress or trauma
    B. Teachers have few expectations
    C. Caregivers present them with tasks that are slightly too difficult to accomplish independently
    D. No adult assistance is available

31. Multisystemic therapy, and the home-based service model within which it is delivered, differs from intensive, home-based family preservation programs that employ the crisis intervention model in several ways. These differences include:
    A. Individual treatment of each family member
    B. Master's level clinicians supervised by doctoral-level clinicians
    C. An assigned family aid who is from the same community as the family
    D. Flexibility of theoretical framework
    E. Inflexibility of treatment framework

32. In defining the clinical skills essential for infant assessment, three techniques are central. Which of the following is NOT one of the techniques?
    A. Basic psychometric statistics
    B. Interviewing skills
    C. Observation of children and caregiver–child interactions
    D. Synthesis of the information gathered during the evaluation

33. A child with deafness is likely to experience delays in ALL of the following areas EXCEPT:
    A. Cognitive/academic
    B. Social
    C. Emotional
    D. Gross motor
    E. Language

34. Which of the following is a side effect of FK506, an immunosuppressant?
    A. Delirium
    B. Akinetic mutism
    C. Seizure
    D. Auditory hallucinations
    E. All of the above

35. Which of the following is most likely to be a direct prevention-minded treatment?
    A. Family therapy
    B. Couples therapy
    C. Individual therapy
    D. Group therapy

36. A survey conducted by the National Association of State Fire Marshals in the late 1990s determined that children were responsible for roughly how many fires set annually?
    A. 1,000
    B. 5,000
    C. 10,000
    D. 25,000
    E. 100,000

37. True or False: According to available evidence, group cognitive-behavioral therapy (CBT) involving other family members is as effective as individual CBT.
    A. True
    B. False

38. As a child psychiatrist, when you receive a subpoena you should provide any documents requested:
    A. If the patient (or guardian) who holds the privilege to the health information has consented to its release
    B. If there is a court order to release the information
    C. As soon as possible, as a court order is presumed in the subpoena
    D. After consulting with your attorney
    E. A or B

39. True or False: In the group of individuals with mental retardation who have no known "organic" cause, disproportionately more persons are poor, from minority backgrounds, and of low intelligence quotient (IQ) parents.
    A. True
    B. False

40. True or False: In middle and high school students with ADHD, the inattentive subtype is more common.
    A. True
    B. False

41. True or False: Boys with gender identity disorder (GID) seem to have an aversion for rough and tumble play.
    A. True
    B. False

42. Drummond conducted the first systematic follow-up of girls with GID, evaluating 25 girls with a mean age of 8.8 years with a follow-up mean of 23.2 years. What conclusion was found?
    A. 3 had persistent GID
    B. 6 had persistent GID
    C. 9 had persistent GID
    D. 12 had persistent GID
    E. 15 had persistent GID

43. In contrast to the more clinically oriented, categorical approach, multivariate or dimensional approaches to diagnosis offer ALL of the following advantages in the diagnosis of children and adolescents EXCEPT:
    A. They assess various behaviors and dimensions of behavior rather than single pathognomonic features
    B. They consider a dichotomous understanding of psychopathology
    C. They encompass symptom coding in other than a dichotomous fashion
    D. They utilize various rating scales and checklists based on self, parent, and teacher reports, or direct observation

44. ALL of these situations represent the potential establishment of a doctor–patient relationship with its ensuing fiduciary and legal obligations EXCEPT:
    A. Responding to a nonpatient's e-mail with therapeutic advice
    B. Therapeutic advice given to an acquaintance at a dinner party
    C. Responding to a prospective patient's e-mail with a referral to someone in the patient's geographic area
    D. Working with the parents of a child in separate sessions without the child
    E. Setting up of an appointment with a prospective patient, whom you have never seen, by the office staff for an initial evaluation

45. The Brazelton Neonatal Behavioral Assessment Scale, second edition, a neonatal assessment test, is intended to assess ALL of the following capacities in the neonate EXCEPT:
    A. Neurobehavioral organization
    B. Adjustment to the *ex utero* environment
    C. Whether the neonate can be weaned from supplemental oxygen
    D. Ability to respond to the stress of labor and delivery

46. Prior to initiating a trial of lithium, a child may warrant which of the following?
    A. Physical examination
    B. Complete blood cell count
    C. Electrolyte levels
    D. Blood urea nitrogen level
    E. All of the above

47. How does parental education relate to children's school achievement?
    A. Directly, through parents' drive to succeed
    B. Directly, through parental evaluation of the teaching environment
    C. Indirectly, though reading and providing a warm and supportive environment
    D. Indirectly, through parental knowledge of discipline
    E. Parental education is not related to children's school achievement

48. Which of the following statistics would most likely be used in a randomized experimental study?
    A. Histogram
    B. Correlation
    C. Analysis of variance
    D. Frequency distribution
    E. Multiple regression

49. True or False: Fluoxetine has a metabolite that is psychoactive.
    A. True
    B. False

50. The concerns of young children about privacy are quite different from older children and adolescents. Which TWO of the following notions of privacy are the first to develop in young children?
    A. Informational privacy
    B. Territorial privacy
    C. Possessional privacy
    D. Clique privacy

51. The direct and indirect cost of mental illness for the total population of the United States was estimated in 1996 to be what amount?
    A. $350 million
    B. $2 billion
    C. $780 million
    D. $150 billion
    E. $12 billion

52. ALL of the following should be considered when a child presents with enuresis EXCEPT:
    A. Urinary tract infection
    B. Constipation
    C. Bladder physiology
    D. Thyroid-stimulating hormone between 0.5 and 3.5 mIU/L

53. The period of the day that is the time of greatest risk for youth-on-youth violence during weekdays occurs between:
    A. Early morning and the start of school
    B. After midnight and early morning
    C. After dinner and before midnight
    D. End of the school day and early evening

54. Which of the following statements likely represents the better approach to managing an aggressive patient in the emergency room?
    A. Firmly but gently say: "You are here for a psychiatric evaluation and you will not leave until it is completed"
    B. "You have been here a while, would you like something to eat or drink?"
    C. "You will not use vulgar language here"
    D. "You have to calm down"
    E. "Have you thought about what your mother goes through?"

55. According to the Diagnostic and Statistical Manual of Mental Disorders (DSM)-IV-TR, a person with a diagnosis of mild mental retardation would have which of the following?
    A. IQ of 85
    B. IQ of 75
    C. IQ of 60
    D. IQ of 45
    E. IQ of 30

56. True or False: There have been two randomized, placebo-controlled trials for selective serotonin reuptake inhibitors in the treatment of trichotillomania. At least one trial demonstrated significant improvement over placebo.
    A. True
    B. False

In the following questions, match the defenses commonly exhibited by children in psychodynamic therapy with their appropriate descriptions.

57. Denial

58. Displacement

59. Externalization

60. Reaction formation

61. Repression

62. Suppression

63. Somatization

64. Turning passive to active
   A. The exclusion of unacceptable ideas, fantasies, affects, or impulses from consciousness
   B. The attribution of internal conflicts to the external environment and a search for external solutions
   C. The management of affects and impulses stirred by a passive experience with an active, more powerful "other" by playing out in action or story the active "other's" role; this includes the process of identification with the aggressor
   D. The transfer of tension from drives or affects into disturbances of bodily functions or rhythms
   E. The disavowal of intolerable external reality factors or the disavowal of thoughts, feelings, wishes, or needs that is apparent to an observer
   F. The conscious effort to control and conceal unacceptable impulses; the exception to the rule that defenses are unconscious processes
   G. The transfer of emotions, ideas, or wishes from the original object to a more acceptable substitute
   H. The adoption of affects, ideas, or behaviors that are the opposites of impulses harbored either consciously or unconsciously

65. The diagnostic criteria for bulimia include ALL of the following EXCEPT:
   A. Recurrent episodes of binge eating
   B. A body mass index <3rd percentile
   C. Recurrent inappropriate compensatory behavior to prevent weight gain, such as self-induced vomiting; misuse of laxatives, diuretics, or other medications; fasting; excessive exercise
   D. These symptoms occur at least twice a week on average and persist for at least 3 months
   E. The disturbance does not occur exclusively during episodes of anorexia nervosa

66. When a credible and appropriate referral to mental health services is offered by a pediatrician, how many families follow-up with a mental health clinician?
   A. Three-quarters
   B. Half
   C. Less than half
   D. Nearly all
   E. Nearly none

67. The first structured parent-report diagnostic interview specifically designed for preschool-age children became available in which year?
   A. 1919
   B. 1959
   C. 1978
   D. 1992
   E. 2000

68. Which edition of the DSM officially introduced the category of conduct disorder?
   A. DSM-I
   B. DSM-II
   C. DSM-III
   D. DSM-IV
   E. DSM-IV-TR

69. True or False: Boys have greater innate capability for mathematics than girls do.
   A. True
   B. False

70. True or False: Medically unexplained physical symptoms and complaints are exceptionally common in children and adolescents.
   A. True
   B. False

71. There are approximately 7,000 child and adolescent psychiatrists in the United States. What is the estimated number of psychiatrists needed to provide care for seriously psychiatrically ill children and youth?
    A. 35,000
    B. 30,000
    C. 20,000
    D. 15,000
    E. 5,000

72. "I will never lose any weight because I just ate a cookie" is an example of which of the following cognitive errors:
    A. Catastrophizing
    B. Overgeneralization
    C. Arbitrary inference
    D. Absolutism
    E. Personalization

73. ALL of the following individual risk factors are associated with the development of disruptive behavior disorders EXCEPT:
    A. Depression
    B. Below average IQ
    C. Difficult temperament
    D. Reading problems
    E. Language impairment

74. Which of the following represents a well-known epidemiological survey in the United States?
    A. The Blue Ridge Mountain Surveys
    B. The Great Plains Surveys
    C. The California Coast Surveys
    D. The Mid-Atlantic Surveys
    E. The Great Smoky Mountains Surveys

75. ALL of these are generally sound principles in the management of functional somatic symptoms EXCEPT:
    A. When the diagnostic formulation is clear it should be discussed frankly with the patient and family together
    B. Once the diagnosis is made additional medical workup should be avoided in the absence of new information or change in clinical status
    C. Do not emphasize that functional somatic symptoms are reactions to adversity and stress
    D. The judicious use of placebo treatment can help limit doctor shopping
    E. Avoid communicating any sense of unease about the diagnosis

76. Which of the following statements is TRUE regarding disorders of communication?
    A. A speech disorder is a disruption in oral communication, whereas a language disorder is a disruption in written communication
    B. Delays in language development are the least common presenting symptom in preschool children
    C. The prevalence estimate of language difficulty is higher for boys than for girls
    D. The prevalence of primary language disorders is higher in school age than in preschool children
    E. There are several biological markers of specific-language impairments (SLI) that have been identified

77. Trichotillomania was a term first coined:
    A. In 2000 BC
    B. In 50 BC
    C. In the 17th century
    D. In the late 19th century
    E. In 1956

78. True or False: Sleepwalkers are able to perform complex behaviors, such as leaving the house and taking a drive.
    A. True
    B. False

79. True or False: A screening measure in speech and language evaluation should focus one area of concern.
    A. True
    B. False

80. True or False: In infant assessments, age equivalent scores represent an estimate of the chronological age at which the typically developing infant would demonstrate the skills being assessed.
    A. True
    B. False

81. True or False: One major focus in resilience research is to identify vulnerability and protective factors that modify the negative effects of adverse life circumstances.
    A. True
    B. False

82. A clinical interview in which the questions are prespecified and the presence or absence of psychopathology lies with the person being interviewed is called what?
    A. Semistructured interview
    B. Fully structured interview
    C. Respondent-based interview
    D. Interviewer-based interview
    E. Glossary-based interview

83. True or False: In order for the diagnosis of PTSD to be given, there must be one symptom involving reexperiencing the traumatic event.
    A. True
    B. False

84. An assessment of factors, supports, or modifications enhancing a child's performance in communication is called what?
    A. Norm-referenced assessment
    B. Assessment of baseline function
    C. Authentic assessment
    D. Dynamic assessment
    E. Criterion-referenced assessment

85. Which of the following is a Phase II metabolic reaction involved in the biotransformation of drugs?
    A. Hydroxylation
    B. Conjugation
    C. Reduction
    D. Hydrolysis

86. A brain state elicited by a threat, a stimulus for which an organism will extend effort to avoid, is called:
    A. Fear
    B. Anxiety
    C. Reverberating limbic loop
    D. Reverberating amygdala loop

87. Which of the following describes variables related to peer relations?
    A. Secure attachment relationships have not been associated with higher levels of social competence
    B. Parental provision of peer play opportunities is associated with more positive peer relationships
    C. Peer-interaction skills are not related to the child's ability to regulate his individual temperament
    D. None of the above
    E. A to C

88. Which of the following treatment programs has significant empirical support as a behavioral and family systems approach for juvenile offenders?
    A. Multisystemic therapy
    B. IPT
    C. Electroconvulsive therapy
    D. Dialectical-behavior therapy
    E. CBT

89. What distinguishes obsessive–compulsive disorder (OCD) in children from other psychiatric diagnoses?
    A. Children are not that ill
    B. Academic achievement is often preserved
    C. Peer relationships are not affected
    D. Parents are quick to seek treatment
    E. There is limited genetic transmission

90. True or False: Synapses change shape as learning proceeds.
    A. True
    B. False

91. True or False: In comparison with positron emission tomography, single photon emission computed tomography can detect slower kinetic processes in the body because of the longer half-life of its tracers.
    A. True
    B. False

92. In psychoanalytic thought, the therapist is considered a model for the child's development of the capacity for self-observation as the therapist acts as an interested and thoughtful observer. Which of the following describes this concept?
    A. Transference
    B. Observing ego
    C. Mechanisms of defense
    D. Internalization
    E. Ego ideal

93. Which TWO of the following choices are the major reasons why IPT has been adapted for work with IPT-A?
    A. Supports integrity
    B. Supports individuation
    C. Supports increased autonomy
    D. Supports identity diffusion
    E. Supports trust

94. A Scandinavian study of 3,206 seven-year-old children found an overall prevalence of enuresis of:
    A. 3%
    B. 5%
    C. 10%
    D. 15%
    E. 20%

95. One study documented the gateways through which youth accessed mental health services. Which of the following was the entry point used by the majority (60%) of children and youth?
    A. Primary care physician
    B. Family friends
    C. Specialized mental health center
    D. School system
    E. Legal system

96. When did Kraepelin propose a comprehensive classification system for psychiatric disorders?
A. 1659
B. 1777
C. 1883
D. 1908
E. 1953

97. True or False: A statistically significant result in a human research study is always clinically important.
A. True
B. False

98. Fonagy, Bleiberg, and others have proposed several elements that account for the developmental trajectory leading to borderline personality disorder, which includes ALL of the following EXCEPT:
A. Infants with an exceptional disposition to mentalization (hypersensitivity to social clues)
B. A disposition to increased affective dysregulation associated with neuropsychiatric vulnerabilities
C. Parents who share similar genetic vulnerabilities or history of maltreatment
D. A parental disposition to respond to their child's distress with distress of their own leading to the capacity to mentalize and accurately match and respond to their child's internal state
E. Children's adaptation to stress and relationship trauma via an inhibition of their capacity to deal with mental states

99. True or False: Central nervous system treatments for childhood cancer can result in significant cognitive impairments.
A. True
B. False

100. Which of the following large studies is currently comparing the efficacy of sertraline, CBT, and combination treatment for children and adolescents with generalized or separation anxiety, or social phobia?
A. Pediatric Obsessive–Compulsive Disorder Treatment Study
B. Multimodal Treatment Study of ADHD
C. Treatment for Adolescents with Depression Study
D. Children and Adolescents Anxiety Multimodal Treatment Study
E. Research Units on Pediatric Psychopharmacology

101. The initiation of substance use in adolescence is best characterized by which of the following?
A. Genetic influence
B. Shared environment
C. Parents
D. Siblings
E. Gene and environment interaction

102. True or False: According to recent research, where domestic violence occurs in families, child maltreatment is rarely present.
A. True
B. False

103. True or False: In resilience studies, male gender can be a vulnerability marker among youth living in a poor urban environment.
A. True
B. False

104. Among the tricyclic antidepressants, which one of the following may have the greatest probability of lowering the seizure threshold?
A. Desipramine
B. Clomipramine
C. Imipramine
D. Amitriptyline
E. Nortriptyline

105. At what age does separation anxiety usually begin to occur in most infants and at what age does it peak?
   A. 6 to 8 months, peaking at 14 to 18 months
   B. 8 to 10 months, peaking at 14 to 18 months
   C. 6 to 8 months, peaking at 12 to 14 months
   D. 8 to 10 months, peaking at 12 to 14 months

106. Infants, toddlers, and young children generally equate death with which of the following?
   A. Disappearance
   B. Separation
   C. Bodily disintegration
   D. Nightmares
   E. A and B

107. What type of variable represents an intervention or treatment that is given to a group of participants but not to another group (that is the control group) within a specified period of time in a study?
   A. Active independent variable
   B. Independent variable
   C. Dependent variable
   D. Attribute independent variable
   E. Extraneous variable

108. The antiepileptic drugs as a group are thought to effect:
   A. Attention, vigilance, and psychomotor speed
   B. Attention, vigilance, and IQ
   C. Attention, IQ, and psychomotor speed
   D. IQ, vigilance, psychomotor speed

109. True or False: Fathers feed their babies less effectively and efficiently compared with mothers.
   A. True
   B. False

110. The definition of rumination disorder includes:
   A. Continuous burping that occurs for a total of more than 1 hour per day
   B. Repeated regurgitation and rechewing of food
   C. Continuation of something (as repetition of a word) usually to an exceptional degree or beyond a desired point
   D. Mid-sternal pain due to gastroesophageal reflux

111. True or False: One exception to the legal requirement that a physician obtain informed consent from a patient is the provision of emergency medical care.
   A. True
   B. False

112. The four basic moral principles that guide medical research and health care include ALL of the following EXCEPT:
   A. Autonomy
   B. Nonmaleficence
   C. Beneficence
   D. Equality
   E. Justice

113. In their influential works regarding the best interests of the child in custody cases, Goldstein, Freud, and Solnit make ALL of the following recommendations regarding custody battles EXCEPT:
   A. The child be kept unaware of the custody battle
   B. Decisions regarding child custody should be made quickly
   C. Whatever decision is made should not be reversible
   D. Full custody should be awarded to the "psychological parent"
   E. An effort should be made to shorten the court proceedings

114. Which of the following is the most effective method in maintaining remission in nocturnal enuresis 6 months after the end of treatment?
    A. Alarm system > desmopressin acetate
    B. Desmopressin acetate > alarm system
    C. Imipramine > alarm system
    D. Desipramine > alarm system
    E. All of the above

115. True or False: Contraindications to family therapy are relative rather than absolute.
    A. True
    B. False

116. True or False: A child who presents with acute suicidal behaviors should be hospitalized.
    A. True
    B. False

117. What is the leading cause of death for youths 10 to 24 years old?
    A. AIDS-related illness
    B. Cardiovascular disease
    C. Cancer
    D. Motor vehicle or other accidents

118. What type of variable intervenes between the independent and dependent variable and helps explain the change in the dependent variable?
    A. Active independent variable
    B. Moderator variable
    C. Extraneous variable
    D. Attribute independent variable
    E. Mediator variable

119. In child custody arrangements, overnight visits for infants with a noncustodial parent are:
    A. Generally harmful
    B. Generally beneficial
    C. Rarely indicated
    D. Never considered by the courts
    E. Indicated when the mother does not have physical custody

120. True or False: The classical Freudian drive theory is a dualistic system composed of a sexual drive and the death drive.
    A. True
    B. False

121. ALL of the following statements is accurate EXCEPT:
    A. Sixty percent of youth suicide victims had parents or adult relatives with suicidal acts, emotional problems, absence from home, and abusive behavior toward their children
    B. Family history of suicide imparts a three- to five-fold greater risk of suicide
    C. Risk of youth suicide can be transmitted in families independent of psychiatric disorders, mediated by the transmission of impulsive aggression
    D. Relatives of adolescent suicide victims have been reported to have a two- to six-fold increase in suicidal behavior
    E. Adolescent boys are more likely to declare their suicide attempt before it happens than adolescent girls

122. Which of the following describes the hypothesized mechanism of action of methylphenidate?
    A. Targets norepinephrine receptors in the striatum
    B. Promotes the release of serotonin in the prefrontal cortex
    C. Selectively promotes the release of newly synthesized dopamine while also blocking dopamine reuptake at the transporter
    D. Promotes the release of stored dopamine and blocks the return of dopamine at presynaptic dopamine transporter sites
    E. Selectively prevents the reuptake of serotonin by the serotonin transporter

123. Children with disruptive behaviors in schools receiving special education may have a "manifestation determination review." What is this?
    A. A process to determine if a student's behaviors are the result of a disability
    B. A process to determine whether a student with disabilities will be promoted to the next grade level
    C. A process to determine the renewal of a 504 Plan
    D. A process to determine whether a reevaluation for special education services is indicated
    E. A process to determine whether a child should go to a therapeutic day school

124. Therapy groups that should accept only single-sex members include those designed to address sensitive issues related to which of the following presentations?
    A. Sexuality
    B. Aggression
    C. Sexual abuse
    D. A and C
    E. All of the above

125. By what age do children first report dreams?
    A. 2 years
    B. 3 years
    C. 4 years
    D. 5 years
    E. 6 years

126. What is the estimated overall prevalence of PTSD in individuals 15 to 54 years of age, according to the National Comorbidity Survey?
    A. 1.2%
    B. 5.6%
    C. 7.8%
    D. 15.1%
    E. 25.5%

127. Which of the following terms defines the sense of belonging and having a rootedness in history that reaches beyond religion, race, and national or geographic origin?
    A. Culture
    B. Ethnicity
    C. Cultural context
    D. Cultural identity
    E. Cultural mask

128. A review article must meet ALL of the following criteria to be considered a systematic review EXCEPT:
    A. Explicitly state inclusion and exclusion criteria regarding studies
    B. Standardize the effect sizes, number needed to treat, and number needed to harm across all studies in a subgroup
    C. Perform a comprehensive search with a transparent search strategy
    D. Summarize results according to explicit rules, including noting varied effects in different subgroups

129. A definable, integrated planning process that results in a unique set of community services (traditional mental health services and natural community supports) that are individualized for a child and family, and which often forms the part of a system-of-care model is known as:
    A. Wraparound services
    B. Family support services
    C. Child and family support services
    D. Community and family support services
    E. Child-centered services

130. ALL the following are examples of speech–language screening measures EXCEPT:
    A. Battelle Developmental Inventory Screening Test
    B. Children's Communication Checklist—2
    C. Early Screening Profiles
    D. Fluharty Preschool Speech and Language Screening Test (Revised)
    E. Kindergarten Language Screening Test—2nd edition

131. True or False: Panic disorder can be diagnosed in the context of an environmental trigger.
    A. True
    B. False

132. Neurobiological findings in autism include ALL of the following EXCEPT:
    A. Decreased peripheral serotonin levels
    B. Persistent primitive reflexes
    C. Macrocephaly
    D. High rates of electoencephalographic abnormalities
    E. Failure to activate the fusiform gyrus

133. Based on prior studies, which one of the following has the greatest antipsychotic efficacy in the pediatric population?
    A. Haloperidol
    B. Risperidone
    C. Clozapine
    D. Olanzapine
    E. Ziprasidone

134. In an extensive review of genetic research, the American Psychological Association concluded that which two forces play a large role in cognitive development?
    A. Genes and caregiver (dyadic) relationship
    B. Genes and onset of early education
    C. Genes and nutritional state
    D. Genes and environment

135. True or False: A comparison of sensory performance and perception on the two sides of the body is significant for obtaining evidence of lateral or bilateral brain impairment.
    A. True
    B. False

136. Which of the following has been correlated with decreased child distress during painful medical procedures?
    A. Parent apologizing for the procedure
    B. Explaining procedural events
    C. Consoling the child
    D. Distracting the child

137. Which of the following statements describes a type I error when testing a null hypothesis?
    A. To reject the null hypothesis when in fact it is true
    B. To not reject the null hypothesis when it is false
    C. To not reject the null hypothesis when it is true
    D. To reject the null hypothesis when it is false
    E. None of the above

138. True or False: Drugs are transported in the general circulation bound to plasma proteins in a greater percentage than found in unbound or free form.
    A. True
    B. False

139. Which captures the suicide rate in descending order of frequency?
    A. White males, white females, nonwhite males, nonwhite females
    B. White males, nonwhite males, white females, nonwhite females
    C. White males, nonwhite males, nonwhite females, white females
    D. Nonwhite males, white males, white females, nonwhite females

140. Which two instruments have been used with children in the assessment of OCD?
    A. Diagnostic Interview Schedule for Children with Obsessions and Compulsions
    B. Leyton Obsessional Inventory-Child Version
    C. Children's Yale-Brown Obsessive Compulsive Scale
    D. A and C
    E. B and C

141. Which of the following terms describes the most frequent score found in a set of data?
    A. Mean
    B. Median
    C. Mode
    D. None of the above

142. In assessing the structural qualities of a childcare environment, ALL of the following attributes should be considered EXCEPT:
    A. Ratio of males to females
    B. Ratio of children to adults
    C. Group size
    D. Caregiver education and training

143. Which of the following statements about the clinical course of Tourette's Syndrome is TRUE?
    A. Given the slow progression of symptoms, most cases are not identified until after puberty
    B. The onset of TS is characterized by limited motor tics affecting the lower limbs
    C. Motor tics in TS tend to progress in a caudal–rostral progression
    D. Phonic tics usually appear a few weeks after the onset of motor tics
    E. Motor tic progression tends to move from simple tics to more complex tics

144. True or False: Selective serotonin reuptake inhibitors do not cause behavioral activation in children and adolescents.
    A. True
    B. False

145. ALL of the following are true of the Stress-Diathesis Theory EXCEPT:
    A. It is a core concept of Multidimensional Family Therapy
    B. It is a model for conceptualizing biologically based disorders including depression, schizophrenia, and alcoholism
    C. It was first proposed by Rosenthal in 1970
    D. Psychotropic medications function by reducing vulnerability
    E. Family interventions focus on lowering sources of stress and enhancing problem-solving capacities

146. As the goals of child psychodynamic psychotherapy extend beyond symptom relief, ALL of the following statements describe possible additional goals EXCEPT:
    A. Restore psychological development to a normal path
    B. Enhance age-appropriate autonomy
    C. Enhance transference to the therapist
    D. Enhance the child's resilience
    E. Enhance affect regulation

147. You receive a call to evaluate a 9-year-old child whom you diagnose with delirium in the context of lupus. Sedative-hypnotic withdrawal is not a concern. Environmental and psychosocial interventions have been inadequately effective and you worry about self-injury. What is your next step?
    A. Do nothing and evaluate further
    B. Start haloperidol 0.5 mg bid
    C. Start lorazepam 0.5 mg tid
    D. Start diphenhydramine 25 mg tid
    E. Start quetiapine 25 mg bid

148. How are tic disorders and group A beta hemolytic streptococci (GABHS) related?
    A. A child with repeated GABHS infections has an 87% chance of developing a tic disorder
    B. They are not related; movement disorders such as Sydenham's chorea have been observed in post-GABHS infections, which involves neuroanatomical lesions that have little to do with tic disorders
    C. They are not related; tic exacerbations have no correlation with streptococci infections
    D. Having a tic disorder places you at increased risk for GABHS infections because of the immunosuppressive nature of movement disorders, particularly TS
    E. Some studies have shown increased proportion of GABHS infections prior to new onset TS, whereas other studies show no temporal relationship

149. First-line treatment for bulimia nervosa is:
    A. Antipsychotic medication
    B. CBT
    C. Antidepressant medication
    D. Anxiolytic medication
    E. Antiemetic medication

150. True or False: The few studies in children with ADHD suggest that the sleep–wake state organization is unaffected.
    A. True
    B. False

151. The largest community-based study of juvenile borderline personality disorder—Children in the Community Study—assessed a sample of 733 children between the ages of 9 and 19 years and found a prevalence of:
    A. 3%
    B. 6%
    C. 12%
    D. 18%
    E. 24%

152. What does the Civil Rights of Institutionalized Persons Act mandate?
    A. Persons, including youths, in state custody have access to a lawyer within 24 hours
    B. Persons, including youths, cannot be held in solitary confinement if their original charges would not warrant segregation from the general community
    C. States provide adequate mental health services to persons detained on a long-term basis in state custody
    D. States provide a community mental health model within their long-term prisons

153. Cocaine use can be detected in the urine for how long?
    A. Less than 24 hours
    B. 24 to 96 hours
    C. 5 days
    D. 1 week
    E. More than 10 days

154. Absence seizures are part of the differential diagnosis for ADHD, especially inattentive type. Regarding other associations, ALL of the following statements are true EXCEPT:
    A. 25% to 35% of children with epilepsy score in the clinical range on the attention scale of the Child Behavior Checklist
    B. A history of ADHD is 2.5 times more common in children newly diagnosed with epilepsy
    C. The rate of ADHD in complicated epilepsy is 12%
    D. The majority of children with epilepsy and ADHD have predominantly inattentive type of ADHD, followed by combined type
    E. Oppositional defiant disorders have a higher association with ADHD when epilepsy is also present

155. The percentage of patients with tuberous sclerosis who have autism is closest to:
    A. 0.1%
    B. 1%
    C. 3%
    D. 5%
    E. 55%

156. Phonological awareness, familiarity with words, and ability to retrieve words rapidly are relevant components of which academic skill?
    A. Reading and spelling
    B. Mathematics
    C. Written language
    D. Oral language
    E. None of the above

157. A large-scale follow-up study of community-identified youth with the core positive symptoms of mania, but failing to meet the full criteria of bipolar disorder, were more likely to develop what disorder when reevaluated in young adulthood?
    A. Bipolar disorder
    B. Anxiety
    C. Schizophrenia
    D. Depression
    E. B and D

158. Two broad areas of long-standing research merged into the relatively new discipline of child psychiatry. Which TWO below describe these areas of research?
    A. Normative child development
    B. Child conduct studies
    C. Investigation of emotional disturbance and disability
    D. Psychopharmacology
    E. Behavioral genetics

159. A large and representative sample of a population at a given point in time is studied. What type of study is this?
    A. Cohort
    B. Cross-sectional
    C. Case–control
    D. Ecological

160. In the search for human disease genes, linkage analysis results are expressed as a logarithm of odds (LOD) score. For example, a LOD score of 3 indicates that the odds in favor of linkage between marker and disease are 1000:1. What LOD score is taken as the threshold for statistical significance?
    A. 1
    B. 2
    C. 3
    D. 4
    E. 5 or more

161. Which TWO of the following side effects are associated with topiramate?
    A. Fetal neural tube malformation
    B. Cognitive blunting
    C. Word retrieval difficulties
    D. Seizures
    E. Hypothyroidism

162. What is the prevalence rate for learning disabilities of the total school-age population in the United States?
    A. 1% to 2%
    B. 5% to 6%
    C. 10% to 11%
    D. 15% to 16%
    E. 19% to 20%

163. Which of the following terms best describes the study of "what the body does to a drug"?
    A. Pharmacology
    B. Pharmacokinetics
    C. Pharmacodynamics
    D. Psychopharmacology
    E. None of the above

164. Which of the following statements is TRUE regarding interpersonal considerations in children with cancer, according to Chesler and Barbarin's stress and coping model?
    A. Children with cancer experience significant social isolation but very positive attention later in treatment
    B. Relationships outside the family provide a source of consistent peer support
    C. Siblings report feelings of anger, resentment, jealousy, frustration, and isolation from their family
    D. In cases involving death and bereavement, siblings often feel prepared, which helps reduce their guilt and anxiety
    E. Siblings will tend to protect their parents as well as their sibling with cancer by not making them worry

165. Which of the following is true of middle ear effusion (MEE) and deafness in children?
    A. Unilateral deafness affects approximately 1 of 1,000 live births
    B. Hearing impairment as a result of MEE is of the conduction type
    C. Chronic MEE with hearing impairment can cause language delay in children
    D. Undetected hearing impairment should always be considered in children referred for the evaluation of attention deficit
    E. All of the above

166. Among the tricyclic antidepressants, which one is unique in its potent inhibition of serotonin reuptake?
    A. Desipramine
    B. Clomipramine
    C. Imipramine
    D. Amitriptyline
    E. Nortriptyline

167. Most epidemiological surveys have found that psychopathology in young people is common, with most studies estimating the prevalence to be:
    A. 5% to 15%
    B. 10% to 20%
    C. 20% to 30%
    D. 30% to 40%
    E. 40% to 50%

168. Which of the following is the normal milestone for a child's ability to drink from a straw?
    A. 10 months
    B. 16 months
    C. 20 months
    D. 24 months
    E. 30 months

169. One milligram of lorazepam is roughly equivalent to which of the following?
    A. Clonazepam 0.25 mg
    B. Alprazolam 0.5 mg
    C. Clonazepam 0.5 mg
    D. Alprazolam 0.25 mg
    E. A and B

170. What percentage of the genome is being expressed at a given time in higher eukaryotic cells?
     A. 1%
     B. 5%
     C. 15%
     D. 30%
     E. 60%

171. "Cooties" are common around which age?
     A. 4 years old
     B. 8 years old
     C. 14 years old
     D. 18 years old

172. True or False: Clinical issues in infancy or very young children are often classified under the traditional categorical disorders in DSM-IV.
     A. True
     B. False

173. The language of children with autism has ALL of the following characteristics EXCEPT:
     A. Echolalia
     B. Idiosyncratic language
     C. Pronoun reversal
     D. Literalness
     E. Normal prosody

174. In children with specific language impairment (SLI), ALL of the following statements are true EXCEPT:
     A. Children with SLI are late to begin talking
     B. It is not appropriate to make the diagnosis until age 4
     C. Pragmatic skills are generally as equally impaired as skills in language form
     D. The first delay to be seen in syntax is failure to combine words spontaneously at age 18 to 24 months
     E. Vocabulary deficits are the first sign of language delay but typically resolve by age 3 to 4

175. Which of the following behaviors is MOST LIKELY to be suggestive of sexual abuse?
     A. Masturbates with hand
     B. Masturbates with objects
     C. Touches genitalia
     D. Shows interest in nudity
     E. Interacts seductively

176. True or False: Neuropsychological tests have consistently identified deficits in executive functioning in patients with ADHD.
     A. True
     B. False

177. True or False: Multiple controlled studies have shown that tics do not invariably increase when children with TS are treated with stimulants.
     A. True
     B. False

178. Which of the following terms best refers to the meaningfulness or relevance of a neuropsychological test, that is, whether the test measures what it is purported to measure?
     A. Validity
     B. Correlation
     C. Regression
     D. Standardization
     E. Reliability

179. Bariatric surgery for adolescents is an absolute contraindication.
     A. True
     B. False

180. Focused attachment is characteristic of which age range?
   A. 0 to 2 months
   B. 2 to 7 months
   C. 7 to 18 months
   D. 18 to 26 months
   E. >26 months

181. Which of the following describes the purpose of magnetic resonance spectroscopy or magnetic resonance spectroscopic imaging?
   A. To delineate the connectivity of white matter in the brain by reconstructing the pathways of nerve fiber bundles based on the principal direction of water diffusion
   B. To measure the electrical activity of the brain to various stimuli
   C. To measure the concentrations and the distributions of metabolites within the brain
   D. To measure regional cerebral blood flow
   E. To provide volumetric data on various brain structures

182. Noted communication differences between typically developing children and those affected with Asperger's disorder include ALL of the following EXCEPT:
   A. Prosody of speech
   B. Social aspect of language
   C. Vocabulary and syntax
   D. Censoring of speech
   E. Volume of speech

183. True or False: In custody evaluations, it is helpful to have had a prior treatment relationship with the child.
   A. True
   B. False

184. ALL of the following are psychosocial strategies in making aggressive behavior in children irrelevant by changing antecedents EXCEPT:
   A. Modifying demands and ways of communicating them
   B. Avoiding problem situations
   C. Reducing positive outcomes of behavior
   D. Reducing provocation and frustration
   E. Restricting access to peers who promote misconduct

185. True or False: In infant/toddler screening tests used to pick out children who are developmentally at risk, the test's sensitivity is considered more important than its specificity.
   A. True
   B. False

186. When were juvenile courts first created?
   A. 1909
   B. 1879
   C. 1919
   D. 1929
   E. 1945

187. Fragile X is a problem of mRNA _____?
   A. transcription
   B. translation
   C. encoding
   D. elimination
   E. splicing

188. The involvement of mental health services, whether directly or indirectly, in school systems has become more prevalent over the years for ALL of the following reasons EXCEPT:
    A. Refugee students were displaced after World War II, and school-based interventions to assist teachers with these students were developed
    B. Federal education rights legislation led to the increasing identification of students with emotional and behavioral difficulties
    C. Increased social change and the recognition of problem behaviors in the 1960s led schools to turn to mental health clinicians for guidance
    D. Decreased psychiatric hospitalizations and residential placements, along with limited outpatient mental health resources, led to increased mental health utilization in schools
    E. No Child Left Behind legislation mandated the early identification and treatment of children with emotional disturbances in school

189. In the biopsychosocial model of formulation, which of the following components belong in the social realm?
    A. Inborn temperament
    B. Constitution
    C. Emotional development
    D. Family constellation
    E. Intelligence

190. Which one of the following antipsychotics was the first used in children with severe behavioral disturbances?
    A. Benzedrine
    B. Haloperidol
    C. Chlorpromazine
    D. Thioridazine
    E. Pimozide

191. True or False: Slightly higher dosing of valproate is required when transitioning to the extended release formulation.
    A. True
    B. False

192. Unlike an aphasia arising from focal lesions, an aphasia from the Landau-Kleffner syndrome:
    A. Is more common in girls than boys
    B. Is the result of right hemisphere damage
    C. May be permanent
    D. Severely affects reading and writing, but usually spares comprehension
    E. Usually has its onset after 13 years of age

193. Optimally, screening the victims of a disaster for possible mental health problems should be done:
    A. The day of the disaster
    B. The day following the disaster
    C. 1 to 3 months after the disaster
    D. 1 year after the disaster
    E. None of the above

194. Melanie Klein, considered one of the founders of child psychoanalysis, coined the term "play analysis." ALL of the following statements describe her therapeutic approach with children EXCEPT:
    A. Emphasizing the ego mechanisms of defense against intolerable affect states
    B. Emphasizing the child's play as equivalent to free association in adult analysis
    C. Encouraging early and deep interpretations in therapeutic methodology
    D. Minimizing the analyst's contact with parents and teachers

195. Which of the following statements best defines the elimination half-life $(t_{1/2})$?
     A. The time required for the concentration of a drug to increase by one-half
     B. The time required for the body to metabolize one-half of the amount of a drug
     C. The time required for the concentration of a drug to decrease by one-half
     D. The time required for one-half of the psychoactive component of a drug to be made inactive

196. True or False: Lamotrigine undergoes only a Phase I metabolic reaction.
     A. True
     B. False

197. True or False: With regard to therapy group and meeting protocol, omission of any segment of the protocol, regardless of how justified such an omission might seem by events of the moment, will always diminish the group's trust in its leaders and in the structure of the group.
     A. True
     B. False

198. Which criterion of OCD in DSM- IV-TR does not apply to children?
     A. The person recognizes that the obsessional thoughts are the product of his or her own mind
     B. At some point, the person has recognized that the obsessions or compulsions are excessive or unreasonable
     C. The obsessions or compulsions are time consuming (take more than 1 hour a day)
     D. The behaviors or mental acts are aimed at preventing or reducing distress
     E. There is no criterion, which does not also apply to children

199. True or False: The successful treatment of adolescent anxiety with selective serotonin reuptake inhibitors may reduce the risk for subsequent depression.
     A. True
     B. False

200. Institutional deprivation syndrome can result in symptoms similar to which of the following diagnoses?
     A. Kleptomania
     B. Munchhausen syndrome by proxy
     C. Seizure disorder
     D. Sleep deprivation
     E. ADHD

1. **Answer: D.** Values in the range of 0.40 to 0.75 represent moderate levels of agreement, and values below 0.40 represent low levels of agreement. Page 292.

2. **Answer: B.** Page 338.

3. **Answer: B.** Preschool children need help in transitioning and saying good-bye. Visits, phone calls, pictures, and letters can often be helpful, and are certainly more helpful than trying to enforce a "clean break." Page 264.

4. **Answer: B.** Single gene disorders typically exhibit mendelian patterns of inheritance (dominant, recessive, or X-linked). The psychiatric disorders listed in the options cannot be accounted for by the transmission of a single gene. Page 190.

5. **Answer: B.** The child has discomfort for his or her *own* sex, not the sex of his *preference*. Page 670.

6. **Answer: D.** Page 816.

7. **Answer: B.** The remaining noradrenergic neurons are distributed in the tegmental region. Page 241.

8. **Answer: E.** Rett syndrome is a disorder within the autism spectrum with prevalence of 1 in 10,000. Affected children achieve normal developmental milestones within the first year of life. One of the first clinical findings is the loss of purposeful hand movements. Others soon emerge including loss of speech, growth retardation with microcephaly, ataxia and severe disruption in normal cognitive functioning. The disorder almost exclusively affects girls. Pages 208–209.

9. **Answer: C.** The Triple Board was approved as a combined residency on a nationwide basis in 1992. Page 25.

10. **Answer: A.** Adrenarche, the steady increase in adrenally produced androgens, begins as early as age 6 to 8 years old and leads to increased skeletal growth and the initial appearance of body hair. Gonadarche occurs when the pulsatile release of gonadotropin-releasing hormone produces increased pituitary release of follicle-stimulating hormone and luteinizing hormone, in turn, driving the production of gonadal hormones (testosterone in boys, estrogen in girls). Gonadarche is the official marker of puberty. Page 280.

11. **Answer: B.** Children with autism do show some improvements in language and social responsiveness with age and early intervention. Detection by age 2 years can be difficult as the classic signs of autism tend to be detected around age 3 to 4 years. The majority of adults with autism do not achieve personal and occupational independence. Page 392.

12. **Answer: E.** In a large cross-sectional study no differences among Asians, African-Americans, Hispanics, and whites were found in mean rates of any eating disorder symptoms. Page 595.

13. **Answer: A.** Page 519.

14. **Answer: B.** The component of dimension refers to the range of psychological vulnerabilities and their severity in a presenting patient. Page 380.

15. **Answer: A.** Page 83.

16. **Answer: E.** Regardless of whether these phenomena accurately represent the external world, they all are components of psychic reality. Page 828.

17. **Answer: E.** Page 917.

18. **Answer: A.** A retrospective review of 41 cases in which covert video surveillance was used to investigate a possible diagnosis of Munchhausen syndrome by proxy in a pediatric hospital found that 23 diagnoses were actually confirmed. Of these 23, covert video surveillance was seen as crucial to making the diagnosis in 13 (56%) and supportive of the diagnosis in five (28%). Page 724.

19. **Answer: A.** This would warrant a diagnosis of hyperkinetic conduct disorder. Page 456.

20. **Answer: E.** Steroid use can result in shrinking testicles. Page 620.

21. **Answer: E.** There is no set age, but most clinicians and adoptive professionals recommend telling a child early. Giving children information early, even before they can comprehend wholly the information, establishes a process of discussion and openness that leads to developmentally appropriate conversations. For example, when toddlers and preschoolers become aware of pregnancy and childbirth, adoptive parents will face questions about the adopted child's origins and early life, and will need to find ways to answer them honestly and openly. Page 1014.

22. **Answer: A.** What is prohibited is the use of persons solely as a means to this end. Page 140.

23. **Answer: B.** Reexperiencing the trauma is one of the symptoms of posttraumatic stress disorder. Page 701.

24. **Answer: A.** When there appears to be two problem areas for the course of interpersonal therapy, the therapist should identify a primary and possibly secondary area of focus. Page 823.

25. **Answer: B.** 300,000 children under 15 have epilepsy, which represents 1 in 200. Each year 7 in 10,000 children under 15 will develop recurrent seizures. In two-thirds, the etiology is unknown. Page 959.

26. **Answer: B.** Forensic psychiatrists should be aware of the ethical guidelines provided by the American Academy of Psychiatry and the Law, which are more specific to forensics than those of the other organizations. Page 21.

27. **Answer: D.** Patients with childhood onset schizophrenia present with higher rates of early language, social, and motor developmental abnormalities. Page 495.

28. **Answer: D.** This side effect can occur with doses greater than 150 mg daily. Page 766.

29. **Answer: C.** Adolescents will also accelerate separation and individuation from the family. Preschool children can experience regression, intensified anxiety, neediness, sleep disturbances, and increased aggression. Middle-school children may experience anxiety, loneliness, and powerlessness, feel responsible for the divorce, have conflicts of loyalty, and fantasize about reconciliation. Page 1007.

30. **Answer: C.** Children acquire skills best when caregivers present them with tasks that are just a bit too difficult for them to accomplish independently, but are possible with appropriate assistance. Page 262.

31. **Answer: B.** Doctoral-level clinicians trained in evidence-based practice supervise master's level clinicians. Multisystemic therapists typically treat four to six families over 4 to 5 months. Page 880.

32. **Answer: A.** Although these three skills are important for medical diagnosis in general, they have special significance in the assessment of infants as elaborated in Chapter 4.2.1. Page 311.

33. **Answer: D.** There is minimal motor delay, although delay linked to balance may occur. The other areas will have varying degrees of delay, depending on intervention and other factors. Page 74.

34. **Answer: E.** FK506 is metabolized by the P450 system. Page 944.

35. **Answer: A.** In direct prevention-minded treatment, the intervention involves other family members as part of the treatment for the primary patient. The therapist is open to the possibility of providing preventive interventions to other family members. Page 173.

36. **Answer: E.** The fire-settings cause more than $250 million in property damage. Page 484.

37. **Answer: A.** Page 808.

38. **Answer: E.** The patient has to waive confidentiality or the court has to provide an order. If the child psychiatrist is not provided with consent by the patient or a court order, he must still appear and answer questions about himself but he or she would respond that information about the patient is confidential and privileged and follow the direction of the judge in court. Page 1000.

39. **Answer: A.** In years past, the terms sociocultural or cultural–familial retardation reflected the view that nonorganic mental retardation (MR) stemmed from environmental deprivation. Although this theory has generally fallen out of favor as an explanation for the population as a whole, a complicating factor is that disproportionately more persons with sociocultural MR are poor, from minority backgrounds, and of low-intelligence quotient (IQ) parents. Page 405.

40. **Answer: A.** Page 433.

41. **Answer: A.** This is one of the descriptions within criterion B for gender identity disorder in the Diagnostic and Statistical Manual of Mental Disorders (DSM). Page 674.

42. **Answer: A.** Two of them had homosexual orientation; the third was asexual. The remaining 22 had a "typical" gender identity. Page 677.

43. **Answer: B.** Categorical approaches are dichotomous in nature: either you have the disorder or you do not, whereas multivariate approaches are dimensional. Page 306.

44. **Answer: C.** In working with parents or families, the physician may be viewed as taking on a doctor–patient with each parent or family member. Case law is evolving, but when working with patients by e-mail across state lines, the trend is to view the state where the patient resides as the area of practice, which raises the medical–legal risk of practicing without a license in that state. Page 1019.

45. **Answer: C.** The Brazelton Neonatal Behavioral Assessment Scale, second edition, is designed for use with neonates of 37 to 44 weeks' gestational age who do not need mechanical supports or supplemental oxygen. Page 316.

46. **Answer: E.** The physician should also obtain creatinine levels and thyroid indices. Page 769.

47. **Answer: C.** Parental education is related to children's achievement in both white and African-American families. Regardless of race, parental education relates indirectly to children's achievement through reading and by providing a warm and supportive environment. Page 275.

48. **Answer: C.** Randomized experimental studies utilize difference inferential statistics such as analysis of variance and t-tests. Page 109.

49. **Answer: A.** Fluoxetine has an active metabolite, norfluoxetine, with an elimination half-life of 7 to 14 days. Page 763.

50. **Answer: B and C.** Territorial privacy ("This is my room.") and possessional privacy ("This is my bike.") develop in children prior to informational privacy, which involves concerns about others' knowledge of one's activities, interests, and associations. Page 148.

51. **Answer: D.** Page 36.

52. **Answer: D.** Option D provides a normal range for thyroid-stimulating hormone. Page 656.

53. **Answer: D.** On nonschool days, however, the pattern of violent crime is more akin to the timing for adult offenders. Page 468.

54. **Answer: B.** Offering something to eat can be an effective tool, if appropriate; however, the main point here is that all other options represent directive or controlling statements, which are apt to be counterproductive. Page 903.

55. **Answer: C.** Various levels of MR are specified in the DSM-IV-TR: mild (IQ 50–70), moderate (IQ 35–49), severe (IQ 20–34), and profound (IQ < 20). Page 401.

56. **Answer: B.** There was no difference between placebo and active treatment. Open-label studies report rates of improvement of 30% to 60%. Case reports have suggested augmentation with olanzapine, risperidone, pimozide. Page 567.

57–64. Answers: 57- E; 58-G; 59-B; 60-H; 61-A; 62-F; 63-D; 64-C. Page 829.

65. **Answer: B.** Body mass index is not part of the diagnostic criteria for bulimia. Page 593.

66. **Answer: C.** Less than half follow-up. Generally, uncomplicated attention deficit hyperactivity disorder (ADHD) can be managed in the primary care setting but pediatric depression and other disorders are generally seen as the purview of mental health specialists. Page 923.

67. **Answer: E.** This question is intended to impress upon you the very little research on preschool psychopathology as reflected by the dearth of diagnostic interviews for this population. Page 354.

68. **Answer: C.** Page 455.

69. **Answer: B.** The belief that boys are more mathematically capable than girls has been demonstrated to be more an effect of socialization than innate capability. Page 270.

70. **Answer: A.** Approximately half of preschool and school age children report at least one somatic complaint in the previous 2 weeks. Page 635.

71. **Answer: C.** This statistic underlines the great need to recruit and train more physicians in child and adolescent psychiatry, especially to underserved areas. Page 23.

72. **Answer: D.** Page. 803.

73. **Answer: A.** Page 459.

74. **Answer: E.** This survey occurred in North Carolina. Much of our child psychiatric epidemiological data comes from the Great Smoky Mountains Surveys. Page 158.

75. **Answer: D.** Use of placebo, which is tempting for generalists, raises ethical, and practical considerations; it emphasizes an underlying medical etiology and leads to either back tracking to a psychological discussion if the placebo does not work or the search of additional sham interventions. The mind–body connection is worth discussing and the reassurance that symptoms are real, but that there is no tissue damage can be helpful. Page 641.

76. **Answer: C.** The prevalence estimate of language difficulty is 8% for boys and 6% for girls. A language disorder is a disruption in any aspect of verbal communication, whether oral or written. Delays in language development are the most common presenting symptom in preschool children. Estimates of prevalence of language difficulty in preschool children vary between 7% and 15%, and at school age, the prevalence of primary language disorders is thought to be between 4% and 7%. Although biological markers of specific language impairments have not been identified, neurobiological factors are clearly implicated. Pages 418–420.

77. **Answer: D.** Page 566.

78. **Answer: B.** One cannot perform complex behaviors such as these while asleep. Like night terrors and sleep talking, sleepwalking is confined to nonrapid eye movement stage 4 sleep. Page 629.

79. **Answer: B.** A screening measure should not be too focused on only one area of concern; for example, it should assess not only a child's ability to comprehend language but also his or her ability to express language. Page 371.

80. **Answer: A.** Page 314.

81. **Answer: A.** Once this focus is accomplished, resilience research seeks to identify mechanisms or processes that might underlie the associations between the factors and adverse life events. Page 293.

82. **Answer: C.** Page 346.

83. **Answer: A.** This criterion is a cardinal feature of posttraumatic stress disorder. Page 705.

84. **Answer: D.** A dynamic assessment is used to determine what aids, such as prompts, cues, or various scaffolds, best support positive changes in communication for a child with language deficits. This assessment provides important information regarding which techniques or teaching styles are most effective for the child. Page 375.

85. **Answer: B.** All the rest are involved in Phase I metabolic reactions. Page 747.

86. **Answer: A.** Page 539.

87. **Answer: B.** Secure attachment relationships have been associated with higher levels of social competence, greater preschool popularity, and more positive friendships. In addition, parents' role in provision of peer-play opportunities, monitoring of peer interactions, modeling and coaching acceptable behaviors are all associated with more positive peer relationships. The child's ability to regulate his or her individual temperament is associated with peer-interaction skills. Page 263.

88. **Answer: A.** Multisystemic therapy, which has a behavioral and family systems emphasis, has shown empirical evidence for its efficacy for juvenile offenders. Page 790.

89. **Answer: B.** Page 551.

90. **Answer: A.** Learning involves formation of new synapses and strengthening of old ones. This occurs in all parts of the brain where memories are formed and is termed synaptic plasticity. Page 200.

91. **Answer: A.** Page 218.

92. **Answer: B.** For children who have deficits in reflective functioning, the therapist's interest in and respect for the child's mental life helps the child develop the capacity for an observing ego. Page 831.

93. **Answer: B and C.** Interpersonal psychotherapy (IPT) has been modified to IPT for depressed adolescents due to its developmental relevance to the adolescent population in supporting individuation and the independence that accompanies adolescence. Page 820.

94. **Answer: C.** 9.8% to be precise; 6.4% had night wetting, 1.8% day wetting, and 1.6% day and night wetting. Page 656.

95. **Answer: D.** Twenty-seven percent of youth entered through specialty mental health systems and 13% through the general medical sector. Page 49.

96. **Answer: C.** Page 305.

97. **Answer: B.** This is a commonly mistaken assumption as statistical significance is not equivalent to practical or clinical significance. The word significance has a very different meaning scientifically than it has when used in common parlance. Statistical significance can be obtained in large samples even though the differences or associations between groups are very small or weak. Page 116.

98. **Answer: D.** Parents in their distress cannot mentalize and as such do not match their child's internal state. Fonagy and colleagues describe a model with seven elements, of which four are listed in the answer options. Page 685.

99. **Answer: A.** Cognitive impairment is most commonly seen in the areas of attention and concentration. Memory, handwriting, mathematics, and organizing or sequencing skills are also affected. Children who have been irradiated and diagnosed under the age of 6 years are at the greatest risk for difficulties in school functioning. Page 930.

100. **Answer: D.** The Children and Adolescents Anxiety Multimodal Treatment Study is currently underway with a projected sample size of 320 children and adolescents, ages 7 to 17. Pages 762–763.

101. **Answer: E.** Page 617.

102. **Answer: B.** In fact, research shows an incidence of child maltreatment of 30% to 60% in families with domestic violence. Page 38.

103. **Answer: A.** Boys are typically more reactive than girls to negative community influences. Page 295.

104. **Answer: B.** Consequently, clomipramine's dose and potential drug interactions need to be monitored closely. Page 764.

105. **Answer: A.** After its peak, separation anxiety begins to decline. Page 257.

106. **Answer: E.** Some children as young as 2 or 3 years old when faced with the death of a parent have been able to demonstrate a nascent understanding of the major concepts of death (irreversibility, finality, causality, and inevitability), but most view the death as a separation or disappearance. Page 972.

107. **Answer: A.** Page 105.

108. **Answer: A.** It is difficult to disentangle the effects of drugs from epilepsy. The correct answer represents the best state of knowledge. However, it is important to note that some studies have found no effect of antiepileptic drugs on cognitive function. Page 964.

109. **Answer: B.** Although fathers have stylistic differences in feeding their infant children, research of married parents indicates that they are just as effective and efficient in this task as mothers. Page 7.

110. **Answer: B.** The DSM-IV defines rumination as (i) repeated regurgitation and rechewing of food (in the absence of associated gastrointestinal illness) for a period of at least 1 month following a period of normal functioning; and (ii) not due to an associated gastrointestinal or other general medical condition (e.g., esophageal reflux). Page 585.

111. **Answer: A.** Page 142.

112. **Answer: D.** Autonomy is the basis for informed consent and therapeutic privilege; nonmaleficence is derived from the Latin phrase translated as "First do no harm," which has roots in the Hippocratic oath; beneficence refers to the obligation to promote the welfare of the patient; and justice refers to providing fair treatment to all. Page 18.

113. **Answer: A.** There is controversy regarding the recommendation to award full custody to the "psychological parent." Page 40.

114. **Answer: A.** Page 662.

115. **Answer: A.** There are no absolute contraindications to family therapy. An example of a relative contraindication is discussing stressful situations with the family when one or more members are severely destabilized and require hospitalization. Page 855.

116. **Answer: B.** Serious suicide attempts usually require hospitalization, but there is a range of potential dispositions for children with suicidal behaviors. Page 900.

117. **Answer: D.** Three-fourths of deaths for youths 10 to 24 years of age are due to motor vehicle crashes; others are due to unintentional injuries, homicide, and suicide. Page 288.

118. **Answer: E.** Page 119.

119. **Answer: B.** Ample evidence indicates children benefit from maintaining close relationships with both parents, and there is no evidence to indicate overnights are harmful. The key factor in adjusting to transitions is the *predictability* of a child's schedule. Page 1009.

120. **Answer: B.** The classical freudian dualistic theory of drives is composed of an aggressive drive and a sexual drive. Page 828.

121. **Answer: E.** Page 533.

122. **Answer: D.** Option C describes the hypothesized mechanism of action for amphetamines. Page 757.

123. **Answer: A.** A manifestation determination review determines if a student's misconduct is the result of a disability. If it is, the school is obligated to continue programming, as embodied in an Individualized Education Program. If the conduct is not the manifestation of a disability, the school may apply the standard disciplinary sanctions. Children suspected of a disability but who have not been evaluated for special education eligibility are afforded the same protections. Page 987.

124. **Answer: E.** Page 845.

125. **Answer: B.** Page 628.

126. **Answer: C.** Page 702.

127. **Answer: B.** Ethnicity is the correct term. Pages 57–58.

128. **Answer: B.** Page 130.

129. **Answer: A.** Central to this process is the development of a child and family team, which assumes the central role in outlining treatment goals and planning. Ideally, according to this model, such teams should be comprised of fewer than 50% professionals. Page 892.

130. **Answer: B.** This question is primarily intended to display some of the great variety of speech–language screening tests available for the clinician. The Children's Communication Checklist—2 is a parental report regarding their child's communication abilities. Page 372.

131. **Answer: B.** Panic attacks can occur in many conditions, but panic disorder is panic attacks without an environmental trigger. (One can have panic disorder and also have panic attacks triggered by situations, but the panic attacks cannot exclusively be triggered by situations.) Page 541.

132. **Answer: A.** All are true except peripheral serotonin levels are *increased*. Page 386.

133. **Answer: C.** Prior studies have shown that clozapine has the greatest antipsychotic efficacy in the pediatric population, although its toxicity limits its use in all but the most severely treatment-refractory patients. Page 500.

134. **Answer: D.** Genes (G) and environment (E) is the most comprehensive answer and the conclusion of this study by the American Psychological Association. This question indicates the current investigative interest in G × E interaction in determining development, resilience, and psychopathology. Page 253.

135. **Answer: A.** Remember your neurology! Page 358.

136. **Answer: D.** The others have been correlated with increased child distress during procedures. Page 913.

137. **Answer: A.** The type I error is an error of commission, saying there is a difference between groups when there really was no difference. Page 115.

138. **Answer: B.** The two forms are found in dynamic equilibrium with each other. Page 746.

139. **Answer: B.** Page 530.

140. **Answer: E.** In option A, the Diagnostic Interview Schedule for Children is a structured diagnostic interview for psychiatric disorders and it assesses for obsessive–compulsive disorder (OCD) according to the DSM, but is not as comprehensive for the assessment of OCD as are the two other instruments; and there is no "DISC with OCD" as titled in the option. Page 557.

141. **Answer: C.** Page 106.

142. **Answer: A.** Sex ratio in the child care environment does not appear to be a factor. Page 255.

143. **Answer: E.** The clinical course of Tourette's disorder typically begins with simple facial motor tics around age 5 to 7 years, which progress to more complex tics in a head-to-toe fashion (rostral–caudal). This is followed years later by vocal tics. The progression tends to be rapid enough that the diagnosis is given by age 11 years. Page 571.

144. **Answer: B.** Behavioral activation can be a common side effect of selective serotonin reuptake inhibitors in children and adolescents resulting in such symptoms as motor restlessness, insomnia, impulsiveness, disinhibited behavior, and garrulousness. The risk of this side effect underscores the importance of starting at low doses and increasing slowly. Activation may indicate a manic or bipolar diathesis, but does not mean a child has bipolar disorder. Page 763.

145. **Answer: A.** Pages 857 and 861.

146. **Answer: C.** A further goal is to decrease the likelihood of symptom relapse by developing the child's capacity for understanding her feelings as well as the connection between thoughts, feelings, and behavior. Page 832.

147. **Answer: B.** Of course, you also search for the underlying etiology. Page 650.

148. **Answer: E.** The neuroanatomical areas affected in Sydenham's chorea (basal ganglia, cortex, and thalamic sites) are also the same areas affected in tic disorders. One study found an increased proportion of group A beta hemolytic streptococci infections within the preceding 3 months in children newly diagnosed with Tourette's syndrome compared with well matched controls. However, a longitudinal study did not show a temporal relationship above chance alone. Page 575.

149. **Answer: B.** Cognitive-behavioral therapy is the first-line treatment for bulimia nervosa. It has been found to be the most effective treatment in over 35 controlled studies. Page 598.

150. **Answer: A.** This appears true despite complaints from parents. Page 631.

151. **Answer: A.** Page 682.

152. **Answer: C.** Adequate health, mental health, and psychosocial services are mandated. For youths specifically, there have been over 20 class action lawsuits involving juvenile justice across the nation. Page 888.

153. **Answer: B.** Page 619.

154. **Answer: E.** There is no evidence suggesting oppositional defiant disorder has a higher association with ADHD when epilepsy is present. The other statements are true as far as individual studies have demonstrated. Page 967.

155. **Answer: C.** A Wood's lamp examination helps identify tubers. Some sources identify up to 25% of children with tuberous sclerosis as also having autism. Page 342.

156. **Answer: A.** Page 364.

157. **Answer: E.** Page 768.

158. **Answer: A and C.** In the late 19th century, the child studies' movement concerned itself with normative child development with a primary audience of educators and parents, not psychiatrists. Concurrently, child development study in the late 19th century began to focus on deviancy and juvenile delinquency and was influenced by darwinian notions of evolution. Page 11.

159. **Answer: B.** Page 153.

160. **Answer: C.** Page 193.

161. **Answer: B and C.** Page 773.

162. **Answer: B.** Page 412.

163. **Answer: B.** Page 237.

164. **Answer: E.** The other statements are inaccurate. Children with cancer often receive much positive attention initially, but subsequently often feel forgotten and isolated from friends and peers as time goes by. Page 931.

165. **Answer: E.** Pages 66–67.

166. **Answer: B.** Page 764.

167. **Answer: B.** Page 164.

168. **Answer: E.** Page 371.

169. **Answer: E.** Page 782.

170. **Answer: A.** According to some estimates, only about 1% of the genome of higher eukaryotic cells is being expressed at a given time. Different sets of genes are active during development compared to the mature organism. Some genes are expressed continuously, whereas others are required during specific time periods and others are only expressed in response to hormonal or environmentally triggered change. Page 179.

171. **Answer: B.** Around age 8, same-sex groupings become polarized, with the opposite sex having "cooties" and being generally avoided or teased. Moving toward preadolescence, this gradually gives way to admiration of opposite-sex peers from a distance. Page 268.

172. **Answer: B.** Clinical problems involving infants and young children are more likely due to familial and contextual factors; that is, they are more related to the "goodness of fit" between parents and infant, than to a specific disorder in an infant. However, a few traditional categories, such as autism, can be diagnosed in infants and very young children. Pages 303–304.

173. **Answer: E.** Language differences in children with autism include abnormal prosody. Page 389.

174. **Answer: C.** Pragmatic skills are generally better than skills in language form, and this is one of the characteristics that differentiates specific language impairment from acute stress disorder. Page 425.

175. **Answer: B.** Table 5.15.1.1 delineates behaviors that are highly suggestive for a possible sexual abuse history. Page 694.

176. **Answer: A.** Page 439.

177. **Answer: A.** The studies include the multisite Treatment of ADHD in Children with Tourette's syndrome study of 136 children ages 7 to 14. Page 781.

178. **Answer: A.** Page 360.

179. **Answer: B.** Bariatric surgery is increasingly being performed on extremely obese adolescents (body mass index >40 kg/m^2) who have not been able to lose weight through conventional treatment. Nevertheless, the use of surgery is viewed as experimental, but not illegal. Page 611.

180. **Answer: C.** Attachment behavior, characterized by proximity seeking in times of stress, appears in the second half of the first year of life. See Table 5.15.3.1. Pages 711–712.

181. **Answer: C.** Page 225.

182. **Answer: C.** Persons with Asperger's disorder have problems with the social aspect of language, which includes appropriate volume, intonation and content; they typically have preservation of vocabulary and syntax. Page 395.

183. **Answer: B.** The forensic evaluator must avoid conflicts of interest. Page 1008.

184. **Answer: C.** Option C is a strategy on how to make aggressive behavior ineffective by changing consequences. Page 477.

185. **Answer: A.** Although it is desirable to reduce both types of errors, sensitivity appears more important than specificity in screening tests as false positives can be identified with follow-up testing. (Specificity reduces the false-positive rate, whereas sensitivity reduces the false-negative rate.) Page 320.

186. **Answer: A.** Juvenile courts were created to focus on the rehabilitation (rather than punishment) of juvenile delinquents, thus differentiating them from adult courts. Page 999.

187. **Answer: B.** There is a mutation in the protein that regulates translation of messages. Page 181.

188. **Answer: E.** No Child Left Behind requires intervention earlier for those students not progressing as expected, and not identification and treatment of emotional disturbances per se. Page 981.

189. **Answer: D.** Refer to Table 4.2.6.2. Page 378.

190. **Answer: C.** Although its use has declined due to newer atypical antipsychotics, chlorpromazine is still routinely used for the acute management of agitation or aggression. Page 776.

191. **Answer: A.** Between an 8% and 20% increase is required. Page 771.

192. **Answer: C.** Landau-Kleffner syndrome (LKS) usually has its onset between 3 and 6 years of age, although it can occur any time between 2 and 13 years. In general, prognosis is worse the earlier the onset of the syndrome, which is more common in boys than in girls. Unlike aphasias associated with focal lesions, LKS may result in a permanent aphasia. Another difference is that comprehension is more severely affected in LKS and reading and writing may be relatively spared. Page 423.

193. **Answer: C.** Page 732.

194. **Answer: A.** Anna Freud studied the ego mechanisms of defense. Page 827.

195. **Answer: C.** In clinical practice, the elimination half-life is usually assessed by measuring the decay of plasma or serum drug concentration. Page 743.

196. **Answer: B.** Lamotrigine undergoes only a Phase II metabolic reaction as it is transformed only by glucuronidation. Page 750.

197. **Answer: A.** Page 846.

198. **Answer: B.** Criterion B. Page 549.

199. **Answer: A.** This question shows one link between anxiety and depression, and a possible preventative approach to adolescent psychiatry. Page 506.

200. **Answer: E.** Although these symptoms (hyperactivity and inattention) are not part of reactive attachment disorder, some have suggested that the inattention and overactivity seen in children with a history of institutionalization and attachment disturbances may reflect an "institutional deprivation syndrome." Page 714.

1. What TWO distinctly American traditions have contributed their own unique emphasis to the field of dynamic psychotherapy with children, particularly play therapy?
   A. The child guidance movement
   B. Cognitive-behavioral therapy (CBT)
   C. Client-centered therapy
   D. Existential therapy
   E. Rational emotional behavior therapy

2. Findings from large-scale epidemiological studies examining individuals with mental retardation (MR) show ALL of the following EXCEPT:
   A. More boys than girls have MR
   B. Rates of MR are generally low in the early years
   C. Rates of MR peak at around 10 to 14 years
   D. Rates of MR stay constant during adulthood
   E. Individuals of lower socioeconomic status (SES) show higher than expected rates of MR

3. Which of the following learning disabilities (LDs) currently has the most research on relevant genes and brain structure and brain function to support a neurobiological base for LDs?
   A. Disability from emotional disturbance
   B. Disability from traumatic brain injury
   C. Disorder of written expression
   D. Specific reading disability
   E. Specific mathematics disability

4. Approximately what percentage of pediatric patients in primary care have mental health problems?
   A. 5%
   B. 10%
   C. 20%
   D. 30%
   E. 50%

5. Child psychiatry in the United States began with the establishment of child guidance clinics, the first of which was the Juvenile Psychopathic Institute of Chicago established by Dr William Healy in which year?
   A. 1793
   B. 1839
   C. 1872
   D. 1909
   E. 1952

6. Which of the following is accurate about epilepsy?
   A. Epilepsy can be associated with a decrease in intelligence quotient (IQ) for a subset of children
   B. Family factors seem to be stronger predictors of psychopathology than epilepsy factors
   C. Students with epilepsy are retained in school more frequently than controls
   D. Children with epilepsy experience more frequent difficulties in reading, writing, and mathematics than controls
   E. All of the above

7. In one cohort study, young adults with depression were found to have which of the following?
   A. Homozygosity for the long allele of the serotonin transporter gene
   B. Homozygosity for the short allele of the serotonin transporter gene
   C. Homozygosity for the short allele of the serotonin transporter gene and negative life events
   D. Homozygosity for the long allele of the serotonin transporter gene and negative life events
   E. None of the above

8. Which of the following describes the hypothesized mechanism of action of selective serotonin reuptake inhibitors (SSRIs)?
   A. Interferes with the return of serotonin into the postsynaptic neuron
   B. Promotes the release of serotonin in the prefrontal cortex
   C. Selectively promotes the release of newly synthesized dopamine while also blocking dopamine reuptake at the transporter
   D. Promotes the release of stored dopamine and blocks the return of dopamine at presynaptic dopamine transporter sites.
   E. Interferes with the return of serotonin into the presynaptic neuron

9. What type of variable represents a variable that cannot be manipulated, as it is specific to the subject (e.g., gender, age, or ethnic group) under study, or part of the subject's usual environment (e.g., low SES)?
   A. Active independent variable
   B. Independent variable
   C. Dependent variable
   D. Attribute independent variable
   E. Extraneous variable

10. Which of the following medications has shown statistically significant superiority compared with valproate in acute onset depression in adolescents with bipolar disorder?
    A. Quetiapine
    B. Sertraline
    C. Venlafaxine
    D. Mirtazapine
    E. Risperdal

In the following questions regarding types of validity, match the terms to the definitions that best describe them.

11. Construct validity

12. Content validity

13. Face validity

14. Concurrent validity

15. Predictive validity
    A. Whether on the surface of things the test appears to be appropriate for its intended use
    B. A form of criterion-related validation that examines the degree to which the measure predicts some other criterion in the future, such as IQ in relation to later academic success
    C. Examines the extent to which a test measures what it purports to measure
    D. Refers to the degree to which a test covers the behavior, skill, or subject matter being measured, that is, whether the test offers representative coverage of the domain assessed
    E. A form of criterion-related validation in which the current measure is compared with a criterion or outcome to which it is related, such as other test scores

16. True or False: Tricyclic antidepressants are more effective in children with depression compared to adults.
    A. True
    B. False

17. True or False: There is indisputable evidence for the heritability of most early-onset psychiatric illnesses.
  A. True
  B. False

18. What is the most common use of single photon emission computed tomography in the study of psychopathological disorders?
  A. Electrical analysis of the brain to various stimuli
  B. The delineation of white matter tracts
  C. The measurement of regional cerebral blood flow
  D. Volumetric analysis of brain structures
  E. None of the above

19. Attention deficit hyperactivity disorder (ADHD) has generally fallen under which type of disability in the determination of eligibility for special education services?
  A. Developmental delay
  B. Emotional
  C. Other health impaired
  D. Specific learning
  E. Neurological

20. At what age does stranger anxiety begin to occur in most infants and at what age does it peak?
  A. 6 months, peaking at 18 months
  B. 8 months, peaking at 18 months
  C. 6 months, peaking at 24 months
  D. 8 months, peaking at 24 months

21. In the population at large, the estimated prevalence of anorexia nervosa in young women in industrialized countries is:
  A. 0.03%
  B. 0.3%
  C. 3%
  D. 30%

22. True or False: Parents of juveniles who set fires have been found to demonstrate a significantly greater incidence of psychological disturbance including schizophrenia, other psychotic disorders, depression, and substance abuse.
  A. True
  B. False

23. Hospital staff members may deal with the anxiety they experience when a child in their care is dying by:
  A. Withdrawal and a conspiracy of silence
  B. Excessive crying
  C. Acting as a coparent
  D. Excessive benzodiazepine use

24. Which of the following is the greatest limitation of applying electroencephalography (EEG)?
  A. Poor spatial resolution
  B. The potential adverse effects of radioactive tracers
  C. Poor temporal resolution
  D. Indirect method of measuring neuronal activity
  E. None of the above

25. Among the tricyclic antidepressants, which one of the following is used to treat enuresis in children?
  A. Desipramine
  B. Clomipramine
  C. Imipramine
  D. Amitriptyline
  E. Nortriptyline

26. Which of the following models of family therapy is particularly applicable to marital problems and children with chronic conduct disorders?
    A. Structural
    B. Strategic
    C. Behavioral
    D. Psychodynamic
    E. Experiential

27. The "developing theory of mind" refers to:
    A. The ability to understand that one's thoughts, beliefs, and feelings are one's own and that others may feel or believe differently
    B. The interpretation of the behaviors and words of others as being a part of their feelings and thoughts
    C. The recognition of the world in both physical and nonphysical terms, with the latter being invisible or imagined states of thoughts, feelings, and beliefs
    D. All of the above
    E. None of the above

28. ALL of the following are autosomal dominant diseases EXCEPT:
    A. Huntington disease
    B. Myotonic dystrophy
    C. Fragile X syndrome
    D. Parkinson disease
    E. Neurofibromatosis

29. Which of the following statements is most accurate for the United States?
    A. The rates of both AIDS and HIV are increasing
    B. The rates of both AIDS and HIV are decreasing
    C. The rate of AIDS is increasing and the rate of HIV is decreasing
    D. The rate of AIDS is decreasing and the rate of HIV is increasing

30. True or False: Obsessive–compulsive disorder (OCD) is a risk factor for trichotillomania.
    A. True
    B. False

31. Caution should be used when administering chlorpromazine in children via intramuscular routes due to the occurrence of which adverse event?
    A. Hypotension
    B. Seizures
    C. Acute dystonic reaction
    D. Neuroleptic malignant syndrome
    E. Extrapyramidal symptoms

32. One study described how children with serious emotional disturbances received services from more than two mental health delivery systems. What percentage of children did so?
    A. 12%
    B. 32%
    C. 52%
    D. 72%
    E. 92%

33. Which of the following encompasses the broad goals of neuropsychological assessment?
    A. To provide a more complete description and understanding of the child
    B. To provide an understanding of the child's prognosis
    C. To inform strategies for intervention
    D. To serve primarily as a diagnostic instrument
    E. A and C

34. Adolescents have an intense striving for physical, sexual, social, psychological, and intellectual independence and mastery. Life-limiting illness turns this developmental process on its head by:
    A. Bringing physical immobility and dependence, rather than independence
    B. Leading to isolation from peers rather than forging new relationships
    C. Stopping educational progress
    D. Preventing independent work
    E. A, B, and C

35. Which of the following is true about gay and lesbian parented families?
    A. The parenting repertoire of homosexual parents is constricted
    B. The psychological health of children suffers
    C. A child's sexual orientation is influenced
    D. Gay and lesbian families are more likely to divorce
    E. None of the above

36. ALL of the following environmental factors appear to be associated with risk for language delay EXCEPT:
    A. Later birth order
    B. Lower SES
    C. Neglectful home environment
    D. Recurrent otitis media
    E. Smaller family size

37. Early manifestations of developmental difficulties are apparent in children who subsequently develop borderline personality disorder. These may include ALL of the following EXCEPT:
    A. Difficult temperament
    B. High activity levels
    C. Poor adaptability
    D. Oddness of speech
    E. Hard to soothe

38. The recommendations for prevention of pediatric obesity by the American Academy of Pediatrics include ALL of the following EXCEPT:
    A. Calculate and plot body mass index once a year in all children and adolescents
    B. Introduce low fat formulas for at risk infants
    C. Recommend limitation of television and video time to a maximum of 2 hours per day
    D. Routinely promote physical activity
    E. Recognize and monitor changes in obesity-associated risk factors for adult chronic disease

39. G. Stanley Hall, a pioneer psychologist in the late nineteenth century, engaged in a variety of investigations into child development and psychology, and was known for using what method to collect data?
    A. Serum samples
    B. EEG
    C. Hypnosis
    D. Questionnaires
    E. Focus groups

40. An expert witness who testifies in court is:
    A. The clinician who has had the most clinical contact in a case
    B. A witness with at least 3 years experience after board certification
    C. Recognized in her field for her expertise
    D. Permitted to testify about conclusions or opinions
    E. Usually an employee of an academic center

41. True or False: SSRI discontinuation syndrome is characterized by increased suicidal ideation in children and adolescents.
    A. True
    B. False

42. Which of the following is the most common problem that emerges for parents of children with childhood cancer?
    A. Posttraumatic stress disorder (PTSD)
    B. Alcohol abuse
    C. Brief psychotic disorder
    D. Somatization disorder
    E. Factitious disorder by proxy (Munchhausen's syndrome)

43. Based on studies of Romanian children, significant reduction of inhibited behaviors in children with reactive attachment disorder was a response to which of the following?
    A. Recreational therapies
    B. High staff-to-children ratio in institutions
    C. Enrollment in special education
    D. Foster care placement
    E. Psychopharmacology

44. Which of the following terms best describes the study of "what a drug does to the body"?
    A. Pharmacology
    B. Pharmacokinetics
    C. Pharmacodynamics
    D. Psychopharmacology
    E. None of the above

45. Which of the following is an approach used to treat substance use in adolescents?
    A. Motivational interviewing
    B. CBT, individual and group
    C. Multisystemic therapy
    D. Community reinforcement therapy
    E. All of the above

46. In interpersonal psychotherapy with depressed adolescents (IPT-A), a termination date is set with the adolescent and family at the beginning of treatment, and the adolescent is reminded of the number of weeks remaining until the end of treatment. What is the time frame chosen for clinical trials assessing the efficacy of IPT-A?
    A. 20 weeks
    B. 16 weeks
    C. 12 weeks
    D. 6 weeks
    E. 1 week

47. True or False: The addition of valproate can significantly elevate lamotrigine levels in the body.
    A. True
    B. False

48. What proportion of youth in the United States pursues college or postgraduate studies after high school?
    A. Under 20%
    B. 40%
    C. Over 60%
    D. 100%

49. When determining a child's baseline level of communicative functioning, standardized tests that focus narrowly on specific areas of function rather than broad-based batteries are used. ALL of the following are examples of standardized tests for focused assessment EXCEPT:
    A. Peabody Picture Vocabulary Test—3rd edition
    B. Oral and Written Language Scales
    C. Test of Narrative Language
    D. Test of Pragmatic Language
    E. Test of Written Language

50. The incidence rate is calculated as follows:
    A. Number of new onsets of disease divided by sum of observation time across individuals
    B. Number of new onsets of disease divided by sum of individuals
    C. Number of individuals with disease divided by sum of individuals
    D. Number of new onsets of disease divided by sum of observation time multiplied by number of individuals
    E. None of the above

51. Complete the following statement. Puberty in girls...
    A. begins on average at 11 to 13 years of age
    B. begins after puberty in boys
    C. takes approximately 1 to 2 years from start to finish
    D. begins approximately 2 years earlier than the average onset for boys

52. Which of the following is NOT a risk factor for childhood onset schizophrenia?
    A. Advanced paternal age
    B. Familial schizophrenia spectrum disorders
    C. Familial neurocognitive deficits
    D. Familial pervasive developmental disorders
    E. Familial mood disorder

53. The process whereby schools send children to the emergency room for evaluation to obtain psychiatric clearance is commonly known as:
    A. Proactive evaluation
    B. Help our Students 9-1-1
    C. Meeting the standard of care
    D. Let's All Be Safe, Not Sorry
    E. Zero tolerance

54. True or False: The amount of talk that caregivers direct toward their young children is associated with vocabulary growth and preliteracy skills.
    A. True
    B. False

55. True or False: Only females are affected by Rett's disorder.
    A. True
    B. False

56. The literature supports most which treatment for selective mutism?
    A. Anxiolytic medications
    B. Behavioral modification approaches
    C. CBT
    D. Psychodynamic therapy
    E. Speech therapy

57. OCD probands have a family history of:
    A. Tics
    B. OCD
    C. Other anxiety disorders
    D. Tourette's disorder
    E. All of the above

58. Which of the following describes the hypothesized mechanism of action of amphetamines?
    A. Targets norepinephrine receptors in the striatum
    B. Promotes the release of serotonin in the prefrontal cortex
    C. Selectively promotes the release of newly synthesized dopamine while also blocking dopamine reuptake at the transporter
    D. Promotes the release of stored dopamine and blocks the return of dopamine at presynaptic dopamine transporter sites
    E. Selectively prevents the reuptake of serotonin by the serotonin transporter

59. A study in which the unit of observation is the group rather than the individual is known as:
    A. Cohort
    B. Case–control
    C. Ecological
    D. Cross-sectional

60. Internalized homophobia in gay youth functions as a defense mechanism and results from the ego's struggle between rules and desires. It is comprised of a number of defense methods. These include ALL of the following EXCEPT:
    A. Rationalization
    B. Denial
    C. Projection
    D. Identification with the aggressor
    E. Splitting

61. Which of the following is TRUE for the severity of hearing impairment?
    A. Mild hearing impairment: <40 dB in the better ear
    B. Moderate hearing impairment: <70 dB in the better ear
    C. Severe hearing impairment: <95 dB in the better ear
    D. Profound hearing impairment: >96 dB in the better ear
    E. All of the above

62. Which of the following statements describes what clinical assessments of infants and toddlers CANNOT provide?
    A. A measure of fixed intelligence
    B. A trajectory for future development
    C. A window on future adjustment
    D. Potential causal factors for presenting symptoms
    E. All of the above

63. True or False: Tricyclic antidepressants can have a dose-dependent adverse effect on cardiac conduction.
    A. True
    B. False

64. In the process of informed consent which of the following should be discussed with the patient?
    A. The nature and condition that requires treatment
    B. The nature, purpose, and benefits of the proposed treatment and the probability that it will succeed
    C. The risks and consequences of each of the following: the proposed treatment, the alternative treatments, and no treatment
    D. The prognosis with and without the proposed treatment
    E. All of the above

65. True or False: The agreement on childhood psychopathology between different informants is notoriously low and is only moderate at best.
    A. True
    B. False

66. Children, as a class of persons, lack the legal capacity for consent, so other means should be taken to show respect for children in place of consent, which includes which TWO of the following?
    A. Capacity
    B. Permission
    C. Comprehension
    D. Assent
    E. Informed

67. The New Beginnings Program is an example of:
    A. A universal preventive intervention targeting children at risk for substance use
    B. A selective preventive intervention targeting children whose parents had divorced
    C. Ali G's New Year's resolution
    D. A universal preventive intervention targeting children entering high school
    E. None of the above

68. True or False: The biopsychosocial model of formulation offers very little guidance on how to integrate three conceptually different areas of a patient's life other than citing them together in the formulation.
    A. True
    B. False

69. The incidence of childhood stuttering is highest between a child's:
    A. Day of birth and second birthday
    B. Second birthday and fourth birthday
    C. Fourth birthday and sixth birthday
    D. Sixth birthday and eighth birthday
    E. Eighth birthday and tenth birthday

70. ALL of the following are psychosocial strategies in making aggressive behavior in children ineffective by changing the consequences of the behavior EXCEPT:
    A. Behavior does not reap positive outcomes
    B. Incentivize alternatives
    C. Behavior does not visibly rile adults
    D. Reduce provocation and frustration
    E. Negative consequences for problem behavior

71. True or False: Placement of a child in multiple foster care homes may result in major behavioral symptoms.
    A. True
    B. False

72. What is number of children in the United States living in a single-parent family?
    A. 1 in 2
    B. 1 in 3
    C. 1 in 4
    D. 1 in 5
    E. 1 in 10

73. In twin studies of anorexia nervosa, the following has been found:
    A. Monozygotic concordance rates are higher than dizygotic concordance rates
    B. Monozygotic concordance rates are equal to dizygotic concordance rates
    C. Monozygotic concordance rates are lower than dizygotic concordance rates
    D. Monozygotic concordance rates are equal to nontwin sibling concordance rates

74. Which of the following matches the Diagnostic and Statistical Manual of Mental Disorders (DSM) diagnostic criteria for encopresis?
    A. The repeated passage of feces into inappropriate places once a week for at least 1 month
    B. The repeated passage of feces into inappropriate places once a week for at least 3 months
    C. The repeated passage of feces into inappropriate places once a month for at least 3 months
    D. None of the above

75. Between 1960 and 2000 the prevalence of being overweight among children ages 6 to 11 increased by:
    A. No change
    B. Two-fold
    C. Four-fold
    D. Ten-fold
    E. Twenty-fold

76. What is the approximate ratio of suicidal ideation to completed suicide in adolescents?
    A. 2,000:1
    B. 1,000:1
    C. 500:1
    D. 100:1
    E. 50:1

77. In the 1950s, Money and colleagues' research on children with physical intersex conditions showed that a key milestone in gender identity formation was between:
    A. 9 and 18 months of age
    B. 9 and 24 months of age
    C. 18 and 36 months of age
    D. 24 and 36 months of age
    E. 36 and 48 months of age

78. Which of the following is most important to address when working with a child and her family when the child has sleep difficulties?
    A. Her comfort
    B. Her security
    C. Her regularity of sleep habits
    D. Protection from overstimulation
    E. All of the above

79. A child entering first grade should be able to do ALL of the following EXCEPT:
    A. Draw a detailed person with body, arms, legs, hands, and feet
    B. Recite the alphabet
    C. Define right and wrong in terms of punishment and pain
    D. Participate in family rituals and routines around meals and bedtimes
    E. Count beyond 20

80. Reduction of tic severity in Tourette's disorder usually ends by what age?
    A. Age 10
    B. Early 20s
    C. Middle age
    D. Late 50s
    E. Tic severity is chronic

81. True or False: Transference refers specifically to intrapsychic conflicts stirred in the therapist by the patient.
    A. True
    B. False

82. Acidic drugs in the general circulation, when bound to plasma protein, bind to which molecule?
    A. Very low-density lipoproteins
    B. Alpha-1 acid glycoprotein
    C. Platelets
    D. Albumin
    E. High-density lipoprotein

83. True or False: The level of agreement (measured by the kappa statistic) between parents and children in rating their psychiatric symptoms has been found to be high, greater than 0.75.
    A. True
    B. False

84. What does the acronym PANDAS stand for?
    A. Pediatric Anatomic Neurologic Disorders Associated with Streptococci infection
    B. Psychiatric Anatomic Neurologic Disorders Associated with Streptococci infection
    C. Pediatric Autoimmune Neuropsychiatric Disorder Associated with Streptococcal infection
    D. Psychiatric Autoimmune Neuroanatomical Disorders Associated with Streptococci infection
    E. Black and white bears native to central-western and southwestern China

85. True or False: Standard deviation is the most common measure of variability for nominal or categorical data.
    A. True
    B. False

86. Which of the following is the BEST definition of a fiduciary relationship?
    A. A relationship composed of a financial transaction for services provided
    B. A relationship in which one receives the trust of another person and is under duty to act for the benefit of that person
    C. A relationship with a contractual basis
    D. A relationship involving legal services

87. True or False: The rehabilitative approach to the treatment of pediatric somatoform illness encourages the patient to rest from usual activities until symptomatic relief is first provided.
    A. True
    B. False

88. True or False: Guanfacine has a longer half-life than clonidine.
    A. True
    B. False

89. True or False: A 21-year longitudinal study of a community sample followed from childhood to late adolescence or early adulthood reported that risk of suicidal behavior in late adolescence and early adulthood was related to severe family adversity.
    A. True
    B. False

90. True or False: Infants and toddlers account for the largest increase in the use of childcare services in the past 15 years or so.
    A. True
    B. False

91. In the 1950s and 1960s, efforts to treat children who had autism included:
    A. Insulin coma
    B. Cold sheet packs
    C. Child and parent psychotherapy
    D. Chlorpromazine
    E. Past life regression

92. True or False: A 5-year study of the impact of managed behavioral health care revealed that access to health services in general has decreased for young people.
    A. True
    B. False

93. The process of behavioral and attitudinal changes in a cultural subgroup because of exposure to the practices of a different dominant group is referred to as:
    A. Accommodation
    B. Culture bound syndrome
    C. Acculturation
    D. Cultural Mask
    E. Ethnic Identity

94. Groups composed of how many members are ideal for most therapeutic tasks?
    A. 2 to 4
    B. 4 to 6
    C. 6 to 8
    D. 8 to 10
    E. It makes no significant difference

95. For inpatient medical services, which of the following is the most common request for consultation–liaison services?
    A. Adjustment problems
    B. Nonadherence
    C. Depression/suicide
    D. Pain management
    E. Parent coping

96. True or False: In resilience studies, low intelligence can be a vulnerability factor among children experiencing severe and chronic life adversities.
    A. True
    B. False

97. Heinz Hartmann, a psychoanalytic theorist, conceptualized "autonomous" ego functions as relatively resistant to disturbances caused by intrapsychic conflict. ALL of the following are examples of "autonomous" ego functions EXCEPT:
    A. Perception
    B. Motility
    C. Defenses
    D. Intention
    E. Logical thought

98. The Vineland Adaptive Behavior Scale assesses capacities for self-sufficiency in ALL of the following domains of functioning EXCEPT:
    A. Communication
    B. Daily living skills
    C. Socialization
    D. Motor skills
    E. Learning and memory

99. At what point is the plasma steady-state concentration of a drug reached?
    A. Usually in two or three plasma half-lives of the drug
    B. When a fixed amount of the drug is eliminated per unit time regardless of the plasma level
    C. Usually in five or six plasma half-lives of the drug
    D. When there is equilibrium between the amount of drug ingested and the amount of drug eliminated

100. Classic as well as recent studies of psychopathic adults have found greater incidence of ALL the following attributes compared with normal controls EXCEPT:
    A. More tolerant of pain
    B. More in touch with their emotions
    C. Less able to be conditioned
    D. More sensitive to monetary cues

101. ALL of the following is a protective factor for children in divorce EXCEPT:
    A. Good relationship with at least one parent or caregiver
    B. Parental warmth
    C. Support of siblings
    D. Support of peers
    E. Male gender

102. For mild-to-moderate OCD in children and adolescents, which option is generally considered the first line of intervention?
    A. Clomipramine
    B. CBT with flooding and response prevention
    C. CBT with exposure and response prevention
    D. CBT
    E. CBT with clomipramine

103. Some intraspecies differences may depend on which parent passed on a particular piece of genetic material; this is called genetic ___?
    A. Polymorphism
    B. Variation
    C. Phenomena
    D. Imprinting
    E. Mutation

104. Valproate inhibits the glucuronidation (Phase II metabolism) of which of the following medications?
    A. Lamotrigine
    B. Quetiapine
    C. Sertraline
    D. Amoxapine
    E. Lorazepam

105. True or False: Every child who tests low on a standardized test to assess speech and language concerns will be able to receive services for a communication deficit.
    A. True
    B. False

106. What percentage of the U.S. population are adoptees?
    A. 0.5%
    B. 1%
    C. 3%
    D. 5%
    E. 7%

107. Narcolepsy is most likely to appear when a child is:
    A. A toddler
    B. In preschool
    C. In elementary school
    D. In junior or high school
    E. All of the above

108. Self-monitoring is an effective technique for which of the following?
    A. Keeping track of moods and planning for unpleasant events in the treatment of depression
    B. Increasing awareness and developing competing responses in the treatment of Tourette's syndrome
    C. Tracking use of breathing and relaxation procedures in the treatment of anxiety
    D. A and C
    E. All of the above

109. What are basic questions to consider when gathering information regarding a child's communication?
    A. What does the family see as the child's most important problem in communication
    B. Can people outside the family understand the child's speech
    C. Can the child follow verbal directions at home and at school
    D. How does the problem influence the child across various environments, including school and social settings
    E. All of the above

110. Which is the most effective treatment for enuresis?
    A. Desmopression acetate
    B. Imipramine
    C. Behavioral interventions
    D. Tolterodine (Detrol)
    E. None of the above

111. Which diagnosis below pertains to the following description? A "minor" or subsyndromal depression, diagnosed in the presence of depressed mood, anhedonia, or irritability, and up to three symptoms of major depression.
    A. Dysthymic disorder
    B. Depressive disorder, not otherwise specified
    C. Double depression
    D. Bipolar II depressive episode
    E. Adjustment disorder with depressed mood

112. A study using the Great Smoky Mountains database found that children diagnosed with bipolar not otherwise specified, or the "broad phenotype" of bipolar disorder, were more likely to develop what disorder later?
    A. Bipolar
    B. Anxiety
    C. Depression
    D. Schizophrenia
    E. ADHD

113. Secondary enuresis is defined according to the DSM as:
    A. A child with enuresis who had maintained continence for at least 3 months before the onset of enuresis
    B. A child with enuresis who had maintained continence for at least 6 months before the onset of enuresis
    C. A child with enuresis who had maintained continence for at least 9 months before the onset of enuresis
    D. A child with enuresis who had maintained continence for at least 1 year before the onset of enuresis
    E. Enuresis that develops after a period of established urinary continence

114. True or False: ADHD is a genetically predisposed disorder that follows a Mendelian pattern of inheritance.
    A. True
    B. False

115. IPT-A met four conditions of a study that permit its inclusion as an efficacious treatment. Which of the following is NOT one of these conditions?
    A. The treatment is manual based
    B. The treatment was superior to medication management
    C. The sample characteristics were detailed
    D. The treatment was tested in randomized clinical trials
    E. At least two different investigator teams demonstrated the intervention's effects

116. True or False: Children can be classified using the DSM-IV.
    A. True
    B. False

117. The second Tarasoff case in California addressed which of the following in its decision:
    A. The duty to warn a potential victim
    B. The duty to notify the police or hospitalize the patient
    C. The duty to protect the potential victim
    D. The duty to protect the patient from his or her actions
    E. The clinician's liability in breaking confidentiality

118. True or False: The available literature about the effects of marijuana use on other drug use concluded that there is a relationship between marijuana use and progression to other drugs.
    A. True
    B. False

119. A 4-year-old boy in the hospital for a chronic medical illness receives a painful lumbar puncture without distress; however, after an intravenous insertion that results in a small amount of blood at the site, the child becomes inconsolable. Which of the following might be an explanation?
    A. His mother was not present for the lumbar puncture
    B. For some reason, he likes lumbar punctures
    C. For some reason, he dislikes intravenous insertions
    D. He views the body as a fluid filled sac that will leak if the skin is compromised

120. In the United States there are more than 3,600 facilities that house juvenile offenders. On any given day the number of juvenile offenders in these facilities is:
    A. 23,000
    B. 55,000
    C. 110,000
    D. 220,000
    E. 550,000

121. Which is the correct frequency for the respective waveform?
    A. Alpha: 4 to 8 Hz
    B. Beta: 8 to 13 Hz
    C. Alpha: 8 to 13 Hz
    D. Theta: 13 to 30 Hz
    E. Delta: 4 to 8 Hz

122. Which of the following is the normal milestone for speech development regarding a child's ability to babble?
    A. 2 months
    B. 4 months
    C. 6 months
    D. 10 months
    E. 12 months

123. What is a transient side effect of OKT3, an agent used to prevent rejection in the immediate postoperative period after a transplant?
    A. Intense depression
    B. Intense anxiety
    C. Hallucinations
    D. Panic attacks
    E. PTSD

124. True or False: Manualized CBT treatment appears to be superior to pharmacotherapy for trichotillomania.
    A. True
    B. False

125. In McHugh and Slavney's four perspectives in psychiatric assessments that serve as an alternative to the biopsychosocial approach to formulation, which component addresses "what a patient wants"?
    A. Disease
    B. Dimension
    C. Behavior
    D. Life story

126. Which of the following statements correctly describes Carol Gilligan's belief about the relationship between body image and IQ in preadolescent girls?
    A. Recognition of a low IQ leads to improved body image
    B. Body image and IQ are determined solely by genetic factors
    C. A negative body image has been associated with high IQ
    D. Preadolescent girls switch to IQ as the primary way to measure themselves
    E. Body image is not related in any way to IQ

127. ALL of the following SSRIs can have nonlinear pharmacokinetics at higher doses EXCEPT:
    A. Paroxetine
    B. Fluvoxamine
    C. Fluoxetine
    D. Citalopram

128. Four categories of techniques are generally employed in the child psychiatric interview, which include engagement, projective, direct questioning and interactive techniques. Which of the following describes direct questioning techniques?
    A. Techniques to put the child at ease so that the child will provide accurate and meaningful clinical information
    B. Techniques to allow the child to reveal underlying themes or issues that the child may be unable to verbalize directly
    C. Techniques to clarify particular points or to elicit specific information
    D. Techniques to clarify how the child relates to, as well as accepts or integrates, input from others

129. Which of the following is a brain state that is similar to fear that occurs in the absence of a stimulus
    A. It is in fact fear
    B. Anxiety
    C. Reverberating limbic loop
    D. Reverberating amygdala loop

130. Catatonia is defined by:
   A. Cognitive changes
   B. An EEG study
   C. A cluster of motor symptoms
   D. A mood disorder
   E. A type of schizophrenia

131. Which of the following is a clinical interview in which the interviewer is expected to ask questions until he or she can decide whether a symptom meeting the definition provided by the interview battery is present or not?
   A. Semistructured interview
   B. Fully structured interview
   C. Respondent-based interview
   D. Interviewer-based interview
   E. Glossary-based interview

132. True or false: Most preschool children do not recognize that their imaginary friends are not really visible.
   A. True
   B. False

133. True or False: Infant assessments are not only a measure of the child's functional or developmental status, but also a measure of the child's environment.
   A. True
   B. False

134. True or False: A licensed and board certified forensic psychiatrist is free to perform forensic evaluations in any state.
   A. True
   B. False

135. When was the DSM-I, the first official US classification for psychiatric disorders, initially published?
   A. 1776
   B. 1812
   C. 1917
   D. 1952
   E. 1983

136. Infants are able to respond differently to their fathers and mothers by what age?
   A. 8 months
   B. 6 months
   C. 4 months
   D. 2 months

137. What is the key difference between quasiexperimental and randomized experimental designs in research?
   A. The manner by which participants are assigned to groups
   B. The manner by which statistics are used to analyze the outcome data
   C. The quasiexperimental design lacks an independent variable
   D. The randomized experimental design lacks a dependent variable
   E. None of the above

138. The first mental health clinics for children in the United States served:
   A. Children entering the foster care system
   B. Mothers and children struggling with a father's alcoholism
   C. Kinship foster families
   D. Juvenile delinquents
   E. Orphans

139. When is it typical for infants to learn to crawl on hands and knees?
   A. 8 to 9 months
   B. 7 to 8 months
   C. 6 to 7 months
   D. 5 to 6 months

140. What act of Congress was designed to prevent children in foster care from languishing in temporary situations and to facilitate adoptions for children who could not be reunited with their biological families?

A. The Adoption Assistance Act of 1980

B. The Adoption Act of 1980

C. The Adoption Assistance and Child Welfare Act of 1980

D. The Foster Care and Residential Placement Transition Act of 1983

E. The Foster Care Act of 1983

141. An 18-year-old female underwent a deceased donor liver transplant at the age of 2 years. She has been prescribed paroxetine and clonazepam for generalized anxiety disorder. She has a history of stopping her rejection medications. She likes to smoke marijuana but says she stopped after an arrest for possession. Her low FK506—an immunosuppressant—levels are puzzling given her insistence that she is compliant. Which of the following is the most likely explanation?

A. Her parents were diverting the FK506 for other uses

B. The paroxetine reduced her FK506

C. The clonazepam reduced her FK506

D. Stopping the marijuana reduced her FK506

E. She was selling the FK506

142. True or False: Maternal employment has a negative effect on children.

A. True

B. False

143. Which option describes when it is desirable to "explode" a MeSH term in a PubMed search?

A. Alternatives to the MeSH term are desired

B. A more specific search pertaining to the MeSH term is desired

C. All the subheadings under the term are of potential interest

D. Not applicable as MeSH terms are only found on Medline

E. None of the above

144. True or False: To minimize devastating side effects, the use of antiretrovirals for the treatment of HIV infection in children should be reserved for patients who have advanced disease, as evidenced by a decline in CD4+ T lymphocytes.

A. True

B. False

145. Hallucinations in traumatized children tend to be associated with ALL of the following EXCEPT:

A. Impulsive behaviors

B. Aggressive behaviors

C. Self-injurious behaviors

D. Formal thought disorder

E. Trance-like states

146. In the observation of Caregiver's–infant interactions during a clinical assessment of the infant, ALL of the following choices are important sources of information EXCEPT:

A. Caregiver's attunement and responsiveness to child's affective state

B. Security of attachment between caregiver and infant

C. Child's psychological role in family

D. Infant's use of caregiver for support and reassurance

E. Caregiver's affective response to child's efforts during assessment

147. True or False: One relatively new measure of effect size, the number needed to treat ranges from 1 to infinity, and large values indicate a significant treatment effect.

A. True

B. False

148. What is the success rate of the bell and pad method for the treatment of enuresis?

A. 95%

B. 75%

C. 25%

D. 10%

149. Headache appears to be the most common type of pain reported by school-aged children and adolescents, with 10% to 30% reporting "frequent" headaches or headaches on at least a weekly basis. Which of the following statements about migraines is most accurate?
    A. There are at least five headache attacks where the headache lasted 1 to 72 hours
    B. The headache has at least two of the following: unilateral location, pulsating quality, moderate to severe pain intensity, and/or aggravated by routine physical activity
    C. The headache is accompanied by nausea and/or vomiting or photophobia and phonophobia
    D. A and C
    E. All of the above

150. Which of the following statements describe the concept of psychic determinism?
    A. The principle that nothing in the mind happens by chance or in a random way
    B. The attribution of internal conflicts to the external environment and a search for external solutions
    C. All psychic acts and events have meanings and causes and can be understood in terms of earlier psychic events
    D. The principle of prognosis by way of psychoanalytic free association
    E. A and C

151. In a child with acute onset of OCD and/or tics following pharyngitis, ALL of the following laboratory tests might be considered EXCEPT:
    A. Homovanillic acid assay
    B. Antideoxyribonuclease B titer
    C. Antistreptolysin O titer
    D. Serological studies for group A beta-hemolytic streptococcus infection
    E. Throat culture

152. ALL of the following family risk factors are associated with the development of disruptive behavior disorders EXCEPT:
    A. Domestic violence
    B. Excessive parental control
    C. Lack of parental supervision
    D. Older male siblings
    E. Early motherhood

153. Which description best characterizes somatoform disorders?
    A. Mental illness manifested as physical symptoms
    B. Physical symptoms that are the product of psychological symptoms
    C. Physical symptoms that suggest a physical disorder but are not fully explained by the presence of a general medical condition
    D. Physical symptoms that suggest a mental disorder but are not fully explained by the presence of a general medical condition

154. Which of the following rare but serious adverse effects is associated with nefazodone, a potent $5HT_{2a}$ antagonist?
    A. Priapism
    B. Hepatoxicity
    C. Neutropenia
    D. Renal insufficiency
    E. Pulmonary edema

155. True or False: Thyroid-stimulating hormone levels may increase in association with higher lithium levels.
    A. True
    B. False

156. A psychotherapeutic intervention is considered a well established, evidence-based therapy if positive effects are demonstrated in a series of carefully controlled, prospective studies by at least two independent teams of investigators. These clinical trials can be generally defined by which TWO of the following criteria?
    A. All raters of treatment progress are blinded
    B. The therapeutic intervention is considered the independent variable
    C. Efficacy and results are reported by effect size, Cohen's *d*
    D. Participants are randomly assigned to treatment groups
    E. Treatment is compared with a placebo or other established intervention

157. Stress inoculation techniques in the treatment of PTSD include ALL of the following EXCEPT:
    A. Cognitive restructuring of thoughts about the event
    B. Positive imagery and self-talk
    C. Thought stopping
    D. Self-monitoring
    E. Avoiding places that are reminders of the event

158. True or False: The ego's task is to optimize pleasure and gratification of wishes and needs while maintaining internal equilibrium, the health of the body, good relations with the external world, and peace with the superego.
    A. True
    B. False

159. The most commonly reported symptoms of panic attacks in adolescents include ALL of the following EXCEPT:
    A. Trembling
    B. Dizziness/faintness
    C. Pounding heart
    D. Nausea
    E. Fear of dying

160. Treatment of encopresis often consists of a combination of ALL of the following EXCEPT:
    A. Laxatives
    B. Motility agents
    C. Dietary changes
    D. Routine pants checks
    E. Overcorrection procedures

161. In an effort to increase the gene-finding power of linkage studies of common child psychiatric disorders, ALL of the following approaches have been employed EXCEPT:
    A. Increasing the number of well characterized samples through collaboration
    B. Stratification of patients (i.e., based on age, sex, etc.)
    C. Identification of endophenotypes
    D. Increasing genetic heterogeneity in research samples
    E. Unifying inclusion criteria

162. True or False: The ratio of males to females in adult samples of ADHD approximates 2:1 or even close to 1:1.
    A. True
    B. False

163. What are key psychosocial interventions in bipolar disorder?
    A. Emphasizing sleep hygiene
    B. Emphasizing a routine
    C. Reducing expressed emotion
    D. Educating school personnel
    E. All of the above

164. True or False: The DSM-I included childhood disorders among its psychiatric classification.
    A. True
    B. False

165. Which TWO of the following functions should be assessed further when assessing for apraxia in a child?
    A. Sensory perception
    B. Motor function
    C. Expressive language function
    D. Visual motor function

166. True or False: The prevalence of PTSD in women is equal to the rate observed in men as found in the National Comorbidity Survey of individuals 15 to 54 years old.
    A. True
    B. False

167. Which of the following refers to a youth's self-perceived gender, regardless of chromosomal constitution, gonadal or hormonal secretions, or genitalia?
    A. Gender role
    B. Sexual orientation
    C. Gender identity
    D. Gender crisis
    E. None of the above

168. The Surgeon General reports on mental health point to research evidence supporting the effectiveness of ALL of the following community-based services EXCEPT:
    A. Intensive case management
    B. Therapeutic foster care
    C. Partial hospitalization
    D. Intensive in-home wraparound interventions
    E. Respite services

169. Regarding cognitive deficits in autism, ALL of the following are true EXCEPT:
    A. Approximately half of persons with autism have MR
    B. IQ tests are generally stable and show scatter in performance
    C. Lower IQ scores predict a worse outcome
    D. Lower levels of intelligence are associated with a greater risk of developing a seizure disorder
    E. Deficits in abstract thinking and processing information are uncommon

170. Which of the following statements is FALSE?
    A. Children of some cultures are not allowed to communicate their feelings after a disaster
    B. Families often fail to appreciate the severity of children's distress due to disasters
    C. Western therapeutic disaster interventions can be used in nonwestern societies
    D. Debriefing has proven to be mostly helpful immediately after the disaster
    E. Studies have shown a correlation between the reactions of children and their mothers to disasters

171. True or False: Early family relationships are relatively unimportant in shaping long-term resilient trajectories.
    A. True
    B. False

172. In psychodynamic play therapy, children's activities can be classified in ALL of the following general categories EXCEPT:
    A. Games with rules
    B. Physical activities
    C. Creative projects
    D. Progressive exposure to phobias
    E. Imaginary play

173. Which of the following is a characteristic of an effective school?
    A. Administrative personnel taking care of all decision-making
    B. School staff with low expectations of students
    C. An orderly environment
    D. Large school size
    E. Less frequent monitoring of student progress

174. Deficits in working memory are likely to impact which academic skill?
A. Reading and spelling
B. Mathematics
C. Written language
D. Oral language
E. None of the above

175. Which of the following describes a type II error when testing a null hypothesis?
A. To reject the null hypothesis when in fact it is true
B. To not reject the null hypothesis when it is false
C. To not reject the null hypothesis when it is true
D. To reject the null hypothesis when it is false
E. None of the above

176. The basic ethical principles that should underlie the conduct of research with human subjects as identified by the National Commission for the Protection of Human Subjects of Biomedical and Behavioral Research include ALL of the following EXCEPT:
A. Respect for persons
B. Beneficence
C. Goodwill to all
D. Justice

177. True or False: Borderline personality disorder is thought to be an interpersonally driven diagnosis with no biological underpinnings.
A. True
B. False

178. In infant assessments, age equivalent scores used to represent a child's development in comparison with a typically developing child are easy to misinterpret and may lead to erroneous conclusions. ALL of the following choices highlight the weaknesses of age equivalent scores EXCEPT:
A. They imply too much about an infant's development, especially when their skills are highly scattered
B. Due to how the tests are scored, infants who are consistent in their ability to do tasks typical for their age often receive an age equivalent score much higher than their chronological age
C. They do not adequately express the severity of developmental delays
D. The data used to compute age equivalents is too weak statistically to support the calculation of confidence intervals
E. They are expressed vaguely by estimates of equivalent years of chronological age and not in equivalent months

179. Fill in the blanks: Clonidine and guanfacine are potent _____ and tend to _____ noradrenegeric tone?
A. Alpha-1 receptor agonists, increase
B. Alpha-1 receptor antagonists, decrease
C. Alpha-2 receptor antagonists, decrease
D. Alpha-2 receptor agonists, decrease
E. Alpha 2 receptor agonists, increase

180. Phencyclidine can be detected in the urine for how long?
A. Less than 24 hours
B. 3 to 5 days
C. 7 days
D. 1 week
E. 2 to 4 weeks

181. Failure to thrive is an eating disorder of infancy or early childhood defined by:
A. Weight below the 5th percentile
B. Height below the 5th percentile
C. Head Circumference below the 5th percentile
D. Marked deceleration of weight gain and a slowing or disruption of acquisition of emotional and social developmental milestones
E. All of the above

182. True or False: Oppositional defiant disorder symptoms appear earlier than symptoms of conduct disorder.
    A. True
    B. False

183. True or False: The diagnosis of reactive attachment disorder was introduced for the first time as a psychiatric diagnosis in DSM-IV.
    A. True
    B. False

184. The Brazelton Neonatal Behavioral Assessment Scale, second edition , assesses the neonate as the child moves from a sleeping to an alert state using ALL of the following categorical items EXCEPT:
    A. Respiratory function
    B. Neurological intactness
    C. State regulation
    D. Autonomic reactivity
    E. Responsiveness to multiple stimuli

185. Which of the following statements is accurate about the prevalence of subclinical obsessions or compulsions in children?
    A. In children under 6 years of age, the urge to make things just right and preoccupations with symmetry and rules are very common
    B. Sixty percent of 4th graders report engaging in checking behaviors and preoccupations with guilt about lying and 50% report contamination and germ fears
    C. Sixty percent of 8th graders report worries about cleanliness and 50% note intrusive rude thoughts
    D. All of the above
    E. None of the above

186. Participation of the child psychiatrist in managing cases of Munchhausen syndrome by proxy is limited sometimes for the following reason:
    A. Countertransference of the child psychiatrist toward the mother
    B. Initial chief complaints do not seem to have psychiatric features
    C. Pediatricians are reluctant to request a child psychiatry consultation
    D. This is not a psychiatric disorder
    E. Adult psychiatrists are more involved than child psychiatrists are

187. The Youth Risk Behavior Surveillance System, with a nationally representative sample of 1,270 high school students from 9th to 12th grade, found what percentage had serious suicidal thoughts in the 12 months before the survey?
    A. 3%
    B. 8%
    C. 20%
    D. 25%
    E. 30%

188. What is the oldest age for which an adoption is still considered early?
    A. 2 years
    B. 4 years
    C. 6 years
    D. 8 years
    E. 10 years

189. Neurotrophins, including brain-derived neurotrophic factor, are thought to participate in the activity-dependent retraction of pruning of connections and synapses, and are thought to mediate learning and memory formation. These neurotrophins are part of a larger family known as:
    A. Hormones
    B. Amino acids
    C. Peptides
    D. Growth factors
    E. None of the above

190. In which year were the first training programs for child psychiatry accredited?
    A. 1889
    B. 1948
    C. 1959
    D. 1968
    E. 1977

191. Which of the following is NOT TRUE regarding talking time in the group therapy setting?
    A. Allows leaders to make any necessary announcements regarding member absences, upcoming events, or other practical issues
    B. Promotes sustained verbal interaction among group members
    C. May become quite lengthy in some types of groups
    D. Leaders should not allow it to exceed 10 minutes in psychotherapy and clinical support groups
    E. Leaders should always be the ones to announce when talking time is completed

192. Which of the following modalities has been tested extensively with youth at risk of detention and incarceration?
    A. Multisystemic Therapy
    B. Juvenile Justice System Centered Therapy
    C. Adolescent Post Adjudication Therapy
    D. Adolescent Psychosocial Community Treatment
    E. Family-based Support Network

193. True or False: All drugs undergoing hepatic and intestinal biotransformation must be metabolized in a Phase I reaction prior to undergoing conjugation by Phase II enzymes.
    A. True
    B. False

194. In the application of CBT in children and adolescents with depression, the use of behavioral activation techniques is a key feature. One strategy may include:
    A. Teaching patients to monitor their behavior for signs of undue excitement or mania
    B. Encouraging patients to normalize their routine and engage in rewarding activities, even if they do not feel like it at the time
    C. Teaching patients to counteract depressive symptoms by keeping a more positive outlook on life
    D. Encouraging patients to activate and take control of their lives by techniques of mastery and self-control

195. The two most important predictors of adult outcome in autism are:
    A. Intellectual functioning and competence in communication
    B. Level of repetitive behavior and competence in communication
    C. Quality of social and intellectual functioning
    D. Level of repetitive behavior and social skills
    E. Competence in communication and level of repetitive behavior

196. Which of the following is an elevated finding in boys with gender identity disorder?
    A. Increased rates of left-handedness
    B. Increased rates of right-handedness
    C. Increased rates of activity level
    D. Decreased rates of activity level
    E. A and D

197. What is the most common precipitant of PTSD in children and adolescents?
    A. Intrafamilial violence
    B. Neighborhood violence
    C. Automobile accidents
    D. War
    E. Terrorism

198. What percentage of children admitted to psychiatric units have a history of sexual and/or physical abuse during their lifetime:
    A. 15%
    B. 30%
    C. 55%
    D. 75%
    E. 97%

199. Patterns emerge in the psychological testing of children with Asperger's disorder that differ from typical findings. Which of the following statements is TRUE about those differences?
    A. Children with Asperger's disorder have relative weaknesses in auditory and verbal skills
    B. Children with Asperger's disorder have relative weaknesses in visual–perceptual skills
    C. Children with Asperger's disorder have patterns that are strikingly different from the pattern seen for nonverbal LDs
    D. Children with Asperger's disorder have relative strengths in the area of visual-motor skills
    E. Children with Asperger's disorder have relative strengths in the area of conceptual learning

200. True or False: Only a minority of children followed prospectively shows a persistence of gender identity disorder.
    A. True
    B. False

Answers

1. **Answer: A and C.** The child guidance movement and client-centered therapy contributed to the development of dynamic play therapy with children, but it should not be equated with child psychoanalytic therapy. Page 827.

2. **Answer: D.** Additional findings have also recently been reported from large-scale epidemiological studies. For individuals with severe mental retardation (MR), prevalence levels mostly converge on 3 to 4 children per 1,000; for mild MR, rates range wildly from 5.4 to 10.6 children per 1,000. Studies also examine such correlates as gender, age, and socioeconomic status. More boys than girls have MR, and rates of MR are generally low in the early years, peak at around 10 to 14 years, and decrease slightly in the late-school years and markedly during adulthood. Individuals of lower socioeconomic status and of ethnic minority groups (in several cultures) also show higher than expected rates of MR. Page 403.

3. **Answer: D.** Far more research on relevant genes and brain structure and function is available for children with specific reading disability than for any other learning disability. Page 413.

4. **Answer: C.** Approximately 15% to 25% of pediatric patients are thought to have mental health problems. Page 921.

5. **Answer: D.** Page 23.

6. **Answer: E.** It is important to note that some of the above findings reflect group trends, and many individuals with epilepsy do exceedingly well in all areas. Generally, the more severe the diagnosis, the more epilepsy is intractable, and the earlier the age of onset of epilepsy, the more the problems. Page 968.

7. **Answer: C.** This was one of the first examples of the importance of gene–environment interaction. Page 165.

8. **Answer: E.** Selective serotonin reuptake inhibitors (SSRIs) block the serotonin transporter located on presynaptic nerve terminals. Over time, this blockade leads to a desensitization of the serotonin autoreceptors, which typically exert an inhibitory influence on serotonin release; consequently, serotonergic function is enhanced. Page 763.

9. **Answer: D.** Page 105.

10. **Answer: A.** Quetiapine has also shown promising results in high-risk adolescents with bipolar depression. Page 773.

11–15. **Answers:** 11-C; 12-D; 13-A; 14-E; 15-B. Page 304.

16. **Answer: B.** The developmental differences in the maturation of noradrenergic pathways may explain in part why tricyclics are less effective in children with depression compared to adults. Page 742.

17. **Answer: A.** However, the specific genes conveying risk are unknown. Page 189.

18. **Answer: C.** Another common use of single photon emission computed tomography has been to study neurotransmitter systems. Page 218.

19. **Answer: C.** The other categories for special education eligibility are autism; intellectual disability (MR); sensory-hearing, vision, deafness, blindness; neurological; and communication. One or more of the aforementioned must be present and documented by medical evaluation/diagnosis and educational/psychological testing. Page 997.

20. **Answer: D.** After its peak, stranger anxiety tends to decline. Page 257.

21. **Answer: B.** In the population at large, the estimated prevalence of anorexia nervosa in young women in industrialized countries is 0.3%. Page 594.

22. **Answer: A.** Page 485.

23. **Answer: A.** Withdrawal and silence in the face of anxiety and hopelessness when treating a dying child may impair the ability to give the child and his family the best care possible. Each of the other options are possibilities, but less likely. Page 978.

24. **Answer: A.** Although the spatial resolution that can be obtained by electroencephalography (EEG) has improved through the use of over 100 scalp electrodes, poor spatial resolution is caused by the blurring of the EEG signal across electrodes by differences in conductivity of the skull, cerebral spinal fluid and other tissues. Page 228.

25. **Answer: C.** Page 764.

26. **Answer: C.** Page 855.

27. **Answer: D.** By the time children are 4 to 5 years old, they have acquired the ability to understand that their thoughts, beliefs, and feelings are their own and that others may feel or believe differently. Page 262.

28. **Answer: C.** Fragile X is an X-linked disorder and is the second most common cause of MR after Down syndrome. It is the most common inherited genetic cause. It affects as many as 1 in 750 to 1,000 males and 1 in 500 to 750 females. Page 201.

29. **Answer: D.** The rate of HIV has increased or remained the same. The decline in AIDS is the result of available treatment, which slows disease progression. Page 947.

30. **Answer: A.** Page 566.

31. **Answer: A.** Hypotension can occur even at low doses of less than 25 mg. Page 776.

32. **Answer: E.** Moreover, 19% of seriously emotionally disturbed youths received services from more than four mental health systems. Page 49.

33. **Answer: E.** Page 357.

34. **Answer: E.** The process of separation and individuation is impacted severely by a life-limiting illness. Pages 973–974.

35. **Answer: E.** The literature does not suggest any difference. Too few states legally allow nonheterosexual marriages to have adequate data on the divorce rate in gay and lesbian families. Page 1009.

36. **Answer: E.** Some environmental factors appear to be associated with risk for language delay, including lower socioeconomic status, larger family size, recurrent otitis media, neglectful home environment, and later birth order. It appears that the operative mechanism behind these factors is deprivation of enriched linguistic input, occurring at a critical stage in language development. Page 420.

37. **Answer: D.** Page 685.

38. **Answer: B.** The American Academy of Pediatrics recommends "Encourage, support, and protect breastfeeding." Page 610.

39. **Answer: D.** Although the questionnaire method was far from scientifically accurate, it represented progress in understanding child development and their capabilities in learning. G.S. Hall would send out questionnaires on a variety of topics to children at various ages. Arnold Gesell and Benjamin Spock both cite Hall as a significant influence upon the genesis of their work with children. Page 12.

40. **Answer: D.** An expert witness renders an opinion in their area of training and expertise during a court proceeding. A fact witness is one who can testify to the specific facts of a case. Page 1003.

41. **Answer: B.** This flu-like syndrome is characterized by dizziness, moodiness, nausea, vomiting, myalgia, and fatigue, which occur in association with the withdrawal or abrupt discontinuation of shorter acting SSRIs such as paroxetine, fluvoxamine, or sertraline. Page 763.

42. **Answer: A.** Mothers, especially, will experience symptoms of posttraumatic stress disorder. Page 932.

43. **Answer: D.** The Bucharest Early Intervention Project is a longitudinal study that includes baseline data about the children before their placement into foster care. The children who were placed in foster homes showed robust improvement in inhibited patterns of attachment disorder behaviors and somewhat less improvement in indiscriminate patterns. Page 716.

44. **Answer: C.** Page 237.

45. **Answer: E.** Page 621.

46. **Answer: C.** Twelve weeks is a reasonable duration for adolescents who are reluctant to stay in treatment for any significant length of time. Page 824.

47. **Answer: A.** Valproate is a UGT2B7 inhibitor; and as lamotrigine undergoes only Phase II glucuronidation, probably by way of UGT2B7 among other UGTs, its levels can become significantly elevated resulting in the increased risk of life-threatening Stevens–Johnson syndrome. Page 750.

48. **Answer: C.** Page 289.

49. **Answer: B.** The Oral and Written Language Scales is an example of a broad-based battery to assess language. This question is intended to inform the reader of the variety and purposes of different types of standardized testing in language. Page 374.

50. **Answer: A.** Page 150.

51. **Answer: D.** Puberty in girls begins, on average, at 9 to 11 years of age, approximately 2 years earlier than in boys, and takes approximately 4 to 5 years from start to finish. Page 280.

52. **Answer: E.** Familial mood disorder is not a risk factor for childhood onset schizophrenia. Page 495.

53. **Answer: E.** Page 900.

54. **Answer: A.** Page 262.

55. **Answer: B.** Both males and females can be affected by Rett's syndrome, although females are almost exclusively affected. Page 208.

56. **Answer: B.** Although some authors have suggested psychodynamic therapy for selective mutism, the most convincing literature pertains to behavioral modification approaches. Contingency management, stimulus fading, shaping, and response cost procedures have all been reported to be successful in eliciting and maintaining speech in selectively mute children. Page 427.

57. **Answer: E.** 10% to 30% of relatives of probands with obsessive–compulsive disorder (OCD) have OCD. Page 552.

58. **Answer: C.** Option D describes the hypothesized mechanism of action for methylphenidate. Page 757.

59. **Answer: C.** Also called an aggregate study. The level of analysis could be classrooms, schools, neighborhoods, municipalities, states, or countries. Page 153.

60. **Answer: E.** Splitting is not generally considered part of the cluster of defense methods that accounts for internalized homophobia. Page 84.

61. **Answer: E.** Page 67.

62. **Answer: E.** Clinical assessments of infants and toddlers can provide information regarding the child's current developmental level and environmental context, which can help with treatment planning and clinical decision-making. Page 309.

63. **Answer: A.** Hence the close monitoring of vital signs and obtaining an electrocardiogram before treatment, during dose adjustment, and at the maintenance phase of treatment with tricyclic antidepressants as there is the rare possibility of sudden death related to tachyarrhythmias such as *torsade de pointes*. Page 764.

64. **Answer: E.** Courts have held that not all risks need be discussed, only the material ones. A risk is material when a reasonable person would be likely to attach significance to the risk. Page 1025.

65. **Answer: A.** For example in one epidemiological survey of 6 to 11 year olds, only a quarter of children scoring the cutoff on at least one screening measure scored above threshold on both parent *and* teacher questionnaire. Correlation is increased when informants have similar roles (e.g., mother–father) and decreases when mixed pairs are questioned (e.g., parent–teacher or parent–child). Page 159.

66. **Answer: B and D.** In place of informed consent, permission of one or both parents or a legal guardian is required (permission to treat) as well as the agreement (assent) of the child. Page 144.

67. **Answer: B.** In this randomized, controlled trial children whose mothers received either 11 group and two individual sessions or the same exact treatment *plus* 11 sessions for the children did better than their comparison peers at 6-year follow-up on measures of alcohol and marijuana use, number of sexual partners, and psychiatric diagnoses. Page 174.

68. **Answer: A.** How the biological, psychological, and social realms should be integrated has thus far been unresolved. Page 378.

69. **Answer: B.** Incidence of childhood stuttering is highest between a child's second and fourth birthdays, ultimately affecting 4% to 5% of the population. Page 424.

70. **Answer: D.** Option D is a strategy on how to make aggressive behavior irrelevant by changing the antecedents. Page 477.

71. **Answer: A.** Landsverk and colleagues found that initial behavior problems was the strongest predictor of placement changes, but also found that children who showed no evidence of psychopathology at baseline developed significant behavior problems subsequent to multiple changes in placement. Page 695.

72. **Answer: C.** Moreover, one in every two children in African-American families lives in a single-parent household. Page 39.

73. **Answer: A.** In a series of 67 twin probands, Treasure and Holland found that the concordance for restricting anorexia nervosa was markedly higher for monozygotic (66%) than dizygotic twins (0%). Page 596.

74. **Answer: C.** The mental or chronological age must be at least 4 years. Mnemonic: 1 + 3 = 4. The two subtypes are "with constipation and overflow continence" and "without constipation and overflow continence". Page 663.

75. **Answer: C.** The National Health Examination surveys have revealed a four-fold increase among children ages 6 to 11 and a three-fold increase in adolescents ages 12 to 19 between 1960 and the most recent surveys, conducted between 1999 and 2002. Page 606.

76. **Answer: A.** The Youth Risk Behavior Surveillance System study found that 16.9% of high school students have seriously considered suicide in the past year. Page 1021.

77. **Answer: C.** Page 670.

78. **Answer: E.** Page 628.

79. **Answer: A.** Page 269.

80. **Answer: B.** Tic severity peaks between ages 8 to 11 years and tends to reduce in severity after puberty. This reduction usually ends in the early 20s resulting in the majority of persons with Tourette's syndrome having little to no symptoms in adulthood. Page 571.

81. **Answer: B.** Countertransference refers generically to all reactions of the therapist to the patient. Page 831.

82. **Answer: D.** Drugs that are basic in pH bind to alpha-1 acid glycoprotein. Page 746.

83. **Answer: B.** In studies involving psychiatric diagnoses, agreement rates between parents and children have ranged from $k = 0.32$ for a diagnosis of separation anxiety to as low as $k = 0.17$ for attention deficit hyperactivity disorder (ADHD). The kappa statistic between parents and children on dimensional measures is even worse. Pages 292–293.

84. **Answer: C.** Page 575.

85. **Answer: B.** The standard deviation is only appropriate in describing normally distributed data: the measure of spread, which describes the number of possible response categories, is used to describe nominal/categorical data. Page 106.

86. **Answer: B.** Examples of a fiduciary relationship include that of attorney and client, broker and client, as well as physician and patient. Trust is the cornerstone of this kind of professional relationship. Page 18.

87. **Answer: B.** One should discourage illness-related behaviors and focus the family away from finding a "cure" to instead finding a way to cope with and overcome a distressing physical problem. Cognitive-behavioral and operant interventions are often used, emphasizing positive reinforcement for functional improvement and extinction of reinforcement for sick role behaviors. Page 641.

88. **Answer: A.** This longer duration of action could translate into a need for fewer doses per day and a lower risk of rebound hypertension. Page 781.

89. **Answer: A.** Page 533.

90. **Answer: B.** There have been increases of 41% for infants and 53% for toddlers enrolled in child care. Page 255.

91. **Answer: C.** As a result of the case representation in Kanner's original group, it was thought that child pathology was due to "refrigerator" mothers; this notion has since been discredited. Page 386.

92. **Answer: B.** According to the National Health Care Reform Tracking Project, access to health care for children and youth have increased; but with the managed care emphasis on brief, problem-oriented approaches, it has become more difficult for children with serious emotional disorders and the uninsured to obtain the care they require. Page 36.

93. **Answer: C.** Definition of acculturation. Page 58.

94. **Answer: B.** Page 845.

95. **Answer: A.** The options are listed in order of frequency. They will differ from center to center. The purpose of this question is to highlight how commonly nonadherence to recommendations is a concern. Page 918.

96. **Answer: A.** Studies have shown that children with low intelligence are more vulnerable to adjustment difficulties over time than others. Page 295.

97. **Answer: C.** Motility subsumes walking and eye-hand coordination; other "autonomous" ego functions include speech, language, and intelligence. Page 830.

98. **Answer: E.** The Vineland Adaptive Behavior Scale is the most widely used instrument of adaptive functioning, which assesses capacities for self-sufficiency in various domains of functioning, including communication (receptive, expressive, and written language), daily living skills (personal, domestic, and community skills), socialization (interpersonal relationships, play and leisure time, and coping skills), and motor skills (gross and fine). Page 407.

99. **Answer: D.** A steady-state concentration results in no net change in plasma concentration over time, and it is usually attained after four or five plasma half-lives of the drug. Page 743.

100. **Answer: B.** Psychopathic adults also showed significantly less emotional arousal in experimental paradigms compared with normal controls. Page 469.

101. **Answer: E.** The data tends to suggest boys are more vulnerable than girls in both short and long-term consequences. Boys do better with regular paternal contact, if the father is reasonably healthy. Page 1007.

102. **Answer: C.** Page 558.

103. **Answer: D.** Genetic imprinting refers to the process by which one parent may pass on a particular piece of genetic information that does not affect the nucleotide sequence itself, but does alter the structure of the DNA. Prader-Willi and Angelman's syndrome (both due to alterations of DNA in the same chromosomal region on chromosome 15) are examples of imprinting. Page 178.

104. **Answer: A.** This point is important as concurrent therapy could cause an unintended increase in lamotrigine blood levels with an increased risk of developing Stevens–Johnson syndrome. Page 771.

105. **Answer: B.** Despite a child's poor test scores, local, state, and federal regulations determine eligibility for educational services, including speech and language services. Page 373.

106. **Answer: C.** 2.5% to 3.5%. Page 1014.

107. **Answer: D.** Narcolepsy has its peak onset in adolescence and young adulthood. It is characterized by (i) irresistible attacks of rapid eye movement sleep; (ii) cataplexy characterized by sudden loss of bilateral loss peripheral muscle tone; (iii) hypnagogic hallucinations; (iv) sleep paralysis. The adolescent sleeps 20 to 40 minutes and wakes refreshed, in contrast to other sleep disorders. Page 629.

108. **Answer: E.** Page 805.

109. **Answer: E.** The evaluator should also ask if the child attained the normal milestones of speech development. Pages 371–372.

110. **Answer: C.** Behavioral interventions such as a "pad and buzzer" or "moisture alarm" are the most effective; however, desmopressin acetate can be a useful short-term adjunct. Page 782.

111. **Answer: B.** This question considers a diagnosis made on the milder end of the range of depressive disorders. Page 503.

112. **Answer: C.** Page 768.

113. **Answer: D.** Page 655.

114. **Answer: B.** Although ADHD is a genetically predisposed disorder, it does not follow the Mendelian patterns of inheritance and it is also phenotypically complex. Page 433.

115. **Answer: B.** This question emphasizes knowledge of criteria for efficacious psychotherapies and the choices save for choice B, represent the criteria. Page 820.

116. **Answer: B.** Although this may appear to be a tricky question, it is not meant to frustrate you; it is a valid clinical point: disorders, not children, are classified. It is important to refer to the child's disorder, not to the child as the disorder. Page 304.

117. **Answer: B.** The First Tarasoff decision addressed duty to warn. The second case reexamined the first decision (and answer A might be considered correct as well). The court's decision in Tarasoff II found that clinicians must take reasonable care to protect the foreseeable victim. This may obviate the need for a warning, if a patient is hospitalized, say. As mentioned in another question and answer, clinicians must know the standards in their own state. Page 1023.

118. **Answer: A.** This occurs through selective recruitment of heavy users to other drugs; affiliation with drug using peers that allows for more drug using opportunities; and socialization into an illicit culture that creates favorable attitudes toward drug use. Page 617.

119. **Answer: D.** A preschool child can name body parts but will have a limited understanding of the details or internal structure. Page 913.

120. **Answer: C.** This question aims to provide an appreciation of the number of children being held in facilities across the United States. Fewer than 10% of families with children on probation have access to evidence-based programs in their community. Page 881.

121. **Answer: C.** Alpha 8 to 13 Hz, Beta 13 to 30 Hz, Delta 1 to 5 Hz, Theta 4 to 8 Hz. Alpha is the frequency when awake with eyes closed. Opening the eyes will lead to other waveforms appearing. With onset of drowsiness more theta and delta waves appear. Page 960.

122. **Answer: D.** Page 371.

123. **Answer: C.** Page 945.

124. **Answer: A.** Page 568.

125. **Answer: D.** The component of the life story refers to the patient's narratives as based on talk therapy. Page 380.

126. **Answer: C.** Carol Gilligan describes "hitting the cultural wall". This is when preadolescent girls realize that society often values appearance more than accomplishment, and they become more self-critical. Page 270.

127. **Answer: D.** For a discussion of nonlinear pharmacokinetics, refer to Chapter 6.1.1. Page 763.

128. **Answer: C.** Page 338.

129. **Answer: B.** One critical differentiation between normal and developmentally appropriate anxiety or fear is the criterion for functional impairment. Page 539.

130. **Answer: C.** These can include rigid posture, mutism, fixed staring, stereotypic movements, hyperkinetic movements, or stupor. Page 650.

131. **Answer: D.** Page 346.

132. **Answer: B.** Although preschoolers often struggle with the line between fantasy and reality, most children with imaginary friends are able to agree that the imaginary friend is not a real person. Page 264.

133. **Answer: A.** This point was emphasized in Chapter 4.2.1 in multiple ways. Page 321.

134. **Answer: B.** Many states now require licensure for forensic evaluations and failure to obtain a local license may result in civil or criminal liability. Page 21.

135. **Answer: D.** Page 305.

136. **Answer: D.** Research reveals how at 8 weeks infants respond differently to their parents. At 6 weeks, infants hunch their shoulders and lift their eyebrows when they see their fathers, while they appear to expect more routine handling, as in feeding or diapering, when they see or hear their mothers. Page 7.

137. **Answer: A.** Page 110.

138. **Answer: D.** The first juvenile courts were developed at the turn of the 19th to 20th century in Chicago and Boston. Some services were community based and aimed to improve parental supervision. Page 878.

139. **Answer: A.** This timeframe is typical, but as the authors indicate, infants may learn to move primarily in other ways, which by itself is not indicative of underlying problems. Page 253.

140. **Answer: C.** The Adoption and Safe Families Act of 1997 created additional requirements, including planning for permanence for children in foster care within a year of removal, and termination of parental rights for children who have been in foster care for 15 out of the last 22 months. The Adoption Promotion Act of 2003 gave enhanced incentives for adoption of older children. Page 698.

141. **Answer: D.** The marijuana reduced her gastric motility. After stopping, her gastric motility increased and she absorbed less FK506. Page 940.

142. **Answer: B.** Research on this subject has found that maternal employment in and of itself is not necessarily associated with either negative or positive effects. Page 40.

143. **Answer: C.** MeSH terms are the National Library of Medicine's controlled vocabulary for medical subject headings. Exploding a MeSH term means that all the subheadings underneath the term of interest will also be searched by PubMed. Page 132.

144. **Answer: B.** This was formerly the approach. Page 949.

145. **Answer: D.** Page 706.

146. **Answer: C.** Choice C is information obtained from the caregiver interview, and not particularly from observation of caregiver–infant interactions. Page 311.

147. **Answer: B.** Very large values of number needed to treat indicate no treatment effect. Page 119.

148. **Answer: B.** Success rate across studies has ranged from 30% to 87%, with most supporting the 75% vicinity. Page 659.

149. **Answer: E.** Page 635.

150. **Answer: E.** Conscious thoughts and overt behaviors provide observable clues to their underlying psychic determinants. Page 828.

151. **Answer: A.** These laboratory tests are to assess for Pediatric Autoimmune Neuropsychiatric Disorders associated with Streptococcal infection. Page 342.

152. **Answer: D.** Page 459.

153. **Answer: C.** Page 633.

154. **Answer: B.** Nefazodone's sale was discontinued in the United States in 2004 due to this severe adverse event. Page 766.

155. **Answer: A.** Thyroid replacement is not generally recommended unless T4 levels start to decrease or if clinical symptoms of hypothyroidism appear. Page 769.

156. **Answer: D and E.** All of the above answers have degrees of applicability to clinical trials; however, random assignment and treatment comparison with a control group are two standards for defining these empirical trials. Page 791.

157. **Answer: E.** Page 808.

158. **Answer: A.** Page 829.

159. **Answer: E.** Other common symptoms are shortness of breath and sweating. The point is that somatic symptoms are more common than cognitive ones. Page 541.

160. **Answer: B.** Pages 815–816.

161. **Answer: D.** Choices A, B, C, and E have the potential to increase the gene-finding power of linkage studies by identifying a more genetically homogenous group of subjects for study, thereby increasing the power of linkage studies. Increasing the genetic heterogeneity in research samples weakens the power of linkage analyses. Pages 193–194.

162. **Answer: A.** The prevalence of ADHD in adult populations is much more equal than in childhood, where it is more likely four or five to one in clinical samples of boys compared with girls. Page 440.

163. **Answer: E.** Page 520.

164. **Answer: B.** DSM-I included no childhood disorders. Page 455.

165. **Answer: B and D.** Page 368.

166. **Answer: B.** The prevalence in women at 10.4% is double the rate observed in men. Page 702.

167. **Answer: C.** Page 79.

168. **Answer: E.** The rationale behind respite services is not disputed, but this modality has not been studied, except for one quasiexperimental design. Page 893.

169. **Answer: E.** Deficits in abstract thinking and processing information are common in individuals with autism. Page 389.

170. **Answer: D.** The criticism raised against debriefing addresses not only outcome but the issue of timing of the intervention. Hobbs and Mayou think that too early an intervention may disrupt the adaptive defenses. Therefore, several authors have suggested intervening after the victims' recovery from their initial shock. Page 733.

171. **Answer: B.** They are extremely important: in a comprehensive review of the early childhood literature, Shonkoff and Phillips emphasized that "[relationships] that are created in the earliest years ... constitute a basic structure within which all meaningful development unfolds." Page 294.

172. **Answer: D.** The category of imaginary play can be further categorized as either solo play or imaginary play with the therapist as a participant. Page 833.

173. **Answer: C.** A list of characteristics of effective schools includes strong leadership, an atmosphere that is orderly and not oppressive, teachers who participate in decision-making, school staff that has high expectations of students, and frequent monitoring of student progress. In addition, large schools are often overmanned, meaning there are more students than role opportunities. Page 276.

174. **Answer: B.** Page 364.

175. **Answer: B.** A type II error is the error of omission: saying there was no difference between groups when there really was a difference. Page 115.

176. **Answer: C.** Page 140.

177. **Answer: B.** Page 683.

178. **Answer: E.** Page 314.

179. **Answer: D.** Clonidine and guanfacine stimulate presynaptic alpha-2 autoreceptors in the locus coeruleus to decrease noradrenergic tone, but their actions at the postsynaptic alpha-2 receptors in the cortex are likely the reason for the clinical benefits of improved attention and impulse control. Page 241.

180. **Answer: E.** Page 619.

181. **Answer: D.** Failure to thrive is a disorder of infancy and early childhood characterized by a marked deceleration of weight gain and a slowing or disruption of the acquisition of emotional and social developmental milestones. Deceleration of linear growth and head circumference growth are associated but are not primary phenomena. Page 586.

182. **Answer: A.** Page 457.

183. **Answer: B.** The DSM-III-R, introduced reactive attachment disorder and its two subtypes, "inhibited" and "disinhibited." The DSM-IV criteria highlight problems of social relatedness in reactive attachment disorder and require that a child demonstrate these aberrant patterns across settings. The DSM-IV also requires that there be a known history of "grossly pathogenic care." Page 712.

184. **Answer: A.** The Brazelton Neonatal Behavioral Assessment Scale, second edition, is primarily used to describe the range of behavioral responses to social and nonsocial stimuli. Page 316.

185. **Answer: D.** Subclinical phenomena are seen in as much as 80% of the general population. Page 549.

186. **Answer: B.** Although Munchhausen syndrome by proxy is a psychiatric disorder, the clinical presentation is medical, and often the apparent lack of psychiatric symptoms precludes a reason for the psychiatrist's involvement. Once the diagnosis is suspected, however, the child psychiatrist's contribution can be important in a number of ways. Page 724.

187. **Answer: C.** The options A—3% and B—8% represent suicidal injury and attempt, respectively. The Youth Risk Behavior Surveillance System is a regularly conducted survey and these high numbers have remained largely consistent. Page 530.

188. **Answer: A.** There is no set cutoff for "early" or "late"; in the past, adoption was considered early before the age of 5 years. However, studies of Romanian children adopted after the fall of the Ceausescu regime indicated that in children exposed to extreme early global deprivation, the duration of emotional deprivation predicted cognitive outcomes at the time of adoption as well as recovery in the adoptive family, with children under 2 years of age doing best. Page 1016.

189. **Answer: D.** Growth factors have been implicated in a broad range of developmental processes in which cell specification, growth, migration, and survival have to be coordinated across tissues or germ layers. Page 182.

190. **Answer: C.** A total of 11 training programs were accredited in 1959, and as of 2005, there were 114 approved child and adolescent psychiatry residency programs in the United States. Page 29.

191. **Answer: D.** In psychotherapy and clinical support groups, talking time may become quite lengthy as the group moves more deeply into its work. In social skills groups, leaders should limit talking time to approximately 10 minutes to allow sufficient opportunities to engage the group members in fuller social interaction. Page 846.

192. **Answer: A.** The other options are fictitious. Page 888.

193. **Answer: B.** Drugs such as the 3-hydroxybenzodiazepines (lorazepam, oxazepam, and temazepam) as well as lamotrigine are not metabolized by Phase I reactions, but are conjugated by glucuronidation only. Page 747.

194. **Answer: B.** This question refers to two key concepts of cognitive-behavioral therapy treatments for depression: cognitive restructuring, that is, increasing awareness of negative distortions and counteracting them to relieve depression; and behavioral activation techniques, which is based on the observation that depressed persons withdraw from activities that are potentially reinforcing. Page 506.

195. **Answer: A.** Higher intellectual functioning and ability to communicate have been shown to be the most important predictors of outcome but do not guarantee a positive outcome. Page 392.

196. **Answer: E.** Page 674.

197. **Answer: A.** Page 701.

198. **Answer: C.** Victims of abuse comprise a significant proportion of all psychiatric admissions, with lifetime incidence of physical and sexual abuse estimated at 30% among child and adolescent outpatients and as high as 55% among psychiatric inpatients. Page 692.

199. **Answer: B.** Psychological testing in children with Asperger's disorder typically follows a profile similar to that of nonverbal learning disability in that verbal skills are stronger than nonverbal skills which include visual-motor, visual perceptual, and conceptual learning. Page 395.

200. **Answer: A.** If gender identity disorder is present in adolescence, the rate for ongoing persistence is much higher. Page 677.

1. An infant or toddler developmental test may be useful for ALL of the following purposes EXCEPT:
   A. Diagnosis
   B. Assessment of intelligence quotient (IQ)
   C. Screening
   D. Early intervention planning

2. Investigators cured a child's rabbit phobia by systematically exposing the child to a rabbit while pairing the exposures with the incompatible response of eating food. This was one of the earliest demonstrations of which of the following techniques?
   A. Counter conditioning
   B. Operant conditioning
   C. Systematic desensitization
   D. Aversive counterconditioning
   E. Covert sensitization

3. True or False: Disruptive disorders accompanied by Attention Deficit Hyperactivity Disorder (ADHD) feature much more aggression than when ADHD is absent.
   A. True
   B. False

4. True or False: Medications may be administered in an inpatient unit in emergency circumstances, but permission must be obtained by the patient's guardian for standing medications.
   A. True
   B. False

5. What are the dizygotic twin concordance rates for autism spectrum disorders?
   A. 3% to 15%
   B. 16% to 25%
   C. 33% to 45%
   D. 50% to 65%
   E. 70% to 85%

6. Children with a medical illness who are in the early stages of Piaget's concrete operations:
   A. May identify themselves as bringing about their own illness as a punishment for misdeeds
   B. May use abstract reasoning to help them understand their bodies' internal structure
   C. May suck their thumbs
   D. Cry with the approach of an unknown clinical provider

7. Raising a child with cancer may alter a parent's ability to parent effectively. ALL of these are typical issues EXCEPT:
   A. Over protectiveness
   B. Difficulty with maintaining consistent discipline
   C. Difficulty expressing appropriate anger toward the child
   D. Concerns about spoiling the child
   E. Excessive focus on the here and now rather than the future

8. True or False: Compared to a group of children who had committed murder, children ages 10 through 17 who set fires were found to have lower rates of previous violent offenses.
   A. True
   B. False

9. A major conference held in 1944 under the auspices of the Commonwealth Fund provided a standard set of skill areas that should be mastered by psychiatrists who treat children and their families, which included ALL of the following EXCEPT:
   A. Heredity and genetics
   B. Growth and development
   C. Psychodynamics
   D. Working with parents
   E. Community organizations
   F. Administration

10. What is the most frequent complaint made about child and adolescent psychiatrists by pediatricians?
    A. Too deliberative and cogitative without sufficient practical action taken
    B. Prescribe psychotropics too readily
    C. Too talkative during calls to the pediatrician's office
    D. Do not seem to agree as a field on diagnostic entities
    E. Poor communication

In the following questions, match the terms to their proper definition:

11. Face validity

12. Predictive validity

13. Construct validity
    A. Whether the category has meaning in terms of what it purports to assess
    B. A judgment about whether the description of a category appears to represent the diagnostic construct reasonably
    C. Whether some aspect of subsequent course or response to treatment is predicted

14. True or False: Aggressive behaviors such as hitting, biting, and smashing objects are common in 4- to 8-year olds and decrease with age.
    A. True
    B. False

15. True or False: A child's narrative abilities are known to be highly related to success in the school curriculum.
    A. True
    B. False

16. Which person or group is often forgotten when a child is diagnosed with cancer or other serious medical illness?
    A. Grandparents
    B. Siblings
    C. The child himself
    D. Peers
    E. Pets

17. True or False: Epilepsy in children has a lower association with psychiatric disorders than does diabetes, another chronic condition.
    A. True
    B. False

18. ALL of the following have been observed in boys with gender identity disorder, EXCEPT:
    A. Increased rates of left-handedness
    B. Increased rates of blue eyes
    C. Increased sibling ratio of brothers to sisters
    D. Late birth order
    E. Decreased rates of activity level

19. An adolescent who uses substances is most likely to present with which of the following stages of change according to the Motivational Interviewing model?
    A. Precontemplative
    B. Contemplative
    C. Preparation
    D. Maintenance
    E. Action

20. Why does carbamazepine, compared with most other psychotropic medications, generally take a greater time to reach steady-state concentration?
    A. It is dosed initially at lower amounts
    B. It induces its own metabolism
    C. Grapefruit juice inhibits its metabolism
    D. Its plasma half-life is shorter
    E. It takes six or seven half-lives to achieve steady-state concentration

21. A notable finding of psychological autopsy studies is that approximately what percentage of children and adolescents who committed suicide had a psychiatric disorder?
    A. 10%
    B. 30%
    C. 50%
    D. 70%
    E. 90%

22. A chart review by Eland of 25 children undergoing major surgery—traumatic amputation, nephrectomy, cleft palate repair—in the 1970s, found what number of children received NO postoperative analgesia care at any point in their hospital stay?
    A. 0
    B. 4
    C. 7
    D. 10
    E. 13

23. True or False: Forensic psychiatry constitutes the practice of medicine.
    A. True
    B. False

24. Which of the following statements regarding prevalence of tic disorders is TRUE?
    A. Transient tics are rare in children
    B. Girls are more affected than boys by a ratio of 2:1
    C. Estimates of the prevalence of Tourette's syndrome are narrow in range
    D. Studies estimate the prevalence of tic disorders in school age children is between 4% and 24%
    E. Estimates of the prevalence of Tourette's syndrome in studies using Diagnostic and Statistical Manual of Mental Disorders (DSM)-III criteria show higher rates than in studies using DSM-IV-TR criteria

25. True or False: Class activation programs are an example of a type of school-based intervention after disasters.
    A. True
    B. False

26. An example of parallel play is
    A. One child playing with a shovel while another child plays with a truck
    B. Two children playing a board game together
    C. One child copying another child's drawing
    D. Two children playing separately in a sandbox but in close proximity to one another
    E. One child following an older child's example

27. Rapid eye movement never follows a period of wakefulness EXCEPT:
    A. When narcolepsy is present
    B. In an infant
    C. After hypnotic drug use
    D. A and B
    E. A and C

28. To meet the criteria for enuresis a child must display a frequency and duration of:
    A. At least two times per week for 3 months' duration
    B. At least three times per week for 3 months' duration
    C. At least two times per week for 6 months' duration
    D. At least three times per week for 3 months' duration

29. Problems with planning and organizing can greatly affect which academic skill?
    A. Reading and spelling
    B. Mathematics
    C. Written language
    D. Oral language
    E. None of the above

30. According to the US Department of Education, the term "specific learning disability" includes children who have learning problems from ALL of the following conditions EXCEPT:
    A. Developmental aphasia
    B. Dyslexia
    C. Mental retardation
    D. Minimal brain dysfunction
    E. Perceptual handicaps

31. Which of the following is true about the prevalence of ever having had sexual intercourse?
    A. It is about 90% by the ninth grade
    B. It is unrelated to gender or ethnicity
    C. It is about two-thirds by the twelfth grade
    D. It has never been studied

32. ALL of the following laboratory tests should be considered for a child or adolescent patient with an eating disorder EXCEPT:
    A. Complete blood cell count
    B. Electrocardiogram
    C. Throat culture
    D. Electrolytes

33. Comorbidities associated with obesity in children and adolescents include ALL of the following EXCEPT:
    A. Hypertension
    B. Nocturnal enuresis
    C. Type 2 diabetes
    D. Pseudotumor cerebri
    E. All of the above are associated with obesity

34. What is the estimated heritability of ADHD as derived from extensive data gathered from twin and adoption studies over the past 30 years?
    A. 5%
    B. 15%
    C. 25%
    D. 55%
    E. 75%

35. In one psychoanalytic approach to the tripartite model, the functions of the ego are divided into basic categories, which include ALL of the following EXCEPT:
    A. Reality testing
    B. Object relations
    C. Regulation of affect
    D. Defensive activity
    E. Acting as conscience

36. In developmental psychopathology research, risk is defined in terms of statistical probabilities. Accordingly, what is the BEST definition of a high-risk condition?
    A. A condition that results in significant delay during critical periods of development
    B. A condition that prolongs the trajectory of development leading to immature behavior at older ages
    C. A condition that carries high odds for measured maladjustment in critical domains
    D. Risk factors such as community violence, domestic violence, and physical or sexual abuse
    E. All of the above

37. Most typically, prepubertal depression has a set of risk factors and course similar to conduct disorder, which includes ALL of the following attributes EXCEPT:
    A. Family discord
    B. Increased risk of antisocial disorder
    C. Depression in adult life
    D. Parental substance abuse
    E. Parental criminality

38. Which one of the following was the most common comorbid condition seen during the National Institute of Mental Health screening for childhood onset schizophrenia (COS)?
    A. Depression
    B. ADHD
    C. Obsessive-compulsive disorder (OCD)
    D. Bipolar disorder
    E. Alcohol abuse

39. Which of the following is the only imaging modality available that provides a quantitative index of intraneuronal current flow?
    A. Electroencephalography
    B. Magnetoencephalography
    C. Diffusion tensor imaging
    D. Functional magnetic resonance imaging
    E. Single photon emission computed tomography

40. Which of the following is the BEST definition of resilience?
    A. A phenomenon or process reflecting relatively positive adaptation despite experiences of significant adversity or trauma
    B. A phenomenon or process that plots the trajectory of productivity and success in life despite overwhelming odds
    C. A phenomenon or process that allows certain individuals to be immune to dysthymia, depression or other internalizing disorders despite adversity
    D. A phenomenon or process that nurtures a proactive approach to life's problems
    E. None of the above

41. Interpersonal psychotherapy (IPT) is a brief, time-limited psychotherapy developed in the late 1960s for the treatment of what type of patient?
    A. Bipolar outpatients
    B. Psychotic inpatients
    C. Depressed outpatients
    D. Bipolar inpatients
    E. Depressed inpatients

42. The diagnosis of trichotillomania requires both behavioral and psychological components, including tension prior to hair pulling and gratification during or after it. Hair pulling without psychological components has what prevalence in the general population?
    A. 1%
    B. 4%
    C. 8%
    D. 12%
    E. 16%

43. What is one factor that delayed the development of in-home, community, and family-based services?
    A. The psychoanalytic movement
    B. The lack of trained clinicians in family theory
    C. McCarthyism and the fear that community-based services represented socialist principles
    D. The lack of a federalist approach
    E. The increased availability of health insurance, which did not pay for community-based services

44. The most up-to-date current legal principle guiding child custody and placement in divorce as described in the Uniform Marriage and Divorce Act is:
    A. The tender years doctrine
    B. Psychological parent determination
    C. Best interests of the child
    D. DNA verification
    E. Assignment and weighing of a number of genetic and psychosocial risk and protective factors

45. Of the following, which one is most likely to be considered a "normal dysfluency" which, by itself, would not be considered a red flag for persistent stuttering:
    A. Repetition of a sound
    B. Repetition of a syllable
    C. Repetition of a word
    D. Silent blocks
    E. Sound prolongations

46. Over the last decade, as a proportion of all pediatric emergency visits, the number of child psychiatric emergencies presenting to hospitals has:
    A. Increased
    B. Remained the same
    C. Decreased
    D. Increased for adolescents and decreased for children
    E. Increased for children and decreased for adolescents

47. How many symptoms from each domain (inattentive and hyperactive-impulsive) are required to meet the DSM-IV criterion for criterion for ADHD, Combined Type?
    A. 2 and 4
    B. 4 and 4
    C. 6 and 6
    D. 5 and 7
    E. 8 and 8

48. What is the suspected prevalence for Gender Identity Disorder?
    A. 1% or less
    B. 2%
    C. 3%
    D. 4%
    E. 5%

49. Which of the following is the normal milestone for speech development regarding a child's ability to speak his first words?
    A. 24 months
    B. 18 months
    C. 14 months
    D. 12 months
    E. 8 months

50. Neuropsychological investigations of OCD suggest impairment is strongest for ALL of the following EXCEPT:
    A. Executive functions of set shifting and motor inhibition
    B. Nonverbal memory
    C. Visual motor integration
    D. Visual–spatial memory
    E. Auditory memory

51. Which cluster of symptoms of posttraumatic stress disorder (PTSD) is the LEAST frequently endorsed in young children?
    A. Avoidance cluster
    B. Reexperiencing cluster
    C. Hyperarousal cluster
    D. None of the above

52. Which of the following is NOT TRUE of fragile X syndrome?
    A. All males who carry the abnormal gene are mentally retarded
    B. The disorder is the second most common cause of mental retardation
    C. Clinical symptoms include facial abnormalities
    D. Abnormal speech patterns are present in a majority of cases
    E. The disorder is a result of a triple repeat expansion

53. True or False: Most abused children develop borderline personality disorder in adulthood.
    A. True
    B. False

54. True or False: Compared to the low potency antipsychotics, haloperidol is much less likely to cause extrapyramidal symptoms.
    A. True
    B. False

55. The Accreditation Council for Graduate Medical Education is responsible for setting training requirements for all specialties and subspecialties that have been approved by the American Board of Medical Specialties and consists of representatives from ALL of the following organizations EXCEPT:
    A. American Medical Association
    B. Association of American Medical Colleges
    C. American Hospital Association
    D. Council of Medical Specialty Societies
    E. American Psychiatric Association

56. The "three-way interaction" model proposed by Kaufman to explain the elevated risk for depression among abused children includes: maltreatment, the 5-HTTLPR, genotype, and:
    A. Monoamine oxidase-A genotype
    B. Monoamine oxidase-B genotype
    C. Alcohol dehydrogenase genotype
    D. Brain-derived neurotrophic factor genotype
    E. Small hippocampal volume

57. True or False: The age at which an infant begins to walk is a good predictor of developmental outcomes.
    A. True
    B. False

58. A child with absence or petit mal seizures may have:
    A. Abnormal glial cell architecture in the limbic system
    B. Inconsistent frequency but typical spike and wave morphology
    C. Abnormal background with 5 Hz spike and wave morphology
    D. A normal background and with onset of hyperventilation 3 Hz spike and wave morphology

59. True or False: Interpersonal conflicts with parents are the most common antecedent to adolescent suicide attempts.
    A. True
    B. False

60. Drugs that are basic in pH in the general circulation, when bound to plasma protein, bind to which molecule?
    A. Very low-density lipoproteins
    B. Alpha-1 acid glycoprotein
    C. Platelets
    D. Albumin
    E. High-density lipoprotein

61. What is the prevalence of OCD in adults?
    A. 0.5% to 3%
    B. 1% to 5%
    C. 2% to 8%
    D. 5% to 10%
    E. Over 10%

62. What is a potential known side effect of oxcarbazepine?
    A. Elevated creatinine
    B. Decreased urine output
    C. Enuresis
    D. Nightmares
    E. Hyponatremia

63. ALL of the following are programs that have been shown to prevent behavioral disorders EXCEPT:
    A. The Incredible Years
    B. Good Behavior Game
    C. Nurse-Family Partnership
    D. Stop and Think

64. Which of the following statements is FALSE?
    A. Persons with severe mental retardation come to diagnosis at a younger age than those with mild mental retardation
    B. Persons with severe mental retardation more frequently have related medical conditions than those with mild mental retardation
    C. Persons with mild mental retardation are usually of typical appearance without dysmorphic features
    D. Persons with mild mental retardation have increased rates of psychopathology relative to nondisabled populations
    E. Persons with mild mental retardation have a wider range of behavioral and psychiatric problems relative to those in normative samples

65. By the end of fifth grade, which of the following is typical?
    A. Creative play is imitative
    B. Egocentricity
    C. Secondary sexual changes
    D. Mild synkinesis
    E. Self-referential drawings

66. True or False: Communication disorders in children are frequently associated with a variety of conditions, deficits, or disorders.
    A. True
    B. False

67. True or False: The legal term of privilege refers only to the patient's right to bar disclosure of information obtained during treatment in judicial or quasijudicial proceedings.
    A. True
    B. False

68. Concrete operations include the following:
    A. Conservation
    B. Classification
    C. Centration
    D. A and B
    E. None of the above

69. Which of the following approaches were used that led to the determination of a lack of an association between autism and the measles, mumps, and rubella vaccine?
    A. Patient registry
    B. Cohort
    C. Case–control
    D. Ecological
    E. All of the above

70. True or False: In the percentile score format of reporting psychological and neuropsychological test scores, the scores between the 25th and 75th percentile are all within the average range.
    A. True
    B. False

71. Which of the following rare but serious adverse effects is associated with trazodone, a potent 5HT2a antagonist?
    A. Priapism
    B. Hepatoxicity
    C. Neutropenia
    D. Renal insufficiency
    E. Pulmonary edema

72. Genetic association studies most closely resemble
    A. Cohort studies
    B. Ecological studies
    C. Naturalistic studies
    D. Case–control studies

73. What is content validity?
    A. The extent to which an instrument is representative of the universe of empirical indicators that are related to the concept measured
    B. The most empirical form of validity, which allows an index to be compared to an independent external criterion thought to assess the same concept
    C. The extent to which individual items or measures intercorrelate or group together to produce derived higher order constructs
    D. None of the above

74. Behavioral differences in children with autism may include ALL of the following EXCEPT:
    A. Stereotypies such as hand flapping and toe walking
    B. Desire for variety in the environment
    C. Preoccupation with inanimate objects or parts of objects
    D. Sensitivity to nonspeech sounds
    E. Attachment to unusual objects

75. Which of the following statements best describes objective countertransference as termed by Winnicott?
    A. Natural reactions to a patient's provocative behavior
    B. Intrapsychic conflicts stirred in the therapist by the patient
    C. Reactions to the patient arising from the therapist's unresolved conflicts
    D. Reactions in the patient toward the therapist as earlier, important relationships are reactivated and projected upon the therapist

76. What is the population-based prevalence of encopresis?
    A. 4% of 5- to 6-year olds
    B. 10% of 5- to 6-year olds
    C. 1.5% of 11- to 12-year olds
    D. A and C
    E. B and C

77. Which edition of the DSM for mental disorders first came out with a multiaxial diagnostic classification?
    A. DSM-I
    B. DSM-II
    C. DSM-III
    D. DSM-III-R
    E. DSM-IV

78. True or False: Meta-analysis reviews of clinical trials involving therapeutic interventions for adolescent youth provide a better interpretation of data if the possible confounding factor of large numbers of adolescent girls enrolled in studies is considered and addressed.
    A. True
    B. False

79. True or False: All children with Munchhausen syndrome by proxy are sensitive to separation from their perpetrators.
    A. True
    B. False

80. Statistical power describes the probability of which scenario in null hypothesis testing?
    A. To reject the null hypothesis when in fact it is true
    B. To not reject the null hypothesis when it is false
    C. To not reject the null hypothesis when it is true
    D. To reject the null hypothesis when it is false
    E. None of the above

81. Which one of the following is true of children with both deafness and blindness?
    A. Approximately 3% to 6% have Usher's syndrome
    B. 75% have intellectual impairment
    C. Rubella accounts for 75% of cases
    D. Brain abnormalities are found in 75% of children
    E. All of the above

82. Self-regulatory disturbances in an infant or toddler can compromise their normal development. Which of the following is NOT an example of a disturbance in self-regulation?
    A. Sleep disturbance
    B. Apathetic, withdrawn, and no expression of affect
    C. Excessive crying or irritability
    D. Low frustration tolerance
    E. Self-stimulatory or unusual movements such as head banging

83. Which treatment has the best available evidence in increasing cognitive, communicative, and social skills in autism?
    A. Psychotherapy
    B. Family therapy
    C. Social skills group
    D. Psychopharmacology
    E. Educational intervention

84. True or False: Bupropion can be effective in children and adolescents with ADHD.
    A. True
    B. False

85. During the termination phase of interpersonal psychotherapy for depressed adolescents (IPT-A), the tasks of this phase include ALL of the following EXCEPT:
    A. Clarification of warning symptoms of future depressive episodes
    B. Identification of successful strategies that were used in therapy
    C. Generalization of skills to future situations
    D. Discussion of the links between thoughts and emotions
    E. Emphasis on mastery of new interpersonal skills

86. ALL of the following confers risk for or is associated with suicidal behaviors EXCEPT:
   A. Physical abuse
   B. Sexual abuse
   C. Homosexual orientation of females
   D. Family adversity
   E. Low levels of cerebral spinal fluid 5-hydroxyindoleacetic acid in adolescents

87. The correlation coefficient, r, often used to evaluate reliability of tests or measures, indicates the strength of a relationship between two variables. The values of the correlation coefficient, r, range between which two numbers?
   A. 0 and 100
   B. 0 and +1
   C. −1 and +1
   D. 0 to 7
   E. −10 to +10

88. In the management of attachment disorders, the model of Circle of Security refers to:
   A. Play therapy
   B. Group therapy
   C. Seclusion intervention
   D. Group safe home
   E. Case management

89. Which of the following is NOT true of culture-bound syndrome?
   A. It consists of disturbances in mood, behavior, or belief systems that appear restricted to a particular cultural context
   B. Symptoms are frequently viewed as exotic or as covert illness phenomena occurring in the context of a local culture
   C. It is a pattern of behavior that is understood locally as a meaningful manifestation of distress, acceptable within the cultural context
   D. Such symptoms signal distress and activate a culturally specific response to the situation
   E. It represents an uncommon socialization process for that cultural subgroup

90. An interviewer-based interview which provides extensive sets of definitions of symptoms and/or detailed guidance on the conduct of the interview is called what?
   A. Semistructured interview
   B. Fully structured interview
   C. Respondent-based interview
   D. Interviewer-based interview
   E. Glossary-based interview

91. N-Methyl-D-aspartate receptors bind which of the following neurotransmitters?
   A. Serotonin
   B. Glutamate
   C. γ-Aminobutyric acid
   D. N-Methyl-D-aspartate
   E. B and D

92. If you are to serve as an expert witness in a court proceeding, who may make initial contact to request an evaluation?
   A. An attorney
   B. A parent
   C. The court
   D. The patient/client
   E. All of the above

93. Four categories of techniques are generally employed in the child psychiatric interview, which include engagement, projective, direct questioning and interactive techniques. Which of the following describes interactive techniques?
    A. Techniques to put the child at ease so that the child will provide accurate and meaningful clinical information
    B. Techniques to allow the child to reveal underlying themes or issues which the child may be unable to verbalize directly
    C. Techniques to clarify particular points or elicit specific information
    D. Techniques needed to clarify how the child relates to, as well as accepts or integrates input, from others

94. Stereotypies in children should be considered in the differential diagnosis of tics. Stereotypies differ from tics in what way?
    A. Stereotypies have an earlier onset than tics
    B. Stereotypies tend to be unilateral whereas tics tend to be bilateral
    C. Tics tend to be consistent over time, whereas stereotypies wax and wane
    D. Tics have an earlier onset than stereotypies
    E. Stereotypies and tics are identical and impossible to clinically separate

95. The average reading comprehension level for adolescents with hearing impairment without cochlear implants is:
    A. First to second grade
    B. Third to fourth grade
    C. Fifth to sixth grade
    D. Seventh to eight grade
    E. Ninth to tenth grade

96. In a neuropsychological examination of patients with trichotillomania and controls, the only differences that emerged were:
    A. Patients with trichotillomania showed increased perseveration errors
    B. Patients with trichotillomania showed increased concept learning
    C. Patients with trichotillomania showed increased attention errors
    D. Patients with trichotillomania had decreased memory
    E. Patients with trichotillomania did less well on visual spatial tasks

97. True or False: Methylphenidate and amphetamines target only the norepinephrine system.
    A. True
    B. False

98. Having a student repeat directions back to the teacher, affixing materials to a student's desk, giving a student duplicate materials, keeping a sample model of a correctly formatted paper, and defining classroom expectations in a positive way are interventions that address the needs of children with which of the following problems?
    A. Bipolar disorder
    B. Psychotic disorder, not otherwise specified
    C. PTSD
    D. ADHD
    E. Generalized anxiety

99. How many children in the United States suffer from life-limiting illness?
    A. 100,000
    B. 500,000
    C. 1,000,000
    D. 5,000,000
    E. 10,000,000

100. True or False: Studies in resilience identify supportive and responsive parenting as being among the most robust predictors of resilient adaptation.
    A. True
    B. False

101. True or False: The most rigorous study to date of Cognitive-behavioral therapy (CBT) in children with OCD was performed in the Pediatric OCD Treatment Study. The response rate was 75%.
    A. True
    B. False

102. In twin studies of bulimia, the following has been found:
    A. Monozygotic concordance rates are higher than dizygotic concordance rates
    B. Monozygotic concordance rates are equal to dizygotic concordance rates
    C. Monozygotic concordance rates are lower than dizygotic concordance rates
    D. Monozygotic concordance rates are the same as nontwin sibling concordance rates

103. A psychic event, such as a symptom, that is typically caused by more than one factor and may serve more than one purpose in the psychic framework is called what in psychoanalytic thought?
    A. Psychic determinism
    B. Overdeterminism
    C. Psychic reality
    D. Multideterminism
    E. B and D

104. Which of the following treatments has been rejected by health and mental health professional organizations?
    A. Reparative therapy
    B. Interpersonal therapy
    C. CBT
    D. Psychodynamic psychotherapy
    E. Flooding

105. Arnold Gesell, one of the great child developmental researchers of the first half of the 20th century, based his research on what primary presupposition?
    A. Children are mainly products of their environment
    B. Child development follows from a biological timetable
    C. Genes are the primary influence upon child behavior
    D. Children follow a series of discrete stages in cognition

106. ALL of the following are psychosocial strategies in making aggressive behavior in children inefficient by developing sufficient alternatives EXCEPT:
    A. Anger management skills training
    B. Improved communication of needs
    C. Avoidance of problem situations
    D. Involvement in positive activities that emphasize strengths
    E. Using alternatives such as chill-out time

107. True or False: Tertiary amine tricyclic antidepressants have low anticholinergic properties.
    A. True
    B. False

108. Pick the answer with the correct descending order of the most common types of pain complaints in children.
    A. Headache, abdominal pain, chest pain
    B. Abdominal pain, headache, chest pain
    C. Chest pain, abdominal pain, headache
    D. Abdominal pain, chest pain, headache
    E. Headache, chest pain, abdominal pain

109. ALL of the following have been or are related to the management of drug and alcohol use in the United States EXCEPT:
    A. The 1914 Harrison Narcotic Act
    B. The Prohibition Amendment of 1919
    C. The US Federal Bureau of Narcotics
    D. The Drug Enforcement Agency
    E. The Americans with Disabilities Act

110. Which of the following statements regarding Medicaid is NOT TRUE?
    A. A governmental program supporting low-income individuals
    B. Covers all senior citizens as well as children
    C. Financed jointly by the federal government and the states
    D. Covers a substantial proportion of child mental health expenditure in the nation

111. In which of the following situations is a psychiatrist typically immune from liability?
    A. Consulting to a school for a school-based evaluation of a child.
    B. Consulting for a court-ordered evaluation
    C. The attending on-call who is not contacted by the resident for a patient discharged from the emergency room
    D. Consulting physician who writes orders
    E. Outrageous actions of a secretary

112. ALL of the following social and school risk factors are associated with the development of disruptive behavior disorders EXCEPT:
    A. Poverty
    B. Association with deviant peers or siblings
    C. Rejection by peers
    D. Intense exposure to media violence
    E. Lack of opposite sex relationships

113. Reversal of roles in a child–caregiver interaction may be an example of what type of reactive attachment disorder?
    A. Emotionally withdrawn/inhibited
    B. Indiscriminately social/disinhibited
    C. Mixed
    D. Other forms of reactive attachment disorder, such as secure base distortions
    E. None of the above

114. True or False: A recent multisite study of children with pervasive developmental disorders accompanied by hyperactivity, impulsiveness, and distractibility showed an equal rate of positive response to stimulants compared to typically developing children with ADHD.
    A. True
    B. False

115. True or False: Neurogenesis occurs in adults.
    A. True
    B. False

116. True or False: In psychodynamic psychotherapy of children, the child's play is equivalent to free association in adult psychoanalysis.
    A. True
    B. False

117. As preschoolers begin to separate from parents, which of the following is true?
    A. They feel more and more independent with little anxiety around separation
    B. Temper tantrums may begin as a result of feeling dependent and powerless
    C. Aggressive behavior is always an expression of fear
    D. Children displaying aggressive behavior generally have extremely high frustration tolerance

118. The following statement: "Apparently normal development for the first 2 years of life followed by significant loss of previously acquired skills in communication, motor, and social areas" describes:
    A. Autism
    B. Asperger's disorder
    C. Rett's disorder
    D. Childhood Disintegrative disorder
    E. Landau-Kleffner syndrome

119. When a 4-year-old protests, "No I don't want to be stuck with a needle!" in response to a nontherapeutic intervention, this wish must be respected even though the child is under the age considered capable for assent. What is the 4-year-old's response called?
    A. Nonconsent by proxy
    B. Legal capacity
    C. Nonbinding resolution
    D. Deliberate objection
    E. Temper tantrum

120. Early studies on the efficacy of psychotherapy for children and adolescents had a number of methodological errors that weakened the internal validity of their study design and made it very difficult to interpret results. These methodological errors include ALL of the following EXCEPT:
    A. Failure to randomly assign children to treatment and control conditions
    B. Specifying what therapeutic procedures were used in the intervention being tested
    C. Using nonequivalent comparison groups, such as therapy dropouts, as the control group
    D. Allowing therapists or other raters who were not blinded to assess outcome
    E. Enrolling heterogeneous samples of children (including different diagnoses and developmental levels) into the same group undergoing intervention

121. Which of the following statements regarding the age range of group therapy members is NOT TRUE?
    A. In actual clinical life, age ranges are rarely absolute
    B. The span of years should be contained within one developmental phase of life
    C. Age range tends to be influenced and sometimes extended by developmental and school grade levels
    D. A general age range of 4-5 years between group members is the most appropriate
    E. All are true

122. As a member of the consultation and liaison service you are asked to evaluate a child on the medical floor for possible depression. He has a chronic illness and has been on the floors several weeks. What diagnosis should be part of your differential?
    A. Conduct disorder
    B. ADHD
    C. Delirium
    D. Conversion disorder
    E. Somatization disorder

123. At this point, the most widely discussed and evidence-supported model of learning disorder identification is which of the following?
    A. Discrepancy between ability and achievement
    B. Individual with Disabilities Education Act model
    C. Identification of cognitive deficits
    D. Responsiveness to intervention model
    E. Use of IQ tests

124. Approximately, what percentage of children with enuresis successfully treated with the bell-and-pad method remain dry after termination of treatment?
    A. 90%
    B. 75%
    C. 50%
    D. 25%
    E. 10%

125. What type of variable represents the outcome or criterion that measures or assesses the effect of the antecedent or presumed cause? This kind of variable comprises scores from a test, ratings on questionnaires, or other research modalities.
    A. Active independent variable
    B. Independent variable
    C. Dependent variable
    D. Attribute independent variable
    E. Extraneous variable

126. CYPs are heme-containing enzymes located primarily in the intestine and liver that metabolize ALL of the following substrates EXCEPT:
  A. Lipids
  B. Toxins
  C. Carbohydrates
  D. Fatty acids
  E. Endogenous steroids

127. The psychiatric assessment of children commonly differs from the assessment of adults in ALL of the following ways EXCEPT:
  A. The child's behavior may cause greater distress to the adults than to the child
  B. Children may not recognize their behaviors as problematic to others
  C. Children often seek out psychiatric assessment or treatment for themselves
  D. Children may attribute problems to others and be unwilling to accept their own personal contribution to the problem
  E. The adult's expectations for the child may exceed the child's abilities

128. What is one of the best replicated neuroimaging findings in adults with PTSD?
  A. Increased amygdala volume
  B. Decreased amygdala volume
  C. Decreased density of neurons in the prefrontal cortex
  D. Reduced hippocampal volume
  E. Increased activation in the orbitofrontal cortex

129. While external population validity depends on the sampling design or how a representative sample is obtained from the target population, internal validity partly depends on what factor?
  A. How the results of the study apply to the target population
  B. If the effect size indicates a measurable benefit for the intervention in the target population
  C. If the number needed to treat is small enough to validate the intervention as practical
  D. How the participants are allocated into groups
  E. None of the above

130. Which of the following symptoms of ADHD is most likely to be outgrown when a child matures into adulthood?
  A. Inattention
  B. Hyperactivity
  C. Impulsivity
  D. Distractibility
  E. Both hyperactivity and impulsivity

131. ALL of these are a specific somatoform disorder listed in DSM-IV-TR EXCEPT:
  A. Conversion disorder
  B. Pain disorder
  C. Hypochondriasis
  D. Body dysmorphic disorder
  E. Differentiated somatoform disorder

132. Regarding dismissal of a group, leaders can help members learn more adaptive ways to manage the ending transition by:
  A. Instituting additional group rituals
  B. Providing "social scripts"
  C. Modeling appropriate departure behavior
  D. B and C
  E. All of the above

133. Clozapine was introduced in what year?
  A. 1914
  B. 1927
  C. 1960
  D. 1971
  E. 1983

134. What percentage of children in foster care are returned to their parents?
    A. 10%
    B. 20%
    C. 40%
    D. 75%
    E. 90%

135. True or False: Valproate is not associated with birth defects.
    A. True
    B. False

136. What is the typical starting dose of fluoxetine for school-age children?
    A. 5 to 10 mg
    B. 10 to 15 mg
    C. 15 to 20 mg
    D. 20 to 30 mg
    E. 30 to 40 mg

137. Which of the following agents may be used in the treatment of nicotine dependence?
    A. Bupropion
    B. Naltrexone
    C. Topiramate
    D. Acamprosate
    E. All of the above

138. True or False: Working memory is fundamental to most aspects of problem solving.
    A. True
    B. False

139. Psychological testing of a child with borderline personality disorder may reveal:
    A. Impairment in formal thought processes in unstructured tests
    B. Recurrent disturbances in ego functions, such as frustration tolerance, attention, and goal-directedness
    C. Marked disturbances in interpersonal relationships and in the experience of self and others
    D. Rigid and tenuous defenses coexisting with primitive defenses
    E. All of the above

140. Which of the following serves as the BEST description of mentalization?
    A. The ability to reflect upon one's experience to devise alternate ways to navigate through everyday life
    B. The internalization of a positive representation of the parent by the child
    C. The ability to take account of one's own and others' mental states in understanding why people behave in specific ways
    D. The capacity to understand what others are thinking

141. Culturally underwritten masculine and feminine behaviors, attitudes, and personality traits, which are in part biologically driven and in part shaped by environment, refer to which of the following?
    A. Gender role
    B. Sexual orientation
    C. Gender identity
    D. Gender crisis
    E. None of the above

142. Fill in the blanks: Mothers tend to facilitate _____ development in their infant while fathers tend to show more involvement in their infant's _____ development.
    A. Gross-motor; fine-motor
    B. Fine-motor; gross-motor
    C. Receptive language; expressive language
    D. Expressive language; receptive language

143. True or False: In infant assessments, asking caregivers to describe a day in the life of their child can serve as a productive method in gathering developmental and family data.
    A. True
    B. False

144. IPT for depressed adolescents (IPT-A) is designed for use with adolescents, ages 12 to 18 years, with ALL of the following diagnostic conditions EXCEPT:
    A. Acute onset of major depression
    B. Dysthymia
    C. Adjustment disorder with depressed mood
    D. Recurrent major depressive disorder
    E. Depression not otherwise specified

145. IPT-A is an adaptation of IPT, which begins by taking an interpersonal inventory of important relationships to determine appropriate treatment targets. The types of problems typically targeted by IPT-A are ALL of the following EXCEPT:
    A. Loss
    B. Transference distortions
    C. Role disputes
    D. Role transitions
    E. Interpersonal skills deficits

146. Currently, what is the percentage of children under 18 years of age living in the United States who are immigrants?
    A. 5%
    B. 10%
    C. 15%
    D. 20%
    E. 25%

147. In divorce and custody determinations, which of the following describes an alternative to dispute resolution through the courts?
    A. Collaborative law
    B. Cooperative law
    C. Mediation
    D. Single judge decision-making
    E. A and C

148. What is the order of the decrease in growth parameters in children who have failure to thrive due to caloric deficiency, from the first to decline to the last to decline?
    A. Weight, head circumference, height
    B. Height, head circumference, weight
    C. Head circumference, weight, height
    D. Weight, height, head circumference
    E. Height, weight, head circumference
    F. Head circumference, height, weight

149. The Tanner stages:
    A. Are most accurately determined by adolescent self-report
    B. Include pubic hair, breast development, penile and testicular growth, and femur length in boys
    C. Are classified into stages A through E
    D. Describe stages of psychosocial development
    E. Include pubic hair, breast development, height spurt, and menarche in girls

150. In the Four Ps model of psychiatric formulation, which domain of factors is concerned with features such as family history, psychiatric history, and chronic social stressors that render a patient vulnerable to their presenting symptoms?
    A. Predisposing
    B. Precipitating
    C. Perpetuating
    D. Protective

151. A child wakes up suddenly, which is accompanied by screaming and thrashing uncontrollably in bed. The likely diagnosis is:
    A. Nightmare
    B. Pavor nocturnus
    C. Somnambulism
    D. A dysomnia
    E. None of the above

152. Which of the following is TRUE regarding puberty?
    A. Breast development begins earlier in African-American girls than in white girls
    B. Ovulation and full fertility are present beginning at menarche
    C. Body weight and fat/muscle ratio are not important for menarche
    D. The age of menarche has remained constant for the past century

153. Two cities listed below are major sites for the evaluation of children with gender identity disorder and have been able to gather prospective data. Please select one of the two.
    A. New York, NY
    B. San Francisco, CA
    C. Toronto, Canada
    D. Utrecht, Netherlands
    E. Los Angeles, CA

154. Which modality has the strongest evidence for the treatment of juvenile offenders?
    A. Functional Family Therapy
    B. Intensive In-home Child and Adolescent Psychiatric Services
    C. Multisystemic Therapy
    D. Multidimensional Treatment Foster Care
    E. Mental Health Services Program for Youth

155. Which of the following assessment team structures is a team made up of professionals from different disciplines, where each completes an independent evaluation of the patient and comes up with a separate set of recommendations that are reported to the team and the client's family?
    A. Multidisciplinary
    B. Interdisciplinary
    C. Transdisciplinary
    D. Subdisciplinary
    E. Postdisciplinary

156. In patients with anorexia nervosa who abuse laxatives or diuretics, which electrolyte disturbance can result in cardiac conductance abnormalities?
    A. Hypokalemic alkalosis
    B. Hyperkalemic alkalosis
    C. Hypokalemic acidosis
    D. Hyperkalemic acidosis

157. In which edition were formal diagnostic criteria for PTSD first introduced into the DSM?
    A. DSM-I
    B. DSM-II
    C. DSM-III
    D. DSM-IV

158. Which of the following is true about lithium in children?
    A. It is rarely used for bipolar disorder
    B. One must keep the level well below 1.0 mmol/L
    C. Children have shown lower brain-to-serum lithium concentration ratios
    D. Maintaining hydration is less of a concern with children given their glomerular filtration rate
    E. In children lithium acts as an anion

159. In school-age children what is the starting dose of clonidine in milligrams?
    A. 0.05
    B. 0.1
    C. 0.15
    D. 0.2
    E. None of the above

160. Animal studies indicate that selective serotonin reuptake inhibitor (SSRI) promotion of enhanced serotonergic function appears mainly in what region of the brain?
    A. Hippocampus
    B. Prefrontal cortex
    C. Limbic cortex
    D. Amygdala
    E. Thalamus

161. True or False: The criterion of effectiveness corresponds to the success of an intervention in experimental conditions.
    A. True
    B. False

162. The ethical principle of "respect for persons" when conducting research on human subjects includes which TWO of the following?
    A. Individuals should be treated as autonomous agents
    B. Individuals should be treated beneficently
    C. Individuals with diminished autonomy are entitled to protection
    D. Individuals should be treated with justice

163. Munchhausen by proxy is generally an example of which TWO forms of abuse?
    A. Psychological abuse
    B. Neglect
    C. Sexual abuse
    D. Physical abuse
    E. Verbal abuse

164. The evaluation to obtain services under Individuals with Disabilities Education Act consists of a comprehensive analysis by school-based professionals of all suspected areas of disability. The components of an assessment usually include ALL of the following EXCEPT:
    A. Cognitive abilities
    B. Communication abilities
    C. Academic performance
    D. Occupational therapy evaluation
    E. Health status

165. True or False: An increased white count between 12,000 and 15,000 cells/mm^3 is common and clinically insignificant when a child is on lithium.
    A. True
    B. False

166. What is the only FDA-approved medication for the treatment of bipolar disorder in youth older than 13 years?
    A. Risperidone
    B. Valproate
    C. Lamotrigine
    D. Lithium
    E. Carbamazepine

167. What region of the brain is implicated in catatonia?
    A. Occipital cortex
    B. Parietal cortex
    C. Frontal cortex
    D. Hippocampus
    E. Amygdala

168. Each of these is a side effect of corticosteroids EXCEPT:
   A. Affective lability
   B. Hypomania or mania
   C. Weight loss
   D. Easy bruising
   E. Hirsutism

169. True or False: Cumulative incidence is generally used for a closed population observed over a fixed period.
   A. True
   B. False

170. Heroin can be detected in the urine for how long?
   A. Less than 24 hours
   B. 24 to 72 hours
   C. 3 to 5 days
   D. 1 week
   E. More than 10 days

171. All of the following community-based interventions show promise EXCEPT:
   A. School-based interventions
   B. Crisis mobile outreach teams
   C. Time-limited hospitalization with coordinated community services
   D. Family support services
   E. CBT

172. A lack of "central coherence" is defined as:
   A. Inability to keep groups of similar items together
   B. A cognitive processing style that makes the integration of parts into wholes problematic
   C. Difficulty with auditory processing
   D. Repetitive behaviors
   E. Inability to remain impartial to outcomes

173. Which part of the serotonergic neuron is the primary target site for SSRIs?
   A. 5-HT2 receptor
   B. 5-HT1A receptor
   C. Serotonin transporter
   D. 5-HT3 receptor
   E. None of the above

174. Pervasive developmental disorders are characterized by delays in all three of the following developmental areas:
   A. Learning, communicative, motor
   B. Social, sensory, cognitive
   C. Social, motor, sensory
   D. Communicative, social, cognitive
   E. Learning, sensory, motor

175. Pharmacokinetics can be conceptualized as having four functionally distinct phases, which include ALL of the following EXCEPT:
   A. Absorption
   B. Distribution
   C. Activation
   D. Metabolism
   E. Excretion

176. A review study on OCD suggested discontinuation of SSRI treatment after a relatively symptom-free period of how long?
   A. 1 to 2 months
   B. 3 to 6 months
   C. 6 to 8 months
   D. 8 to 12 months
   E. 4 years

177. In the United States, the current rate of perinatal transmission of HIV from an infected mother to her child is closest to:
    A. 75%
    B. 50%
    C. 25%
    D. 10%
    E. 5%

In the following questions, match the databases listed to their relative strengths and weaknesses as a consideration of which one to choose for a literature search.

178. PubMed

179. PsycINFO

180. Journal of the American Academy of Child & Adolescent Psychiatry

181. Cochrane Library
    A. Retrieves many references for medications but omits significant journals in psychology
    B. Offers a complete source for data on randomized-controlled trials
    C. Includes an extensive array of psychology journal articles of variable quality
    D. Offers members full-text access to articles published since its inception but only from a single, albeit highly relevant journal for child and adolescent psychiatry

182. Hydrocortisone is secreted in response to stressful events. Where is it secreted?
    A. Neocortex
    B. Hypothalamus
    C. Pituitary gland
    D. Hippocampus
    E. Adrenal cortex

183. Superego functions, as found in the psychoanalytic tripartite model, are predominantly unconscious, or out of an individual's awareness. Which of the following attributes is NOT considered a superego function?
    A. Conscience
    B. Repression
    C. Morality
    D. Critical self-observation
    E. Holding up of ideals

184. True or False: One of the problems in implementing prevention programs for childhood mental illness is that there are no well validated prevention intervention programs for this population.
    A. True
    B. False

185. True or False: The idea for measuring intelligence capacities in infants and toddlers grew out of the intent to find a metric for intelligence to establish admission criteria for schools for children with intellectual deficiencies.
    A. True
    B. False

186. The validity of The Brazelton Neonatal Behavioral Assessment Scale, second edition, has been demonstrated in a number of studies to correctly identify neonates who are potentially ALL of the following EXCEPT:
    A. Underweight
    B. Experiencing respiratory difficulties
    C. Exposed *in utero* to drugs or alcohol
    D. Exposed *in utero* to maternal malnutrition
    E. Exposed *in utero* to maternal gestational diabetes

187. In Rett syndrome the genetic disorder is:
   A. Autosomal dominant
   B. Imprinted
   C. Autosomal recessive
   D. X-linked
   E. Mitochondrial

188. True or False: Separation anxiety disorder is a risk factor for the development of OCD.
   A. True
   B. False

189. Which of the following groups of children who were adopted had the highest rate of adolescent problems?
   A. Children adopted as babies
   B. Children adopted older who had good care as babies
   C. Children adopted older who had poor care as babies
   D. The groups had the same rates of problems

190. True or False: After adjusting for family characteristics, childcare accounts for up to a quarter of the effect that parents have on child development.
   A. True
   B. False

191. True or False: Exposure to domestic violence can account for a significant variation in a child's IQ.
   A. True
   B. False

192. Although DSM-II did not have the category of conduct disorder, it listed three categories that were close equivalents of the category of conduct disorder, which included ALL of the following EXCEPT:
   A. Juvenile Delinquency
   B. Unsocialized Aggressive Reaction of Childhood
   C. Group Delinquent Reaction
   D. Runaway Reaction

193. The core concepts of Strategic Family Therapy include ALL of the following EXCEPT:
   A. Repeated patterns of interaction
   B. Power/control struggles
   C. Flexibility
   D. Boundaries and subsystems
   E. Large behavioral repertoire for problem-solving and life-cycle passage

194. Which term denotes the early experimental paradigm used in functional magnetic resonance imaging studies in which a series of trials in one condition is presented for an extended period of time?
   A. Event-related design
   B. Blocked design
   C. Region of Interest
   D. Parcellation
   E. Subtraction paradigm

195. Regarding specific genetic contributions to generalized anxiety disorder, which of the following has been found in the promoter region of the serotonin transporter gene (5HTT) involving a 44 base pair insertion or deletion?
   A. Individuals with the short form of the gene, *ss* only, have been shown to have higher neuroticism, harm avoidance, and anxiety
   B. Individuals with the short form of the gene, *ss* or *sl*, have been shown to have higher neuroticism, harm avoidance, and anxiety
   C. Individuals with the long form of the gene, *ll* only, have been shown to have higher neuroticism, harm avoidance, and anxiety
   D. Individuals with the long form of the gene, *ll* or *sl*, have been shown to have higher neuroticism, harm avoidance, and anxiety
   E. None of the above

196. Which of the following describes a phenomenon found in divorce and custody conflicts?
    A. Absentee father
    B. Deadbeat dad
    C. Gassner's syndrome
    D. Parental alienation syndrome

197. What are TWO fundamental issues that have challenged the discipline of intelligence testing?
    A. How to administer intelligence tests
    B. The definition of intelligence
    C. How IQ changes as we mature
    D. The use and interpretation of measures of intelligence
    E. The gradual decline of IQ in the general population over the last half-century

198. ALL of the following social and/or environmental risk factors are implicated in the onset of mental dysfunction in increasing numbers of children EXCEPT:
    A. Extended school commutes
    B. Prolonged separations between parent and child
    C. Physical or sexual abuse
    D. Poverty
    E. Marital discord

199. Common exclusion criteria for a transplant include ALL of the following EXCEPT:
    A. Active substance abuse
    B. Active psychotic symptoms
    C. Any Axis II disorder in the cluster B category
    D. Suicidal ideation with intent and plan
    E. Self-injurious behavior

200. In what year did the White House have a Conference on Children with the conclusion that the need for childcare services was the number one priority for the nation to address?
    A. 1970
    B. 1980
    C. 1992
    D. 1998
    E. 2002

Answers

1. **Answer: B.** Infant IQ tests are no longer used in infant assessments. Page 315.
2. **Answer: A.** Page 805.
3. **Answer: A.** Page 471.
4. **Answer: A.** In emergency circumstances, medications may be given, but typically, this is discussed with the family upon admission. Permission for standing medications can be oral or by signature of a form, but must be written in the patient's chart. Page 871.
5. **Answer: A.** Dizygotic concordance rates have been found to be relatively low, about 3% to 15% depending on the diagnostic criteria used. By contrast, monozygotic concordance for autism spectrum disorders approaches 60% for the full syndrome and 90% for the broad spectrum. Page 192.
6. **Answer: A.** Page 914.
7. **Answer: E.** Mothers of survivors of childhood cancer continue to worry about their child's medical and social futures, especially when they perceive that their child worries about these issues. This suggests that parental concerns and well-being along with those of the child have reciprocal influences on one another. Page 931.
8. **Answer: B.** They had higher rates of prior violent offenses. Moreover, children who set fires were more likely than the homicidal group to carry a diagnosis of conduct disorder. Page 486.
9. **Answer: A.** Page 23.
10. **Answer: E.** The other answers are inventions, although they might represent real views. Collaborating with pediatricians for patients with somatic disorders is usually indicated. Page 642.
11–13. **Answers:** 11-B; 12-C; 13-A. In general, child psychiatric disorder classification has face validity but not necessarily predictive or construct validity. Page 304.
14. **Answer: A.** However, severely aggressive acts typically start after puberty. Page 457.
15. **Answer: A.** Likewise, a child's narrative abilities have been documented to represent weaknesses in various kinds of language problems. Page 375.
16. **Answer: B.** All of these could be correct, and are at times, but this question aims to remind you of the children in the child's life, his or her siblings. Siblings can feel anger, resentment, jealousy, frustration, and isolation from their family, overwhelmed with fear of their brother or sister's health, fear contagion, guilt for not being sick themselves, and of being treated differently by their parents. They also report concerns about change in peer relationships, in that peers might react negatively to their sibling's illness. Page 931.
17. **Answer: B.** Children with epilepsy appear to have psychiatric disturbances at three times the rate of controls. Children with diabetes also have elevated rates of psychiatric disturbances compared with controls, but at a lower rate than children with epilepsy. Page 966.
18. **Answer: B.** Page 675.
19. **Answer: A.** It is often a parent or caregiver who is concerned, not the child. Still, an early strong alliance can be facilitated by using motivational interviewing techniques. Page 618.
20. **Answer: B.** Page 743.

21. **Answer: E.** Page 531.

22. **Answer: E.** The 12 children who did receive analgesia were given a total of 24 doses of analgesic drugs, compared with 372 opioid and 299 nonopioid doses in a comparison series of adult patients. Clinicians in the 1970s had the prevailing attitude that children tolerated discomfort well. More recently, in a study covering the period 1990 to 1997, parents of children who died of cancer indicated that 80% of patients were treated for pain in the last month of life, but only 30% were treated successfully. In 1999 the Joint Commission on Accreditation of Healthcare Organizations developed the standard that policies and procedures must be in place to assess and manage pain in every patient. Page 974.

23. **Answer: A.** The American Medical Association has issued an affirmative decision upon this point. Consequently, many states require local licensure for forensic evaluations. Page 21.

24. **Answer: D.** All answers but D are true in reverse. Transient tics are common in children with boys being more affected than girls. Estimates of prevalence have been broad partially due to differences in DSM-III and DSM-IV-TR criteria. Page 572.

25. **Answer: A.** School-based interventions include single session debriefing, small group programs and class activation programs. Class activation programs, which are programs implemented in the classroom itself, may vary in focus, scope, and depth but are all intended to minimize stigma, encourage normality, and reinforce the expectations that the children will soon resume their roles as students. Page 734.

26. **Answer: D.** Parallel play is simply two or more children playing by themselves but close to each other. They do not necessarily play the same game, and they do not play with one another. Parallel play is typical of children 3 years of age and younger. Option A could also be parallel play, if there is little interaction, but D is the best answer among the options. Page 263.

27. **Answer: D.** Page 629.

28. **Answer: A.** Mnemonic: I need to pee, 2 plus 3 = 5, and 5 is the chronological or mental age required. Page 656.

29. **Answer: C.** Page 364.

30. **Answer: C.** According to this definition, specific learning disability includes such conditions as perceptual handicaps, brain injury, minimal brain dysfunction, dyslexia, and developmental aphasia. The term does not include children who have learning problems, which are primarily the result of visual, hearing, or motor handicaps, mental retardation (MR), emotional disturbance, or of environmental, cultural, or economic disadvantage. Page 411.

31. **Answer: C.** Page 286.

32. **Answer: C.** A complete blood cell count assesses for anemia. Page 342.

33. **Answer: E.** Page 606.

34. **Answer: E.** Page 433.

35. **Answer: E.** The superego conceptualizes the conscience. Page 829.

36. **Answer: C.** The possible risk factor of community violence can constitute high risk if children experiencing it show significantly greater maladjustment than those who do not. Page 292.

37. **Answer: C.** Prepubertal depression is different from adolescent-onset depression and conduct disorder, both of which have a higher risk of depression in later stages of life. Page 504.

38. **Answer: A.** Depression was the most common comorbid diagnosis seen during the national Institute of Mental Health screening. Page 496.

39. **Answer: B.** While electroencephalography (EEG) provides a measure of extraneuronal current flow, magnetoencephalography provides the only measure of intraneuronal current flow. Page 229.

40. **Answer: A.** Inherent in the definition are two fundamental conditions: the existence of significant risk and adversity, and positive adaptation. Page 293.

41. **Answer: C.** The underlying assumption of interpersonal psychotherapy is that the quality of interpersonal relationships can cause, maintain, or buffer against depression. Page 819.

42. **Answer: B.** For trichotillomania it is up to 1%. Prevalence questions such as these are not worth memorizing, but it is good to have a ballpark idea of the prevalence rates for different disorders. Page 566.

43. **Answer: A.** The psychoanalytic movement contributed to an individually oriented treatment approach in social work practice and less focus on the social context in childhood problems. Page 879.

44. **Answer: C.** The "best interests of the child" is the generally accepted principle in child custody and placement. Page 1007.

45. **Answer: C.** Although many children go through periods of dysfluency through the developmental period, these "normal dysfluencies" tend to occur in the large linguistic units (words, phrases, and sentences). Page 424.

46. **Answer: A.** Page 900.

47. **Answer: C.** Page 430.

48. **Answer: A.** According to the chapter, no contemporary epidemiological studies have examined gender identity disorder. The answer reflects an estimate based on rather unsophisticated approaches. Page 670.

49. **Answer: B.** Page 371.

50. **Answer: E.** Obsessive–compulsive disorder (OCD) is associated with impairment in prefrontal lobe functions. Page 552.

51. **Answer: A.** Only 2% of highly traumatized young children endorse sufficient avoidance symptoms for the diagnosis of posttraumatic stress disorder (PTSD) according to the DSM-IV criteria. Page 706.

52. **Answer: A.** Approximately 20% of males who carry the abnormal gene are not mentally retarded and are called "normal transmitting males." These males pass the abnormal gene to their daughters, who may also be unaffected; however, their grandsons are at high risk for the syndrome (anticipation). Fragile X is the second most common cause of MR after Down syndrome. Additional clinical symptoms include facial, testicular and connective tissue abnormalities. Page 203.

53. **Answer: B.** Page 683.

54. **Answer: B.** However, haloperidol is much sedating than low potency antipsychotics. Page 776.

55. **Answer: E.** In addition, representatives from the American Board of Medical Specialties also sit on the Council. Page 29.

56. **Answer D.** Kaufman and colleagues were able to document a significant three-way interaction between brain-derived neurotrophic factor genotype, 5-HTTLPR, and maltreatment history in predicting depression. See Figure 5.15.1.2. Page 696.

57. **Answer: B.** This criterion by itself is not a good predictor as it only considers one aspect of one domain, that of gross motor skills. Page 253.

58. **Answer: D.** The EEG findings occur in the context of behavioral arrest, which lasts 10 to 30 seconds. After the seizure, the child picks up where they left off. Absence epilepsy peaks in children from the age of 5 to 10 then declines, being quite rare by the age of 30. Pages 960–961.

59. **Answer: B.** Interpersonal conflicts with peers are the most common antecedents in this age group. Family conflicts are often present and are the key trigger for younger children. Page 810.

60. **Answer: B.** Acidic drugs bind to albumin. Page 746.

61. **Answer: A.** Page 549.

62. **Answer: E.** This is not in the textbook but is a rare side effect of oxcarbazepine according to the package insert and worth knowing. The other side effects are less likely or unlikely. The data on oxcarbazepine has not been favorable for use in pediatric bipolar and that is in the book. Page 965.

63. **Answer: D.** The Incredible Years emphasizes parent training and includes watching standardized videotapes of parents and their children engaging in both problematic and desirable behaviors. The Good Behavior Game is aimed at improving the classroom management skills of teachers. In the Nurse-Family Partnership, nurses follow mothers prenatally until the child is 24 months of age. Page 174.

64. **Answer: E.** Persons with severe and profound MR come to diagnosis at a younger age, more often exhibit related medical conditions, may exhibit dysmorphic features, and have a range of behavioral and psychiatric disturbances. In contrast, persons with mild MR often come to diagnosis much later (typically when academic demands become more prominent in school), are less likely to have medical conditions that could account for the MR, and usually are of normal appearance without dysmorphic features. In this latter group, although rates of psychopathology are increased relative to nondisabled populations, the range and nature of problems seen are fundamentally similar to those in normative samples. Persons with moderate levels of MR are intermediate between these two extremes. Page 403.

65. **Answer: C.** Page 269.

66. **Answer: A.** Although poor development in speech and language may be a child's presenting problem, oftentimes an evaluation uncovers deficits in other areas of development, including cognitive abilities, hearing, motor and social skills, which contribute to the determination of a diagnostic label. Page 373.

67. **Answer: A.** Oftentimes, there is confusion between the terms confidentiality and privilege. In contrast to the definition of privilege, confidentiality refers to the disclosure or nondisclosure of information learned in a patient's treatment to third parties. Page 18.

68. **Answer: D.** The two crucial elements of concrete operations are classification (the ability to group objects or concepts) and conservation (the ability to recognize constant qualities/quantities of material even when the material undergoes change in morphology). In general, concrete operations allow a child to deal with things systematically. Page 270.

69. **Answer: E.** A patient registry is a data collection system that allows for an easily accessible sampling source and from which hypotheses can be rapidly tested. Page 154.

70. **Answer: A.** This question is meant to highlight the weakness of this popular means of reporting test performance. Percentile rank is a way of positioning the child's performance relative to the norm group, however the numbers can be deceptive as they may overemphasize or underemphasize differences between standard scores. Page 362.

71. **Answer: A.** It warrants consideration that children or even adolescents may not report this side effect as readily. Page 766.

72. **Answer: D.** Affected individuals are compared to unaffected controls, with common genetic polymorphisms (markers) investigated near the predetermined gene of interest (candidate genes). Genetic association studies are also susceptible to false-positive results. Page 194.

73. **Answer: A.** Page 160.

74. **Answer: B.** Children with autism typically become quite anxious when the environment to which they have become accustomed changes. Page 389.

75. **Answer: A.** Countertransference is considered objective if virtually everyone would find a patient's behavior provocative. Answers B and C are definitions of countertransference but not as specific. Page 831.

76. **Answer: D.** From a Dutch study involving 20,000 children. One-fourth to one-third had not been taken to a physician for evaluation. Page 663.

77. **Answer: C.** Page 305.

78. **Answer: A.** Investigators have found that adolescent girls (as a group, not as individuals) were especially likely to improve under psychotherapeutic treatment such that studies that include large numbers of adolescent females have stronger findings than those that do not. Page 790.

79. **Answer: B.** Preliminary findings from investigation of the consequences of separation from the perpetrator suggest that many children are "quite indifferent" to separation when it does occur and they go on to embrace their own wellness and engage with others around them. Page 726.

80. **Answer: D.** One wants to reject the idea that there is no difference (null hypothesis) if in fact there is a difference. The statistical power is inversely related to a type II error. Conventionally, the desired statistical power of a study is 0.80. Page 115.

81. **Answer: A.** Page 70.

82. **Answer: B.** Apathetic and withdrawn behavior is classified under disturbances in social development and/or the care-giving environment. Page 253.

83. **Answer: E.** Continuous educational interventions have been shown to improve long-term outcomes. Social skills groups and psychopharmacological agents also have a role in treating target problems. Page 392.

84. **Answer: A.** A placebo-controlled trial of bupropion in 72 children with Attention Deficit Hyperactivity Disorder (ADHD) showed its greater effectiveness over placebo; however, the treatment effect was smaller than that with stimulants. Page 766.

85. **Answer: D.** In the termination phase of IPT-A, the therapist needs to balance the tasks of this phase with the concluding work on the identified problem area that was previously identified. Page 824.

86. **Answer: C.** Population-based studies have indicated a risk for males but not females concerning sexual orientation. Page 532.

87. **Answer: C.** A value of 0 indicates no relationship between two variables, while values close to either -1 or +1 indicate a very strong relationship between two variables. Page 107.

88. **Answer B.** Attachment-based interventions can also be provided in a group setting. The circle of security model integrates attachment theory and object relations theory. Using group discussions about video clips of each dyad, this treatment model focuses on enhancing parents' reflective functioning, observational skills of their children's exploration and attachment cues, emotional regulation, and empathy. Page 717.

89. **Answer: E.** The symptoms are recognized and interpreted through the appropriate attribution, which is part of the common socialization process for the cultural subgroup. Page 58.

90. **Answer: E.** Page 346.

91. **Answer: E.** Page 243.

92. **Answer: E.** Any of the parties may make the request, however most often the attorney or court makes the request. This is the better approach, as it allows for the clarification of roles, makes clear the purpose is not clinical evaluation and care, and to clarify the specific questions to be addressed in the evaluation. Page 1003.

93. **Answer: D.** Page 338.

94. **Answer: A.** Stereotypies tend to have an earlier age of onset—age 2 or 3—are bilateral, and are consistent rather than waxing and waning as tics usually are. Page 576.

95. **Answer: B.** Average reading comprehension level for adolescents without cochlear implants is third to fourth grade. Language and reading outcomes for children who receive cochlear implants are generally higher. Page 421.

96. **Answer: A.** Page 567.

97. **Answer: B.** The primary mechanism of action of these stimulants are the striatal (and at least indirectly) the prefrontal dopaminergic neurons; however, they affect the norepinephrine system as well, and the combined effect is most likely essential for the clinical effects of stimulants. Page 757.

98. **Answer: D.** Table 7.2.6 lists interventions useful for a variety of symptoms. The table is derived from suggestions found at www.schoolpsychiatry.org. Page 991.

99. **Answer: B.** 50,000 children die annually, and a large number—500,000—suffer from an illness that is chronic and terminal. Page 971.

100. **Answer: A.** In particular, early family relationships are identified as extremely important in shaping long-term resilient trajectories. Page 294.

101. **Answer: B.** It was 40%. The Pediatric OCD Treatment Study also examined the use of sertraline. Page 558.

102. **Answer: A.** In a large population-based twin-registry study, Kendler et al., showed that concordance for bulimia nervosa was significantly higher in monozygotic than dizygotic twin pairs. Page 596.

103. **Answer: E.** The multidetermined nature of symptoms provides the psychodynamic therapist with more than one way to approach a symptom. Page 828.

104. **Answer: A.** So called Reparative Therapy, which claims to "cure" homosexuality, is embraced by groups who view homosexuality as pathological or sinful, which is not the view of professional mental health organizations. Page 84.

105. **Answer: B.** Gesell represents one pole of the two competing schools of thought in America on child development (environmental vs. biological). Gesell emphasized the innate biological processes in child development whereas others such as Dr. William Healy emphasized the more environmental vectors of child behavior and delinquency. Page 14.

106. **Answer: C.** Option C is a strategy on how to make aggressive behavior irrelevant by changing the antecedents. Page 477.

107. **Answer: B.** Tertiary amine tricyclic antidepressants, such as imipramine and amitriptyline, have highly anticholinergic properties. Page 764.

108. **Answer: A.** Pain appears to be the most common specific somatoform disorder in children. Fatigue is also a very common physical symptom in children. Page 635.

109. **Answer: E.** In the late 19th century and early 20th century the recognition that certain substances could lead to abuse resulted in increased regulation. The Harrison Act limited the sale of opiates and cocaine to licensed physicians and pharmacists. Page 615.

110. **Answer: B.** Medicare covers senior citizens; Medicaid is for low-income individuals. Page 52.

111. **Answer: B.** Psychiatrists in court-ordered evaluations are considered agents of the courts and are typically found immune from liability. The courts have had mixed views on school consultations, with some courts finding that the evaluator has a duty to the employer and others to the identified child. In consulting relationships, the liability depends on whether a doctor-patient relationship is formed; if orders are written or care is directed by the consultant, the liability increases. Page 1019.

112. **Answer: E.** Page 459.

113. **Answer: D.** Investigators and clinicians have noted severely disordered attachment behaviors in children who appear to have a focused attachment figure, albeit in the context of a disturbed relationship. The distortions can be of four major types: role reversed behaviors, provocative self-endangering behaviors, excessive clinginess and restriction in exploration, and excessive vigilance and hypercompliance. In the role reversed pattern, a child takes on a directive, parent-like role in his or her relationship with a primary caregiver. Page 714.

114. **Answer: B.** Children with pervasive developmental disorder showed a lower rate of positive response to stimulants. Page 755.

115. **Answer: A.** New neurons have been identified that originate in the subventricular zone and then migrate through the white matter to the neocortex, where they extend axons, and become functionally active. Page 185.

116. **Answer: B.** It is not equivalent to free association as in adult psychoanalysis because the child's capacity for insight is limited and the child is not instructed to say whatever comes to mind. Page 834.

117. **Answer: B.** Developmentally, temper tantrums start as children begin to experiment with separation from their parents. The more they move away from the emotionally secure base of the parent, the more dependent and small they may feel, and the more vulnerable to frustration and tantrums they may become. Page 265.

118. **Answer: D.** Childhood disintegrative disorder is a very rare condition that is defined by the loss of clearly acquired developmental skills in areas of motor, social, and communication abilities. Some children also lose bladder or bowel control. The hand wringing motion associated with Rett disorder is not present. Landau-Kleffner syndrome is also associated with regression, epilepsy, and aphasia; however, other skills and social interest are preserved. Page 397.

119. **Answer: D.** The term deliberate objection recognizes that even children too young for meaningful assent are able to communicate their disapproval of a nontherapeutic procedure, that is, a procedure with research purposes only. Page 145.

120. **Answer: B.** In fact, early efficacy studies on child psychotherapy failed to specify what therapeutic procedures were used in the tested intervention, further weakening the internal validity of the studies. This question explores some of the crucial components of internal validity. Page 789.

121. **Answer: D.** Page 845.

122. **Answer: C.** All of the diagnoses could of course be considered, however delirium, especially if hypoactive, often presents as depression and can be overlooked. The Lewis text does not address this issue specifically but the chapter section describes the evaluation process in consultation and liaison. Page 919.

123. **Answer: D.** At this point, the most widely discussed and evidence supported model of learning disabled identification is the responsiveness to intervention model. Page 414.

124. **Answer: C.** Page 659.

125. **Answer: C.** Page 105.

126. **Answer: C.** CYPs also metabolize drugs, which happens to be quite an important point in psychopharmacology. Page 747.

127. **Answer: C.** In most cases, parents or adults provide the impetus to initiate treatment. Page 323.

128. **Answer: D.** However, multiple pediatric studies have failed to detect hippocampal atrophy in children with PTSD. Page 702.

129. **Answer: D.** Random assignment of participants into groups contributes to high internal validity whereas self-selection of participants based on knowledge of the treatment contributes to low internal validity. Page 114.

130. **Answer: B.** Adults with ADHD may have an inner feeling of restlessness only. Page 441.

131. **Answer: E.** The three other somatoform disorders in the DSM are undifferentiated somatoform disorder, somatization disorder, and somatoform disorder, not otherwise specified. Page 633.

132. **Answer: E.** Page 847.

133. **Answer: C.** After reports of agranulocytosis, clozapine was withdrawn by its manufacturer in the mid-1970s. In 1989 the FDA approved its use for treatment resistant schizophrenia, given its efficacy, but with intense blood monitoring. It has also been approved for the reduction of suicidal behavior in patients with schizophrenia. Page 773.

134. **Answer: E.** Page 889.

135. **Answer: B.** False! Mothers taking valproate during pregnancy have a 20-fold increase in the risk for their fetus to contract a variety of malformations including neural tube defect, cleft lip and palate, cardiovascular abnormalities, genitourinary defects, and others. Prior to initiating treatment in sexually active female adolescents, a negative pregnancy test and a reliable method of contraception should be documented. Page 771.

136. **Answer: A.** Smaller children may start at 2.5 mg per day. Page 763.

137. **Answer: A.** Page 623.

138. **Answer: A.** Working memory encompasses the ability to simultaneously attend to, recall, and act upon information held in the mind. Page 368.

139. **Answer: E.** Pages 685–686.

140. **Answer: C.** Choice B is a brief description of object constancy as put forth by Margaret Mahler and others. Page 827.

141. **Answer: A.** Gender role is the correct answer. Page 79.

142. **Answer: B.** As mothers tend to respond to their infants on a more intimate level, they appear to facilitate affective differentiation and fine-motor development; fathers tend to be more active with their infants, showing more involvement in their gross-motor skills. Such findings are generalizations, of course. Page 7.

143. **Answer: A.** Sally Provence initially suggested this method. Page 312.

144. **Answer: D.** IPT-A is probably most effective for adolescents with acute onset depressive feelings, normal intelligence, not actively suicidal, and without chronic or severe interpersonal problems. Page 821.

145. **Answer: B.** Transference distortions refer to a more psychodynamic outlook; the other targets are explicitly within the domain of interpersonal therapy for adolescents. Page 508.

146. **Answer: D.** This percentage is likely to increase; furthermore, immigrants in the United States are arriving from increasingly diverse countries of origin. Page 39.

147. **Answer: E.** Collaborative law and mediation, which are mandated in some jurisdictions, reflect approaches that are alternatives to adversarial litigation. Page 1011.

148. **Answer: D.** Milestones are lost in weight first, then height, and then head circumference. Page 588.

149. **Answer: E.** Tanner stages I through V describe stages of puberty. Tanner stage is most accurately determined by direct physical examination, although self-report can be an alternative method. Page 280.

150. **Answer: A.** Page 379.

151. **Answer: B.** Pavor nocturnus is night terror, which is a parasomnia not a dysomnia. The child may appear glassy-eyed and may stare without seeing, and is unresponsive to visual or verbal cues. The event usually terminates spontaneously after 3 to 5 minutes. The experience is not recalled. The EEG shows continuous high-voltage delta waves. Page 628.

152. **Answer: A.** Menarche is the clearest marker of puberty in girls. Periods remain irregular for some time, and ovulation and full fertility may require up to 2 years to develop. A critical body weight and fat/muscle ratio appears to be necessary for menarche. In addition, likely because of improved nutrition and body weight, there has been a steady decrease in the age of menarche since the Industrial Revolution. Page 280.

153. **Answer: C or D.** Page 679.

154. **Answer: C.** Multisystemic therapy, an in-home community-based service, developed as an alternative to incarceration for serious juvenile offenders, is known for its strong evidence in the treatment of this population and substance abusing youth. The data are less robust for psychiatrically ill populations. The other programs listed among the options have a community-based, in-home component. Page 881.

155. **Answer: A.** Page 372.

156. **Answer: A.** In patients with anorexia nervosa who engage in self-induced vomiting or abuse laxatives and diuretics, hypokalemic alkalosis may develop. These electrolyte disturbances are associated with physical symptoms of weakness, lethargy, and at times cardiac arrhythmias. Page 594.

157. **Answer: C.** PTSD criteria were introduced in 1980 in the DSM-III. Page 702.

158. **Answer: C.** This suggests youth may need higher serum lithium concentrations. Page 521.

159. **Answer: A.** Page 781.

160. **Answer: A.** Page 763.

161. **Answer: B.** Effectiveness is based on the performance of an intervention under naturalistic, or real-world, conditions. Page 127.

162. **Answer: A and C.** These are at least two of the basic principles associated with the tenet 'respect for persons' when involved in human research. Page 141.

163. **Answer: A or D.** Psychological abuse can be caused by repeatedly taking a child for unnecessary medical treatment. Other forms of abuse may be present. Page 692.

164. **Answer: D.** Social/emotional status, vision/hearing screening, and motor abilities are often assessed as well. Occupational therapy, along with other specialized evaluations, such as intelligence testing, neuropsychological testing, and psychiatric assessments are added when deemed necessary. Page 987.

165. **Answer: A.** Page 769.

166. **Answer: D.** Page 766.

167. **Answer: C.** Page 651.

168. **Answer: C.** Weight gain is a side effect of steroids. Page 945.

169. **Answer: A.** For example, if 9 of 100 siblings of probands with autism develop autism from birth to age 3 the cumulative incidence would be reported as 9% over the first 3 years of life. Page 151.

170. **Answer: B.** Page 619.

171. **Answer: E.** Not fair, a tricky question, as cognitive-behavioral therapy is not a community-based intervention but a psychotherapeutic modality. Page 894.

172. **Answer: B.** Some symptoms of autism have been attributed to a lack of ability to integrate parts into wholes. This has been consistent with neuroimaging studies that demonstrate abnormal patterns of "functional connectivity." Page 387.

173. **Answer: C.** Page 239.

174. **Answer: D.** Pervasive developmental disorders are a group of neuropsychiatric disorders that share developmental delays in language, social, and cognitive areas. Page 384.

175. **Answer: C.** These four phases help to determine the duration of drug activity in the body. Page 743.

176. **Answer: D.** A long-term follow-up study of 54 children and adolescents with OCD found that 70% remained on medication for more than 2 years. Page 763.

177. **Answer: E.** With antiretroviral drugs available for prevention, it is less than 5%, down from a rate of 25% before such drugs were used perinatally. The rate is 35% in resource poor countries. Page 947.

178–181. **Answers:** 178-A; 179-C; 180-D; 181-B. The Cochrane Library's Central Register of Controlled Trials is the full moniker of the database providing full randomized controlled trial data. Page 131.

182. **Answer: E.** Page 182.

183. **Answer: B.** Repression is a defense mechanism of the ego. Self-punishment is also under the influence of the superego. Page 830.

184. **Answer: B.** There is a number of well-validated programs, and hindrances to implementation lie elsewhere, including political, economic and other considerations. Page 171.

185. **Answer: A.** In response to the French state's request for a study of special education, Binet and Simon developed the concept of mental age and a test for measuring it in 1905. Page 310.

186. **Answer: B.** Page 316.

187. **Answer: D.** X-linked with mutation of the MeCP2 gene. Page 208.

188. **Answer: B.** There is some evidence, not conclusive, that separation anxiety disorder, however, is a risk factor for the development of panic disorder or agoraphobia as an adolescent or adult. Page 539.

189. **Answer: C.** Even in the older group with poor care as babies, only one-fourth had problems, which included difficulties with peers and the lower likelihood of having a special friend. Page 1017.

190. **Answer: B.** The effect is actually higher, at about half the magnitude of parenting. As can be expected, a child's parents have a greater effect, but childcare can be an influential factor, the details of which should be considered and investigated by clinicians in their assessment, considering its effect. Page 255.

191. **Answer: A.** Koenen and colleagues have shown that even after controlling for genetic factors and externalizing and internalizing problems, exposure to domestic violence accounted for a significant variation in children's IQs. Page 295.

192. **Answer: A.** Page 455.

193. **Answer: D.** Page 856.

194. **Answer: B.** The signal acquired during the one blocked condition is compared with the data acquired under another blocked condition. As the images in blocked conditions are temporally integrated, only the average differences in brain activity between the two conditions can be compared. Page 222.

195. **Answer: B.** Page 543.

196. **Answer: D.** First coined by Dr. Richard Gardner in the 1980's this has been a controversial topic. A more up-to-date formulation by Kelly and Johnston focuses on the alienated child, which they describe as "one who expresses, freely and persistently, unreasonable negative feelings and beliefs toward a parent that are significantly disproportionate to the child's actual experience with that parent." Page 1010.

197. **Answer: B and D.** Page 357.

198. **Answer: A.** Included among the risk factors are parental psychopathology and instability in the family environment. Pages 36–37.

199. **Answer: C.** Different centers use different exclusionary criteria. Page 941.

200. **Answer: A.** This question reveals how long the issue of quality childcare has been a nationwide issue. However, two obstacles have impeded policy action on the issue: ideological arguments regarding the use of childcare and the lack of public awareness of the need for childcare services. Page 40.

Appendix

For those interested in focusing on a single topic or chapter, this appendix lists all the pertinent questions in the seven tests ordered under the chapter number and title.

1.1 The Art of the Science
Test One: 7, 41
Test Two: 20, 73
Test Three: 130, 188
Test Four: None
Test Five: 109
Test Six: 136
Test Seven: 142

1.2 Prevailing and Shifting Paradigms: A Historical Perspective
Test One: 32
Test Two: 26
Test Three: 82
Test Four: 108
Test Five: 158
Test Six: 39
Test Seven: 105

1.3 Ethics
Test One: 125, 154
Test Two: 47, 195
Test Three: 31, 44
Test Four: 65, 84
Test Five: 26, 112
Test Six: 86, 134
Test Seven: 23, 67

1.4 Education and Training
Test One: 87, 187
Test Two: 82
Test Three: 48, 75
Test Four: 8, 56
Test Five: 9, 71
Test Six: 5, 190
Test Seven: 9, 55

1.5 Child and Family Policy
Test One: 14, 107, 167
Test Two: 34, 46, 85, 167
Test Three: 14, 62, 156, 162
Test Four: 42, 49, 76, 195
Test Five: 51, 102, 113
Test Six: 72, 92, 142
Test Seven: 146, 198, 200

1.6 Money Matters: Funding Care
Test One: 60
Test Two: 181
Test Three: 69
Test Four: None
Test Five: 95
Test Six: 32
Test Seven: 110

1.7.1 Cultural Child and Adolescent Psychiatry
Test One: 162
Test Two: 80
Test Three: None
Test Four: 20
Test Five: 127
Test Six: 93
Test Seven: 89

1.7.2 The Hearing or Visually Impaired Child
Test One: 198
Test Two: 63
Test Three: 12, 15
Test Four: 17, 47
Test Five: 33, 165
Test Six: 61
Test Seven: 81

1.7.3 Sexual Minority Youth
Test One: 42, 62
Test Two: 62
Test Three: 55
Test Four: 191
Test Five: 15
Test Six: 60, 167
Test Seven: 104, 141

1.8 International Child and Adolescent Mental Health
Test One: None
Test Two: 29, 64
Test Three: 91, 194
Test Four: 6
Test Five: None
Test Six: None
Test Seven: None

3.1.3 Development of School-Age Children

Test One: 47, 89, 101
Test Two: 50, 114, 143
Test Three: 24, 144, 200
Test Four: 3, 34, 109
Test Five: 47, 60, 69, 171
Test Six: 79, 126, 173
Test Seven: 65, 68

3.1.4 Adolescence

Test One: 155, 200
Test Two: 41, 125
Test Three: 132, 163
Test Four: 7, 113
Test Five: 10, 117
Test Six: 48, 51
Test Seven: 31, 149, 152

3.2 Developmental Psychopathology

Test One: 13, 26, 68, 69
Test Two: 23, 130, 194
Test Three: 68, 181, 195
Test Four: 73, 74, 106
Test Five: 1, 81, 103
Test Six: 83, 96, 171
Test Seven: 36, 40, 100, 191

4.1 Classification

Test One: 20, 126
Test Two: 2, 42, 185
Test Three: 131, 140, 191
Test Four: 80, 156
Test Five: 43, 96, 172
Test Six: 116, 135
Test Seven: 11–13, 77

4.2.1 Clinical Assessment of Infants and Toddlers

Test One: 24, 146, 160, 161
Test Two: 8, 84, 141, 200
Test Three: 53, 58, 71, 192
Test Four: 28, 55, 142, 147
Test Five: 32, 45, 80, 185
Test Six: 62, 133, 146, 178, 184
Test Seven: 1, 143, 185, 186

4.2.2 Clinical Assessment of Children and Adolescents: Content and Structure

Test One: 133, 165
Test Two: 68, 175
Test Three: 79, 107
Test Four: 53, 179
Test Five: 2, 155
Test Six: 128, 151
Test Seven: 32, 93, 127

4.2.3 Structured Interviewing

Test One: 27, 189
Test Two: 101, 133
Test Three: 109, 178
Test Four: 41, 171
Test Five: 67, 82
Test Six: 131
Test Seven: 90

4.2.4 Psychological and Neuropsychological Assessment of Children

Test One: 9, 31, 106, 135
Test Two: 65, 88, 102, 178
Test Three: 50, 104, 109, 179
Test Four: 14, 16
Test Five: 135, 156, 178
Test Six: 11–15, 33, 174, 165
Test Seven: 29, 70, 138, 197

4.2.5 Assessing Communication

Test One: 39, 112, 159
Test Two: 32, 112, 188
Test Three: 6, 57, 196
Test Four: 72, 159, 163
Test Five: 79, 84, 130, 168
Test Six: 49, 105, 109, 122
Test Seven: 15, 49, 66, 155

4.2.6 Formulation and Integration

Test One: 12, 79
Test Two: 11, 30
Test Three: 4, 145
Test Four: 61, 174
Test Five: 14, 189
Test Six: 68, 125
Test Seven: 150

5.1.1 Autism and the Pervasive Developmental Disorders

Test One: 11, 94, 108, 140, 152
Test Two: 67, 93, 153, 186
Test Three: 61, 97, 139, 180
Test Four: 36, 96, 154, 173
Test Five: 11, 132, 173, 182
Test Six: 91, 169, 195, 199
Test Seven: 74, 83, 118, 172, 174

5.1.2 Mental Retardation

Test One: 51
Test Two: 142, 179
Test Three: 122, 193
Test Four: 23, 180
Test Five: 39, 55
Test Six: 2, 98
Test Seven: 64

5.1.3 Learning Disabilities

Test One: 25, 90
Test Two: 27, 95
Test Three: 51, 113
Test Four: 176
Test Five: 162
Test Six: 3
Test Seven: 30, 123

5.1.4 Disorders of Communication

Test One: 100, 185
Test Two: 51, 157
Test Three: 7, 111
Test Four: 90, 152, 189
Test Five: 76, 174, 192
Test Six: 36, 56, 69
Test Seven: 45, 95

5.2.1 Attention Deficit Hyperactivity Disorder

Test One: 54, 136, 164
Test Two: 45, 168
Test Three: 34, 124, 190
Test Four: 5, 11, 75
Test Five: 40, 176
Test Six: 114, 162
Test Seven: 34, 47, 130

5.2.2 Oppositional Defiant and Conduct Disorder

Test One: 117, 145, 177–182
Test Two: 104, 105, 127
Test Three: 22, 40
Test Four: 44, 182
Test Five: 19, 68, 73
Test Six: 152, 164
Test Seven: 14, 112, 192

5.2.3 Aggression in Children: An Integrative Approach

Test One: 5, 81
Test Two: 149
Test Three: 47, 155
Test Four: 164, 194
Test Five: 53, 184
Test Six: 70, 100
Test Seven: 3, 106

5.2.4 Fire Behavior in Children and Adolescents

Test One: 132
Test Two: 87, 108
Test Three: 168
Test Four: 27
Test Five: 36
Test Six: 22
Test Seven: 8

5.3 Childhood Onset Schizophrenia and Other Early-Onset Psychotic Disorders

Test One: 188
Test Two: 5
Test Three: 5, 65
Test Four: 170, 188
Test Five: 27, 133
Test Six: 52
Test Seven: 38

5.4.1 Depressive Disorders

Test One: 172
Test Two: 155
Test Three: 17
Test Four: 158
Test Five: 199
Test Six: 111, 194
Test Seven: 37, 145

5.4.2 Bipolar Disorder

Test One: 59, 83
Test Two: 169, 180
Test Three: 9, 157
Test Four: 160
Test Five: 13
Test Six: 163
Test Seven: 158

5.4.3 Suicidal Behavior in Children and Adolescents: Causes and Management

Test One: 44, 70
Test Two: 109, 163
Test Three: 127, 183
Test Four: 33, 140
Test Five: 121, 139
Test Six: 89, 187
Test Seven: 21, 86

5.5.1 Anxiety Disorders

Test One: 35, 119
Test Two: 110, 152
Test Three: 126, 189
Test Four: 25, 46, 135
Test Five: 86, 131
Test Six: 129, 159
Test Seven: 188, 195

5.5.2 Obsessive–Compulsive Disorder

Test One: 46, 58, 72
Test Two: 12, 38, 75
Test Three: 77, 150, 165
Test Four: 60, 87, 199
Test Five: 89, 140, 198
Test Six: 57, 102, 185
Test Seven: 50, 61, 101

5.5.3 Trichotillomania

Test One: 184
Test Two: 40
Test Three: 26
Test Four: 193
Test Five: 56, 77
Test Six: 30, 124
Test Seven: 42, 96

5.6 Tic Disorders

Test One: 55, 105, 116
Test Two: 43, 144, 160
Test Three: 37, 186
Test Four: 145, 153
Test Five: 143, 148
Test Six: 80, 84
Test Seven: 24, 94

5.7.1 Eating and Growth Disorders in Infants and Children

Test One: 52
Test Two: 119
Test Three: 11, 66
Test Four: 150
Test Five: 110
Test Six: 181
Test Seven: 148

5.7.2 Anorexia Nervosa and Bulimia Nervosa

Test One: 92, 166
Test Two: 13, 164
Test Three: 88, 99
Test Four: 111, 115, 165
Test Five: 12, 65, 149
Test Six: 21, 73
Test Seven: 102, 156

5.7.3 Obesity

Test One: 84
Test Two: 99
Test Three: 115
Test Four: 137
Test Five: 179
Test Six: 38, 75
Test Seven: 33

5.8 Substance Use Disorders

Test One: 8, 82, 114, 197
Test Two: 19, 146, 190
Test Three: 92, 114, 198
Test Four: 10, 68, 141
Test Five: 20, 101, 153
Test Six: 45, 118, 180
Test Seven: 19, 109, 137, 170

5.9 Sleep Disorders

Test One: 17, 73
Test Two: 9, 15, 94

Test Three: 23, 27, 108
Test Four: 85, 130, 183
Test Five: 78, 125, 150
Test Six: 78, 107
Test Seven: 27, 151

5.10 Somatoform Disorders

Test One: 93
Test Two: 14, 96
Test Three: 45, 85
Test Four: 9, 70
Test Five: 70, 75
Test Six: 87, 149, 153
Test Seven: 10, 108, 131

5.11 Delirium and Catatonia

Test One: 139, 151
Test Two: 7, 132
Test Three: 20, 116
Test Four: 162
Test Five: 147
Test Six: 130
Test Seven: 167

5.12 Elimination Disorders: Enuresis and Encopresis

Test One: 48, 64, 99
Test Two: 28, 103, 150
Test Three: 137, 199
Test Four: 38, 117, 167
Test Five: 52, 94, 114
Test Six: 74, 113, 148
Test Seven: 28, 76, 124

5.13 Gender Identity Disorder

Test One: 141, 147, 158
Test Two: 36, 37
Test Three: 39, 76, 187
Test Four: 78, 82, 151
Test Five: 5, 41, 42
Test Six: 77, 196, 200
Test Seven: 18, 48, 153

5.14 Personality Disorders in Children and Adolescents

Test One: 75, 194
Test Two: 22, 121, 176
Test Three: 42, 64, 185
Test Four: 63, 86, 131
Test Five: 98, 151
Test Six: 37, 177
Test Seven: 53, 139

5.15.1 Child Abuse and Neglect

Test One: 124, 156
Test Two: 39, 74
Test Three: 36, 95
Test Four: 185

Test Five: 175
Test Six: 71, 198
Test Seven: 56, 163

5.15.2 Posttraumatic Stress Disorder

Test One: 37, 77, 153
Test Two: 33, 61, 136
Test Three: 54, 129, 153
Test Four: 102, 132, 149
Test Five: 23, 83, 126
Test Six: 145, 166, 197
Test Seven: 51, 128, 157

5.15.3 Reactive Attachment Disorder

Test One: 34, 191
Test Two: 17, 151
Test Three: 184
Test Four: 71, 136
Test Five: 180, 200
Test Six: 43, 183
Test Seven: 88, 113

5.15.4 Munchhausen Syndrome by Proxy

Test One: None
Test Two: None
Test Three: 110
Test Four: 58
Test Five: 18
Test Six: 186
Test Seven: 79

5.15.5 Children Exposed to Disaster: The Role of the Mental Health Professional

Test One: 10, 111
Test Two: 158, 171
Test Three: 121, 164
Test Four: 66
Test Five: 193
Test Six: 170
Test Seven: 25

6.1.1 Clinical and Developmental Aspects of Pharmacokinetics and Drug Interactions

Test One: 121, 138, 183, 186
Test Two: 56, 57, 72, 92
Test Three: 43, 106, 138, 197
Test Four: 62, 67, 89, 177, 186
Test Five: 85, 138, 195, 196
Test Six: 16, 47, 82, 99, 193
Test Seven: 20, 60, 126, 175

6.1.2 General Principles, Specific Drug Treatments, and Clinical Practice

Test One: 19, 29, 49, 53, 66, 85, 127, 148, 149, 192, 195
Test Two: 10, 60, 66, 81, 91, 97, 113, 115, 126, 156, 165, 173, 189, 191

Test Three: 2, 16, 29, 32, 33, 67, 72, 86, 90, 94, 96, 100, 148, 158
Test Four: 12, 45, 69, 77 83, 114, 116, 146, 148, 169, 181, 184, 196
Test Five: 28, 46, 49, 100, 104, 122, 144, 157, 161, 166, 169, 177, 190, 191
Test Six: 8, 10, 25, 31, 41, 58, 63, 88, 104, 110, 112, 154, 155
Test Seven: 54, 71, 84, 97, 107, 114, 133, 135, 136, 159, 160, 165, 166, 176

6.2.1 Psychotherapy for Children and Adolescents: A Critical Overview

Test One: 67
Test Two: 192
Test Three: 143
Test Four: None
Test Five: 88
Test Six: 156
Test Seven: 78, 120

6.2.2 Cognitive and Behavioral Therapies

Test One: 56, 76, 169
Test Two: 16, 177, 193
Test Three: 10, 13, 161
Test Four: 26, 57, 100
Test Five: 6, 37, 72
Test Six: 108, 157, 160
Test Seven: 2, 59

6.2.3 Interpersonal Psychotherapy

Test One: 61, 78
Test Two: 198, 199
Test Three: 89, 118
Test Four: 1, 94
Test Five: 24, 93
Test Six: 46, 115
Test Seven: 41, 85, 144

6.2.4 Psychodynamic Principles in Practice

Test One: 63, 86, 104, 109, 123, 129, 143
Test Two: 4, 35, 49, 78, 98
Test Three: 28, 78, 84, 125, 151
Test Four: 52, 64, 99, 155, 168, 187
Test Five: 16, 57–64, 92, 120, 146, 194
Test Six: 1, 81, 97, 150, 158, 172
Test Seven: 35, 75, 103, 116, 140, 183

6.2.5 Group Therapy

Test One: 40, 80
Test Two: 120, 123, 161
Test Three: 60, 80
Test Four: 43, 93
Test Five: 124, 197
Test Six: 94, 191
Test Seven: 121, 132

6.2.6 Family Therapy

Test One: 16
Test Two: 70
Test Three: 70, 98
Test Four: 172
Test Five: 115, 145
Test Six: 26
Test Seven: 193

6.3.1 Milieu-Based Treatment: Inpatient and Partial Hospitalization, Residential Treatment

Test One: 118, 137
Test Two: 31
Test Three: None
Test Four: None
Test Five: None
Test Six: None
Test Seven: 4

6.3.2 Intensive Home-Based Family Preservation Approaches, Including Multisystemic Therapy

Test One: 144, 199
Test Two: 79, 135
Test Three: 103
Test Four: 107
Test Five: 31
Test Six: 120, 138
Test Seven: 43, 154

6.3.3 Community-Based Treatment and Services

Test One: 97, 102, 171
Test Two: 3, 53
Test Three: 41, 46, 166
Test Four: 18, 19, 51
Test Five: 129, 152
Test Six: 168, 192
Test Seven: 134, 171

6.4 Child and Adolescent Psychiatric Emergencies

Test One: 2, 88, 128
Test Two: 48, 154
Test Three: None
Test Four: 73, 194
Test Five: 54, 116
Test Six: 53
Test Seven: 46

7.1.1 The Consultation and Liaison Processes to Pediatrics

Test One: 98, 174
Test Two: 128
Test Three: 56
Test Four: 88, 178

Test Five: 17, 136
Test Six: 95, 119
Test Seven: 6, 122

7.1.2 Integrating Behavioral Services into Pediatric Care Settings: Principles and Models

Test One: 33
Test Two: 107
Test Three: 1, 19
Test Four: 92, 133
Test Five: 66
Test Six: 4
Test Seven: None

7.1.3.1 Cancer

Test One: 38, 65, 150, 187
Test Two: 69, 90, 136
Test Three: 128, 167
Test Four: 79, 95, 112
Test Five: 99, 164
Test Six: 42
Test Seven: 7, 16

7.1.3.2 The Role of the Child and Adolescent Psychiatrist on the Pediatric Transplant Service

Test One: 157
Test Two: 106, 145
Test Three: 87
Test Four: 97, 105
Test Five: 34
Test Six: 123, 141
Test Seven: 168, 199

7.1.3.3 Psychosocial Aspects of HIV/AIDS

Test One: 131
Test Two: 111, 117
Test Three: None
Test Four: None
Test Five: None
Test Six: 29, 144
Test Seven: 177

7.1.3.4 Epilepsy

Test One: 3, 142
Test Two: 25, 111, 129
Test Three: 73, 120, 147, 182
Test Four: 13, 103
Test Five: 25, 108, 154
Test Six: 6, 121
Test Seven: 17, 58, 62

7.1.4 Life-Limiting Illness, Palliative Care, and Bereavement

Test One: 120, 122
Test Two: 100, 116
Test Three: 102, 152
Test Four: 15, 110, 144
Test Five: 106

Test Six: 23, 34
Test Seven: 22, 99

7.2 Schools

Test One: 30
Test Two: 131, 196
Test Three: 18
Test Four: 161
Test Five: 123, 188
Test Six: 19
Test Seven: 98, 164

7.3.1 The Child and Adolescent Psychiatrist in Court

Test One: 168
Test Two: 159
Test Three: None
Test Four: 91
Test Five: 38, 186
Test Six: 40
Test Seven: 92

7.3.2 Divorce and Child Custody

Test One: 113
Test Two: 184

Test Three: 105, 133
Test Four: 54, 81
Test Five: 29, 119, 183
Test Six: 35, 101
Test Seven: 44, 196

7.3.3 Adoption

Test One: 6, 175
Test Two: 118, 183
Test Three: 63
Test Four: None
Test Five: 21
Test Six: 106, 140, 188
Test Seven: 189

7.3.4 Malpractice and Professional Liability

Test One: 115, 173
Test Two: 58, 59, 197
Test Three: None
Test Four: None
Test Five: 44
Test Six: 64, 76, 117
Test Seven: 111

Index